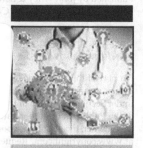

T0312640

Do No Harm

Protecting Connected Medical Devices, Healthcare, and Data from Hackers and Adversarial Nation States

Matthew Webster

WILEY

To Katherine

About the Author

Matthew Webster is the Chief Information Security Officer at Galway Holdings. He has more than 25 years of experience in IT and cybersecurity—including multiple cybersecurity officer positions. Matthew clearly has a passion for cybersecurity, which is evidenced by the fact he has earned more than 20 IT and cybersecurity certifications including the coveted Certified Information Systems Security Professional (CISSP).

Matthew has worked in and around many companies throughout the northeast in a variety of capacities, and he has built many cybersecurity programs from the ground up. As a skilled professional, Matthew has spoken in a range of contexts, including in person and at online events.

Acknowledgments

If there is one adage that best describes writing a book of this nature it is that Rome was not built in a day. I could not begin to thank each person who helped me lay the foundation for this book. The hundreds if not thousands of conversations around cybersecurity and leadership have influenced my thinking in both large and small ways.

Many of the people are probably completely unaware of how they have helped me over the years. I have learned from others at numerous conferences and webinars and from cybersecurity tool vendors. Each technology, each person, has helped to provide me with greater background and knowledge in order to gain a better context and understanding.

In terms of writing this book I would like to thank Peter Gregory, a very experienced author, who introduced me to Carole Jelen, the vice president of Waterside Productions, who helped to mentor me through the ABCs of writing a book of this magnitude. Without their help, I never would have had the opportunity to write such a book.

I also want to thank both Wiley and my editors who have been very patient making corrections, asking questions, and making recommendations throughout the whole process. Their patience and understanding has been greatly appreciated.

Finally, I want to thank my lovely wife, Sumiko, who has been extremely patient with me as I spent an enormous number of hours writing this book. Without her patience this would have been a much more difficult endeavor.

—Matthew Webster

Contents at a Glance

Preface   xviii

Introduction   xxi

Part I   Defining the Challenge   1

Chapter 1   The Darker Side of High Demand   3

Chapter 2   The Internet of Medical Things in Depth   27

Chapter 3   It Is a Data-Centric World   53

Chapter 4   IoMT and Health Regulation   73

Chapter 5   Once More into the Breach   85

Chapter 6   Say Nothing of Privacy   97

Chapter 7   The Short Arm of the Law   123

Chapter 8   Threat Actors and Their Arsenal   135

Part II   Contextual Challenges and Solutions   151

Chapter 9   Enter Cybersecurity   153

Chapter 10   Network Infrastructure and IoMT   171

Chapter 11   Internet Services Challenges   185

Chapter 12   IT Hygiene and Cybersecurity   201

Chapter 13   Identity and Access Management   227

Chapter 14   Threat and Vulnerability   247

Chapter 15   Data Protection   263

Chapter 16   Incident Response and Forensics   275

Chapter 17   A Matter of Life, Death, and Data   287

Part III   Looking Forward   311

Chapter 18   Seeds of Change   313

Chapter 19   Doing Less Harm   329

Chapter 20   Changes We Need   343

Glossary   351

Index   367

Contents

Preface	xviii
Introduction	xxi

Part I	Defining the Challenge	1

Chapter 1	The Darker Side of High Demand	3

Connected Medical Device Risks	4
Ransomware	4
Risks to Data	7
Escalating Demand	10
Types of Internet-Connected Medical Devices	11
COVID-19 Trending Influences	12
By the Numbers	13
Telehealth	15
Home Healthcare	15
Remote Patient Monitoring	16
The Road to High Risk	16
Innovate or Die	19
In Summary	26

Chapter 2	The Internet of Medical Things in Depth	27

What Are Medical Things?	28
Telemedicine	29
Data Analytics	30
Historical IoMT Challenges	31
IoMT Technology	36
Electronic Boards	36

Operating Systems 37
Software Development 38
Wireless 39
Wired Connections 43
The Cloud 43
Mobile Devices and Applications 46
Clinal Monitors 47
Websites 48
Putting the Pieces Together 48
Current IoMT Challenges 48
In Summary 50

Chapter 3 It Is a Data-Centric World 53
The Volume of Health Data 53
Data *Is* That Important 55
This Is Data Aggregation? 57
Non-HIPAA Health Data? 59
Data Brokers 60
Big Data 63
Data Mining Automation 68
In Summary 70

Chapter 4 IoMT and Health Regulation 73
Health Regulation Basics 73
FDA to the Rescue? 77
The Veterans Affairs and UL 2900 81
In Summary 83

Chapter 5 Once More into the Breach 85
Grim Statistics 86
Breach Anatomy 89
Phishing, Pharming, Vishing, and Smishing 90
Web Browsing 92
Black-Hat Hacking 93
IoMT Hacking 94
Breach Locations 95
In Summary 95

Chapter 6 Say Nothing of Privacy 97
Why Privacy Matters 98
Privacy History in the United States 101
The 1990s Turning Point 103
HIPAA Privacy Rules 104
HIPAA and Pandemic Privacy 104
Contact Tracing 106

Corporate Temperature Screenings 107
A Step Backward 107
The New Breed of Privacy Regulations 108
California Consumer Privacy Act 108
CCPA, AB-713, and HIPAA 109
New York SHIELD Act 111
Nevada Senate Bill 220 111
Maine: An Act to Protect the Privacy of Online
    Consumer Information 112
States Striving for Privacy 112
International Privacy Regulations 113
Technical and Operational Privacy Considerations 114
Non-IT Considerations 115
Impact Assessments 115
Privacy, Technology, and Security 115
Privacy Challenges 117
Common Technologies 118
The Manufacturer's Quandary 119
Bad Behavior 121
In Summary 122

Chapter 7   **The Short Arm of the Law**   **123**
Legal Issues with Hacking 124
White-Hat Hackers 125
Gray-Hat Hackers 125
Black-Hat Hackers 127
Computer Fraud and Abuse Act 127
The Electronic Communications Privacy Act 128
Cybercrime Enforcement 128
Results of Legal Shortcomings 131
In Summary 132

Chapter 8   **Threat Actors and Their Arsenal**   **135**
The Threat Actors 136
Amateur Hackers 136
Insiders 136
Hacktivists 137
Advanced Persistent Threats 138
Organized Crime 138
Nation-States 139
Nation-States' Legal Posture 140
The Deep, Dark Internet 141
Tools of the Trade 143
Types of Malware 144
Malware Evolution 146

	Too Many Strains	147
	Malware Construction Kits	148
	In Summary	148
Part II	**Contextual Challenges and Solutions**	**151**
Chapter 9	**Enter Cybersecurity**	**153**
	What Is Cybersecurity?	154
	Cybersecurity Basics	154
	Cybersecurity Evolution	156
	Key Disciplines in Cybersecurity	158
	Compliance	158
	Patching	160
	Antivirus	161
	Network Architecture	161
	Application Architecture	162
	Threat and Vulnerability	162
	Identity and Access Management	163
	Monitoring	164
	Incident Response	165
	Digital Forensics	166
	Configuration Management	166
	Training	168
	Risk Management	168
	In Summary	169
Chapter 10	**Network Infrastructure and IoMT**	**171**
	In the Beginning	172
	Networking Basics: The OSI Model	173
	Mistake: The Flat Network	175
	Resolving the Flat Network Mistake	177
	Alternate Network Defensive Strategies	178
	Network Address Translation	178
	Virtual Private Networks	179
	Network Intrusion Detection Protection Tools	179
	Deep Packet Inspection	179
	Web Filters	180
	Threat Intelligence Gateways	180
	Operating System Firewalls	181
	Wireless Woes	181
	In Summary	182
Chapter 11	**Internet Services Challenges**	**185**
	Internet Services	186
	Network Services	186
	Websites	187

IoMT Services	189
Other Operating System Services	189
Open-Source Tools Are Safe, Right?	190
Cloud Services	193
Internet-Related Services Challenges	194
Domain Name Services	195
Deprecated Services	197
Internal Server as an Internet Servers	197
The Evolving Enterprise	198
In Summary	199

Chapter 12	**IT Hygiene and Cybersecurity**	**201**
	The IoMT Blues	202
	IoMT and IT Hygiene	202
	Past Their Prime	203
	Selecting IoMT	203
	IoMT as Workstations	204
	Mixing IoMT with IoT	204
	The Drudgery of Patching	206
	Mature Patching Process	207
	IoMT Patching	208
	Windows Patching	208
	Linux Patching	209
	Mobile Device Patching	209
	Final Patching Thoughts	210
	Antivirus Is Enough, Right?	210
	Antivirus Evolution	211
	Solution Interconnectivity	211
	Antivirus in Nooks and Crannies	212
	Alternate Solutions	213
	IoMT and Antivirus	214
	The Future of Antivirus	215
	Antivirus Summary	215
	Misconfigurations Galore	215
	The Process for Making Changes	216
	Have a Configuration Strategy	217
	IoMT Configurations	218
	Windows System Configurations	218
	Linux Configurations	219
	Application Configurations	219
	Firewall Configurations	220
	Mobile Device Misconfigurations	220
	Database Configurations	221
	Configuration Drift	222

		Configuration Tools	222
		Exception Management	223
		Enterprise Considerations	224
		In Summary	224
Chapter 13	**Identity and Access Management**		**227**
	Minimal Identity Practices		228
		Local Accounts	229
		Domain/Directory Accounts	229
		Service Accounts	230
		IoMT Accounts	230
		Physical Access Accounts	231
		Cloud Accounts	231
		Consultants, Contractors, and Vendor Accounts	232
		Identity Governance	232
	Authentication		233
		Password Pain	233
		Multi-factor Authentication	236
		Hard Tokens	236
		Soft Tokens	237
		Authenticator Applications	238
		Short Message Service	238
		QR Codes	238
		Other Authentication Considerations	239
		Dealing with Password Pain	239
		MFA Applicability	240
		Aging Systems	240
	Privileged Access Management		240
		Roles	241
		Password Rotation	242
		MFA Access	242
		Adding Network Security	242
	Other I&AM Technologies		243
		Identity Centralization	243
		Identity Management	244
		Identity Governance Tools	244
		Password Tools	244
	In Summary		245
Chapter 14	**Threat and Vulnerability**		**247**
	Vulnerability Management		248
		Traditional Infrastructure Vulnerability Scans	248
		Traditional Application Vulnerability Scans	249
		IoMT Vulnerability Challenges	249
		Rating Vulnerabilities	250

Vulnerability Management Strategies   251
   Asset Exposure   251
   Importance   252
   Compensating Controls   252
   Zero-Day Vulnerabilities   252
   Less-Documented Vulnerabilities   253
   Putting It All Together   253
   Additional Vulnerability Management Uses   254
Penetration Testing   254
   What Color Box?   255
   What Color Team?   255
   Penetration Testing Phases   256
      Scope   256
      Reconnaissance   256
      Vulnerability Assessments   257
      The Actual Penetration Test   257
      Reporting   258
   Penetration Testing Strategies   258
   Cloud Considerations   258
New Tools of an Old Trade   259
   MITRE ATT&CK Framework   259
   Breach and Attack Simulation   259
   Crowd Source Penetration Testing   260
   Calculating Threats   260
In Summary   261

Chapter 15   Data Protection   263
Data Governance   264
   Data Governance: Ownership   264
   Data Governance: Lifecycle   265
   Data Governance: Encryption   265
   Data Governance: Data Access   267
   Closing Thoughts   268
Data Loss Prevention   268
   Fragmented DLP Solutions   269
   DLP Challenges   270
Enterprise Encryption   270
   File Encryption   271
   Encryption Gateways   271
Data Tokenization   272
In Summary   273

Chapter 16   Incident Response and Forensics   275
Defining the Context   276
   Logs   277
   Alerts   278

SIEM Alternatives   279
Incidents   280
Breaches   281
Incident Response   281
Evidence Handling   282
Forensic Tools   283
Automation   283
EDR and MDR   284
IoMT Challenges   284
Lessons Learned   285
In Summary   285

Chapter 17   A Matter of Life, Death, and Data   **287**
Organizational Structure   288
Board of Directors   288
Chief Executive Officer   289
Chief Information Officer   289
General Counsel   290
Chief Technology Officer   290
Chief Medical Technology Officer   290
Chief Information Security Officer   291
Chief Compliance Officer   291
Chief Privacy Officer   291
Reporting Structures   292
Committees   293
Risk Management   294
Risk Frameworks   294
Determining Risk   295
Third-Party Risk   296
Risk Register   297
Enterprise Risk Management   297
Final Thoughts on Risk Management   298
Mindset Challenges   298
The Compliance-Only Mindset   298
Cost Centers   299
Us Versus Them   300
The Shiny Object Syndrome   300
Never Disrupt the Business   301
It's Just an IT Problem   301
Tools over People   303
We Are Not a Target   303
The Bottom Line   304
Final Mindset Challenges   304

	Decision-Making	304
	A Measured View	305
	Communication Is Key	306
	Enterprise Risk Management	307
	Writing and Sign-Off	308
	Data Protection Considerations	308
	In Summary	309
Part III	**Looking Forward**	**311**
Chapter 18	**Seeds of Change**	**313**
	The Shifting Legal Landscape	314
	Attention on Data Brokers	314
	Data Protection Agency	316
	IoT Legislation	317
	Privacy Legislation	318
	A Ray of Legal Light	318
	International Agreements	319
	Public-Private Partnerships	319
	Better National Coordination	320
	International Cooperation	322
	Technology Innovation	323
	Threat Intelligence	323
	Machine Learning Revisited	323
	Zero Trust	324
	Final Technology Thoughts	325
	Leadership Shakeups	325
	Blended Approaches	326
	In Summary	327
Chapter 19	**Doing Less Harm**	**329**
	What IoMT Manufacturers Can Do	330
	Cybersecurity as Differentiator	332
	What Covered Entities Can Do	332
	Cybersecurity Decision Making	333
	Compliance Anyone?	334
	The Tangled Web of Privacy	335
	Aggregation of Influence	335
	Cybersecurity Innovators	337
	Industrial Control Systems Overlap	338
	What You Can Do	339
	Personal Cybersecurity	339
	Politics	341
	In Summary	342

Chapter 20	**Changes We Need**	**343**
	International Cooperation	344
	Covered Entities	344
	Questions a Board Should Ask	345
	More IoMT Security Assurances	346
	Active Directory Integration	347
	Software Development	347
	Independent Measures	348
	In Summary	348
Glossary		**351**
Index		**367**

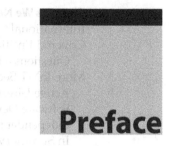

Preface

This is a book specifically focused on the cybersecurity of internet-connected medical devices written by a cybersecurity professional for the general public. It looks at the problem from a broad spectrum of angles, from education, technical, the legal landscape, the threat landscape, through the very management of these devices. It covers why the devices are made the way they are and why not enough attention has been placed on their security. It then goes into possible solutions and directions that we as members of a global society need to take in the wake of a powerful technology like the internet.

This book does not focus on the specific medical challenges from a medical perspective related to internet-connected medical devices. There are already a number of books that talk about the medical challenges related to various types of implants. This was a conscious choice not to focus on challenges that I am simply not qualified to talk about nor provide interesting insights about.

Where I can provide interesting insights is in the realm of cybersecurity, where I have a great deal of experience—an area that I have been involved in and have loved for many years. Through that experience, I hope to show you a bit behind the scenes of what it takes to truly protect those devices—sometimes from a technical angle. I have striven to make these technical concepts more accessible to the average reader so almost everyone can enjoy this book.

It has been very challenging to determine the right amount of content to reach every reader. Each topic in this book can easily be a book unto itself. The book could have been a thousand pages, but it would not have succinctly driven home the important points. Readers within many of the professions could point out obvious shortcomings, which would have taken chapters to explore. In the end, cybersecurity is a complex topic, and I tried to strike the right balance in choosing what to discuss.

I have had the honor to work with people from all walks of life, but cybersecurity is not something that everyone understands. Sometimes, it is important to point out the ABCs of how cybersecurity is built into society. It isn't as ingrained in our thinking as many people might assume. I hope that most readers gain a little insight into the reasons why attackers may go after hospitals, and realize the dangers that IoMT devices and their interconnections with other technologies pose to the security of healthcare organizations.

It should be noted that throughout this book, we use the term *covered entity* quite frequently. In the broader scope of things, there are numerous types of covered entities, but this book refers specifically to covered entities under the HIPAA law—mainly companies that create or produce health data—such as the kind that healthcare professionals create and are often the output from internet-connected medical devices.

It should also be noted that I have no special love for internet-connected medical devices. I recognize their critical value in creating the next generation of medical breakthroughs as we seek to understand at a deeper level the key things that keep us alive. They are a necessity to reduce medical costs and spur future technologies. Like any device on a network, they take diligence and thoughtfulness to protect. I don't consider myself an expert on those devices; the doctors are the experts. But I have seen the challenges related to these devices just by working with people who secure those devices. Understanding the fundamental components of those devices and how they are constructed is also critical to understanding how to protect the overall ecosystem. With each link, a chain is forged in that complex array of relatively new medical devices. Understanding each link has helped to prepare me to write this book. It really does take a sea of understanding to look at the big picture related to topics as large as IoMT. No one perspective really is enough, and each internet-connected medical device needs to be judged on its own with its own quirks and particularities. It is only by exploring the big picture related to internet-connected medical devices that we can hope to see the whole of the challenges related to these devices.

All of this understood, it is my sincere hope that you both enjoy and learn something about the highly complex set of interconnections between privacy, compliance, cybersecurity, and the often-vulnerable internet-connected medical devices—even if there are a few sections that may be slightly too technical for the average reader. This book shows where cybersecurity is placed within organizations and why it is more critical than ever to protect internet-connected medical devices.

Introduction

Along with the expanding challenges of the COVID-19 pandemic was another pandemic hitting our hospitals and healthcare systems in the United States—ransomware. Ransomware is software that cybercriminals use to render a computer or machine unusable. They then demand a ransom for a code that will (ideally) enable the compromised organization to disable the software and restore the machine to a usable state. The vulnerabilities and the weaknesses inherent in internet-connected medical devices helps to enable these cybercriminals.

This book is about the relationships between vulnerable internet-connected medical devices, cybercriminals, and nation-state actors and how they not only take advantage of exceptionally vulnerable devices, but also profit from it.

But the story relating to insecure medical devices is much deeper than this. It is the story of American innovation and ingenuity—a story where cybersecurity often takes a back seat to the needs of saving human lives. That story, through no particular person's or organization's fault, has started to leave our hospitals in a more vulnerable state than ever before. Through the pandemic, the fundamental flawed state of many internet-connected medical devices, along with insufficient global legal protections, has allowed organized crime and nation-state actors to collect trillions of dollars.

If you care about your data, your privacy, and why the situation is so dire from a cybersecurity perspective, this book is worth reading. It also offers a glimpse inside the perspective of a Chief Information Security

Officer regarding the security and privacy of our data as a result of the decisions we have collectively made.

This book leans heavily on the cybersecurity perspective, as that is the perspective I know best. It does dive into the technical aspects of internet-connected medical devices, but then it jumps into law, big data, and other global challenges and ties them together in an overarching story about hospitals, data, and cybercriminals.

This book touches heavily on the technical aspects of protecting internet-connected medical devices, but its scope is much broader than that. It provides a larger legal, privacy, and threat landscape perspective, which completely shapes the context for why having insecure medical devices presents a challenge for today's hospitals.

What Does This Book Cover?

This book covers a broad range of subjects in and around the protection of data and the challenges related to IoMT.

Chapter 1: The Darker Side of High Demand   This chapter sets the stage for why internet-connected medical devices are so insecure. It explores some of the chief drivers for today's healthcare and why healthcare tends not be overly focused on cybersecurity, historically speaking.

Chapter 2: The Internet of Medical Things in Depth   This chapter dives into the technical side of internet-connected medical devices. It defines what is and is not an internet-connected medical device, and explores the larger context of those devices and how they fit together with other technologies.

Chapter 3: It Is a Data-Centric World   This chapter explores many of the different facets of what is and is not medical data. The definition is often blurrier than we might expect, and the ramifications can be large—especially once big data is part of the overarching picture. The ramifications and risks are often not what they may seem.

Chapter 4: IoMT and Health Regulation   This chapter covers how HIPAA and other regulations relate to the deluge of data created as a result of internet-connected medical devices. It also looks at the enforcement mechanisms related to HIPAA through the Office of Civil Rights.

Chapter 5: Once More into the Breach This chapter focuses on the actions of cybercriminals once they take initial steps into an organization. It covers why cybersecurity is so difficult with the vulnerabilities that internet-connected medical devices have and how attackers take advantage of those vulnerabilities.

Chapter 6: Say Nothing of Privacy This chapter explores the history and evolution of privacy and how that privacy relates to both HIPAA data and the proliferation of data relating to internet-connected medical devices. It also brings surprising ties to big data and the challenges to the data market.

Chapter 7: The Short Arm of the Law This chapter explores the global legal landscape and the related enforcement challenges and how that landscape only amplifies the challenges related to vulnerable internet-connected medical devices.

Chapter 8: Threat Actors and Their Arsenal This chapter explores, at a high level, the various threat actors, some of the characteristics of their arsenal, and why they are so effective at their tradecraft.

Chapter 9: Enter Cybersecurity This chapter provides an in-depth introduction to what cybersecurity is. It explores some of the basic tradecraft of cybersecurity and related disciplines.

Chapter 10: Network Infrastructure and IoMT This chapter explores what a network is, how it is set up, and some basic network architectures and tools that can be used to protect internet-connected medical devices from harm.

Chapter 11: Internet Services Challenges This chapter reviews some of the basic services of the internet and how those services relate to internet-connected medical devices.

Chapter 12: IT Hygiene and Cybersecurity This chapter describes the basics of IT hygiene, what it is, and why it is important. IT hygiene is also something that is not possible with internet-connected medical devices, which brings increased risks to those devices.

Chapter 13: Identity and Access Management This chapter explores the complex world of identity and access management. It touches on the technology, the governance, the challenges that many internet-connected medical devices have, and how internet connected medical devices affect the security posture of organizations.

Chapter 14: Threat and Vulnerability This chapter explores the various tools and techniques related to discovering vulnerabilities within an environment and the associated challenges with internet-connected medical devices.

Chapter 15: Data Protection This chapter explores some basic data protection strategies, governance, and tools related to protecting data. It has ties back to privacy, big data, IT, and other considerations.

Chapter 16: Incident Response and Forensics This chapter explores incident response and forensics from a disciplinary perspective and how internet-connected medical devices can be a challenge to the two disciplines.

Chapter 17: A Matter of Life, Death, and Data This chapter takes a step back from the details of cybersecurity to examine how all of the cybersecurity considerations fit into the bigger governance frameworks and why decision-making can be so challenging.

Chapter 18: Seeds of Change This chapter explores some of the changes we need to better protect internet-connected medical devices. It explores everything from decision-making processes to hospitals, supply and demand, and so on.

Chapter 19: Doing Less Harm This chapter covers some strategies that we can focus on to optimize the overall balance between competing needs related to securing internet-connected medical devices.

Chapter 20: Changes We Need Despite the many we have talked about, there are still fundamental changes that need to take place in order to better protect hospitals, data, and internet-connected medical devices.

How to Contact the Publisher

If you believe you've found a mistake in this book, please bring it to our attention. At John Wiley & Sons, we understand how important it is to provide our customers with accurate content, but even with our best efforts an error may occur.

To submit your possible errata, please email it to our Customer Service Team at wileysupport@wiley.com with the subject line "Possible Book Errata Submission."

How to Contact the Author

We appreciate your input and questions about this book! Email me at awakenings@mindspring.com.

Part

I

Defining the Challenge

If we step back and look at the big picture related to insecure internet-connected medical devices, the concerns are primarily around risks to healthcare organizations and risk to data. Fortunately, there have been very few deaths related to these insecure devices, but as adoption of internet-connected medical devices continues to rise, so will the associated risks. If COVID-19 has taught us one thing, it is that tragedy for some is an opportunity for others. From a cybersecurity perspective, it is important to understand who these actors are, what they are motivated by, and how can we stop, or at least reduce, the number and/or effectiveness of these attacks.

Before we can do this, it is extremely helpful to understand why poor security on internet-connected medical devices is such a challenge for IT and cybersecurity practitioners and why the devices have so many challenges to begin with. Looking at poor security as an origin story provides us with the context for understanding how to proceed. The world of IT, and especially internet-connected medical devices, is filled with a complex interrelation of social, technological, and economic challenges. It is important to understand this complex relationship if we are to devise a strategy for best protecting the devices, our hospitals, and the associated data.

As you read this first part of this book, keep the bigger picture in your head in order to more fully understand how we ended up where we are today. We have legal requirements that are not always followed by manufacturers, which creates both challenges and victories for protecting our healthcare, our data, and occasionally our lives.

The Darker Side of High Demand

The road to Hell is paved with good intentions.
—Henry G. Bohn, *A Handbook of Proverbs*, 1855

"First, do no harm" is attributed to the ancient Greek physician Hippocrates. It is part of the Hippocratic oath. The reality is that every day, doctors and hospitals need to make decisions about how to best help patients under the existing conditions. If doctors need to operate, they may harm the patient by making an incision—sometimes to save a patient's life. This is a calculated and acceptable harm from a moral perspective.

What isn't always as obvious to hospitals is the harm introduced by using an internet-connected medical device. In many cases, such as in hospitals, the doctors may have limited input about which devices are chosen for their environment. These devices have critical medical value not only for the hospital or doctor's office, but also from the patient's point of view. They are at the forefront of today's medical transformations. Often the harm that is introduced is unknown, unseen, or downplayed—if it is assessed at all.

This chapter explores, at a high level, the state of internet-connected medical devices and how those devices are impacting hospitals and unfortunately, and indirectly, human life. More importantly, this chapter covers the overall trends related to hospitals, partially as a result of internet-connected medical devices and how businesses evolved to the state they are in today. First, we need to understand the risks that internet-connected medical devices pose.

Connected Medical Device Risks

What exactly are the risks related to internet-connected medical devices? The hit TV show *Homeland* popularized the idea of an attacker assassinating someone by taking over a pacemaker. While this is not beyond the realm of possibility, the most common forms of attack utilizing internet-connected medical devices are ransomware and distributed denial of service attacks (DDOS).[1] In the former case, the attacker takes over a system (often with malware, but sometimes with a password) and prevents (often through the use of encryption) the end user from using the system. In latter case, the attacker will own the device and use it to attack other sites.

Ransomware

Ransomware is essentially software that prevents systems from running. Criminals require that the owners pay to be able to gain access to their own systems. Imagine you had pictures of your family on your home computer and you could no longer access them unless you paid a fee. Now imagine critical medical systems rendered inoperable instead of family pictures. To make matters worse, once attackers are inside of systems, they often leave behind a way to gain access to them over and over again—meaning they are more susceptible to future attacks. This trend has only increased in the time of COVID. Obviously, the attackers do not care about the lives of others enough to not do the attacks.

Ransomware has been evolving tremendously over the last few years, and the number of the ransom demands has gone up significantly from a few years ago. In 2019 alone, 764 healthcare providers in the United States were hit with ransomware.[2] One might be tempted to think that the attackers would not go after hospitals in a time of a global pandemic, but while this is the case for some attackers, the reality is that ransomware attacks are on the rise since COVID-19 hit.[3] What is worse is that while ransom demands used to be a few hundred dollars, now they

---

[1] Nicole Feraro, "Health Prognosis on the Security of IoMT Devices? Not Good," *Dark Reading,* April 25, 2020, https://www.darkreading.com/endpoint/health-prognosis-on-the-security-of-iomt-devices-not-good/d/d-id/1337649.

[2] "The State of Ransomware in the US: Report and Statistics," 2019, https://blog.emsisoft.com/en/34822/the-state-of-ransomware-in-the-us-report-and-statistics-2019/.

are growing and are often more than a million dollars. With so much to gain, it is no wonder that ransomware demands are on the rise. Clearly, hospitals have a great deal of risk related to ransomware.

The effect that ransomware has had on hospitals is crippling. The attackers are well aware that COVID-19 has severely stretched the resources at hospitals. They know that this is a life-and-death situation, which makes hospitals even more likely to pay the ransom,[4] especially the smaller hospitals that may not have as mature of an IT and/or security program in place to protect their environments from the ravages of ransomware.[5] Essentially, they are easier targets. Sadly, even larger, more mature organizations are susceptible to ransomware attacks, but can sometimes respond to them more effectively.

September 10, 2020, unfortunately marks a grim milestone for ransomware—the first indirect death. A patient was rerouted from Duesseldorf University Hospital in Germany as 30 of its internal servers were hit with ransomware. As a result of the subsequent delay getting the much needed medical treatment, the patient died.[6] This particular attack was aimed at Heinrich Heine University and mistakenly hit the hospital because it is part of the same network. In this case, the perpetrators provided the keys to decrypt the systems and withdrew their extortion demands, but despite that, the hospital's systems were disrupted for a week.[7]

That was not the only death associated with ransomware in September 2020, unfortunately. Universal Health Services (UHS) was hit with a massive ransomware attack. UHS is a Fortune 500 company with more

[3] "Covid-19: Ruthless Ransomware Authors Attack Hospitals," 2020, https://securityboulevard.com/2020/06/covid-19-ruthless-ransomware-authors-attack-hospitals/.

[4] Lily Hay Newman, "The Covid-19 Pandemic Reveals Ransomware's Long Game," 2020, https://www.wired.com/story/covid-19-pandemic-ransomware-long-game/.

[5] Jessica Kim Cohen, "Washington hospital refuses to pay $1 million ransomware demand," 2019, https://www.modernhealthcare.com/cybersecurity/washington-hospital-refuses-pay-1-million-ransomware-demand.

[6] Catalin Cimpanu, "First death reported following a ransomware attack on a German hospital: Death occurred after a patient was diverted to a nearby hospital after the Duesseldorf University Hospital suffered a ransomware attack," 2020, https://www.zdnet.com/article/first-death-reported-following-a-ransomware-attack-on-a-german-hospital/.

[7] "German Hospital Hacked, Patient Taken to Another City Dies," *Cleveland Daily Banner*, https://hosted.ap.org/clevelandbanner/article/cf8f8eee1ad-cec69bcc864f2c4308c94/german-hospital-hacked-patient-taken-another-city-dies.

than 400 healthcare facilities in the U.S. and the UK. It provides services to more than 3 million patients yearly. In many cases whole hospitals were shut down and services were rerouted to other hospitals. Because of this rerouting of services, four people died.[8] With the frequency of ransomware growing, these kinds of problems will not only continue, but will likely become worse before they get better.

It is important to note that medical devices are not the only avenue for ransomware attacks, but they are, arguably, the most egregious vector due to the gaps in their fundamental security, inability to patch cybersecurity flaws in some circumstances, and the volume of problems they have—especially in the long run. One report shows that malware against internet-connected devices (not just medical devices) is up 50% from 2019.[9] That being said, they are a unique avenue due to the kinds of flaws they have. For example, the range of flaws in today's internet-connected medical devices is staggering. Take medical imaging devices: 70% of the devices are based on retired operating systems or systems that are under limited support.[10] The potential for vulnerabilities is extremely high. In many cases internet-connected medical devices run on Windows XP, which is no longer supported. There continues to be new vulnerabilities found—many of which allow complete compromise of the whole system. Associated with a compromised system is a whole host of risks, including everything from the system not functioning to data being exfiltrated. Either way, these are risks to both patients and to hospitals.

Now let us think about connectivity. Today's world is also much more connected than ever before. Many systems connect back to something referred to as "the cloud." While I will go into greater depth in later chapters about the cloud, it should be noted here that the cloud aggregates and correlates data in one location. It also comes with a whole new set of risks that adds an extra layer of complexity for IT and cybersecurity teams.

---

[8] Sergiu Gatlan, "UHS hospitals hit by reported country-wide Ryuk ransomware attack," 2020, https://www.bleepingcomputer.com/news/security/uhs-hospitals-hit-by-reported-country-wide-ryuk-ransomware-attack/?utm_medium=email&_hsmi=96262261&_hsenc=p2ANqtz-8L3v0ZVtO4P3wgXU05ReBUHRZfuWMMoaMdTsDri89BURxNP-RVxwkTlH5sJZwmIx-oW7eVuuuTbnGmMcuDQ4DLod179gsRrcB4LfLdQWpIT_7ESHw&utm_content=96262261&utm_source=hs_email.

[9] SonicWall, "2020 Cyber Threat Report," 2020.

[10] Kelly Jackson Higgins, "Over 80% of Medical Imaging Devices Run on Outdated Operating Systems," 2020, https://www.darkreading.com/iot/over-80--of-medical-imaging-devices-run-on-outdated-operating-systems/d/d-id/1337273?_mc=NL_DR_EDT_DR_daily_20200311&cid=NL_DR_EDT_DR_daily_20200311&elq_mid=96222&elq_cid=23133172.

Let's take a ransom in another direction—from a personal perspective. If you had a pacemaker, what would you be willing to pay to save your own life if someone threatened you with turning off the pacemaker? If attackers do not care about the lives of multiple people, they will not care about the life of one person. Attackers typically go for the easiest targets that offer the most reward. If they started targeting the rich who had internet-connected medical implants, that could be a lucrative route going forward. Of course this is not as lucrative as having a hospital pay a ransom.

Risks to Data

What does not often come to mind is the data risk related to internet-connected medical devices. Data can be as potentially deadly a risk as any device. An insulin pump that received the wrong amount of information can potentially kill someone with diabetes. A number of events can cause errors—everything from human error to machine flaws. This too deserves a much deeper dive as the data is far more interconnected than at any point in history, and that interconnection is only going to accelerate with the advent of new internet-connected medical devices.

Some risks are due to existing flaws in medical devices combined with the desire for people to have a better quality of life. For example, diabetics have hacked their own pumps to achieve innovation the manufacturers have not. While many of the devices have been recalled, people have been hurt by insulin overdoses as a result of hacking their own devices.[11] Keep in mind that this was with commercial-grade systems that were attacked. These are not systems purchased off the black market.

Not everyone opts for commercially viable solutions. The cost associated with some of these solutions is too high for many to afford. As a result, they go through alternative sources that may not have the strict quality control that the commercial world has. In some cases, unknowingly, people will work with devices that are actually from the black market, such as insulin pumps that may be even less secure because they are not subject to the stronger regulation that exists today.[12]

[11] Dalvin Brown, "Hacking Diabetes: People break into insulin pumps as an alternative to delayed innovations," 2019, https://medicalxpress.com/news/2019-06-hacking-diabetes-people-insulin-alternative.html.
[12] Serena Gordon, "Medtronic recalls some insulin pumps as FDA warns they could be hacked," 2019, https://medicalxpress.com/news/2019-06-medtronic-recalls-insulin-fda-hacked.html.

While ransomware is taking the spotlight as of late, a host of other attacks are related to internet-connected medical devices. These will be described in greater detail in Chapter 8, but suffice it to say that numerous attacks can be leveraged, many of which could be avoided with sufficient cybersecurity practices. In many of these attacks, the attacker could have complete control of the data on the device. A few of the attacks against connected medical devices are listed in Figure 1-1, but this is far from a complete list. The lesson here is that quite often the vulnerabilities that can physically harm someone can also be leveraged to steal data. Data theft, by far, is much more common than the physical harm that could occur as a result of the internet connection. The stark difference is that the harm of data theft may or may not be known.

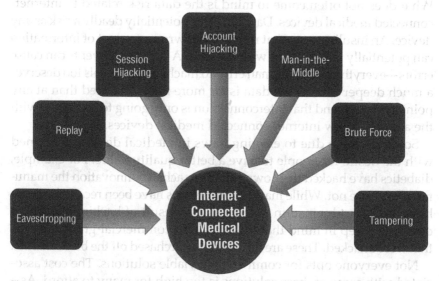

Figure 1-1: Example types of attacks against internet-connected medical devices

The vulnerabilities related to internet-connected medical devices are having an impact on organizations, and these weaknesses are not just trivialities. Nuspire, a managed security services provider, put out a few interesting statistics. The first statistic is that "18% of medical devices were affected by malware or ransomware in the last 18 months."[13] That is not a small number. Roughly 1 out of 5 devices have been affected by

---

[13] "How vulnerable is the internet of medical things to cyber threats?" https://www.nuspire.com/wp-content/uploads/2020/04/Nuspire-IG-Healthcare-Infographic.pdf.

malware. If there is an average of 15 devices around a patient, roughly 3 of them have the possibility of being infected. Further, that malware can often be used to infect other devices. The other statistic that Nuspire mentioned was that "89% of health care organizations have suffered from an IoMT Related Security Breach." IoMT is short for internet of medical things. For our purposes, think of IoMT as internet-connected medical devices. That alone is another concerning statistic. It means that the connected medical devices are a serious concern for healthcare organizations. It makes protecting these critical organizations all the more difficult.

If risks to human life are on one end of the spectrum, the other end of the spectrum relates to data risks. Healthcare data is one of the most sought-after data types on the internet. Security reports over the years have shown the value of a healthcare record to be worth anywhere from $10 to $1,000. By contrast, the typical credit card is worth only a few dollars. The reason is that most credit card companies have robust fraud departments that stop fraudulent transactions relatively quickly. After one or more transactions, the card is usually cut off. This is not typically true for health records. The process of detecting problems can take much more time.

From a patient perspective, the associated fraud can be a painful and lengthy road to deal with. Advisory Board, a leader in the healthcare advisory space, had an article that illustrated this quite clearly. A patient's identity was stolen, and the result was $20,000 worth of medical procedures that the victim was responsible for. It kept up over billing cycles, and the perpetrator was eventually caught and jailed, but there are still serious questions about the integrity of the victim's medical files.[14] Imagine what that can do to the victim. There may be conflicting information about the health information contained in many hospital records. In a worst-case scenario, this can be life threatening.

From a hospital's perspective, it means that they can lose a great deal, too. They can perform procedures essentially for free because they performed surgery on a misauthorized individual. The victims also have a great deal to do because they have to work through the fraud with the hospitals and the insurance companies—at no fault of their own. Health and Human Services, in conjunction with the Office

---

[14] "What hackers actually do with your stolen medical records," 2019, https://www.advisory.com/daily-briefing/2019/03/01/hackers#:~:text=Gary%20Cantrell%2C%20head%20of%20investigations,security%20numbers—which%20is%20enough.

of the Inspector General, put out a report citing they won or negotiated $2.6 billion dollars in fraud adjustments in 2019. There were 1,060 new criminal investigations in 2019.[15] Undoubtedly the numbers are much higher if you consider the cases that were thrown out or were never detected. It takes constant vigilance to detect fraud cases.

The protection of the data related to medical records is absolutely critical. We have only touched the tip of the iceberg finding all the different forces that tie into the safety of information. It is such a complex web of interrelated societal forces that need to be explored more fully to ultimately understand the ripple effect from a few vulnerabilities in connected medical devices and how everything is related to Medicine 2.0—the type of next-generation healthcare we are entering into now.[16]

Escalating Demand

The roots of why there has been such radical transformation in healthcare the last few years are on a few different levels. One of the key drivers is to reduce healthcare costs, which have been escalating. One of the avenues of that change has been as a result of the Patient Protection and Accountable Care Act (PPACA), which President Obama signed into law in March 2010. There were a few key provisions within this bill. The first provision was to create a Patient-Centers Outcomes Research Institute (PCORI), which would compare clinical effectiveness of medical treatments. The goal was to help the healthcare profession determine the most effective strategy for providing treatments. The second provision was a penalty that prohibited payments to states for hospital-acquired infections. Other provisions included reduced payments for hospital readmissions.[17]

As a result, hospitals were more incentivized to stay clean and to improve what they were doing—not just in the cleanliness, but how care would be administered. This required rethinking through many of

---

[15] "The Department of Health and Human Services And the Department of Justice Health Care Fraud and Abuse Control Program Annual Report for Fiscal Year 2019," 2020, https://oig.hhs.gov/publications/docs/hcfac/FY2019-hcfac.pdf.

[16] There are debates about Medicine 2.0 versus 4.0. It could take chapters to debate the difference between the two of them, but it would derail the discussion at hand.

[17] Youssra Marjoua and Kevin Bozic, "Brief history of quality movement in US healthcare," 2012, https://www.ncbi.nlm.nih.gov/pmc/articles/PMC3702754/.

the processes, changing hospitals' approach to technology, and catching medical issues more proactively than reactively. It would involve rethinking how they currently approach treatment and becoming more proactive. It would also involve the use of more connected technology and devices to treat and monitor patients, not just when they come to doctor's offices, but also remotely so conditions could be detected prior to onset of a more serious illness. America needed to revolutionize its way of caring for patients. Doctors would have to rely on a new generation of medical devices for their transformation effort—devices that would be internet connected to provide real-time capabilities or more real-time capabilities than they already do.

America responded as it always does by being innovative and thoughtful about the approach to help the medical community achieve its goals. The new generation of medical devices not only met the goals needed by physicians, but it jump-started continual changes in the technology. These new devices helped to lower per-patient costs, improve efficiency, provide better response care, offer greater convenience, and provide a better overall patient experience. In short, the existing value we are getting from medical devices will fuel the desire for more medical devices. But let us look at these positives, because within the desire for positive changes lies the seeds of the challenges related to the security of internet-connected medical devices.

Types of Internet-Connected Medical Devices

If we step back in time a hundred years, there were only a small number of electronic medical machines. They were bulky, crude, and not able to store or send information. Everything had to be done by hand. By modern standards, this is painstakingly slow and inefficient. Now we have streamlined systems that not only can alert, but help with centralization of alerts meaning that, for example, a nurse does not have to be in physical proximity to a patient and/or device to be aware of a potential problem. While not everything connects together harmoniously, many devices are centralized to create alerts. In a hospital setting this is particularly important because a nurse does not have to hear an alarm from the physical machine in order to know there is an issue with a patient. A random walkthrough of the environment is not required. Nurses can be more focused on patients. Not only that, but patients who need long-term monitoring and want freedom from being at a hospital can get the care they need thanks to remote monitoring. This means the patient has a better quality of life.

Four types of medical monitoring devices are important to consider—wearable, on the skin, ingestible, and implanted. Some of these are sensory in nature, which means they can collect information or detect problems and relay them back to a centralized information source and potentially provide an alert. They are electronic in nature and can have a variety of follow-on actions such as alert for emergency medical systems.

Other systems are more protective and can respond, in a limited way, to the environment. These are referred to as *smart systems*. A good example of this is implanted insulin-releasing needles. If the blood sugar levels are off, the smart system can release the appropriate level of insulin to best protect the patient. In some cases, this can literally transform the lives of those who are diabetic, making it possible for them to have almost near normal lives.

With these kinds of transformations, you can imagine that the demand is very high from the patient. From the hospital's perspective, they can do more with less staff than ever before. The automated alerts mean that they do not necessarily need around-the-clock care watching over the patients if they are not in the hospital. This reduces cost for the hospital and the patient, so all-in-all this is a win-win situation.

COVID-19 Trending Influences

COVID-19 has only accelerated some of the existing trends in the market. For example, prior to the pandemic, telehealth utilization for Medicare patients was roughly 0.1%. By April 2020, visits were up to 43.5%. Some of the changes were due to relaxing the regulations around telemedicine—partially in response to consumer demand.[18] The Center for Medicaid and Medicare Services (CMS) made some significant changes. Since then, it has added some 135 services to be permitted via telehealth.[19] What is more eye-opening is that doctors can treat patients by phone or radio.[20]

---

[18] "HHS Issues New Report Highlighting Dramatic Trends in Medicare Beneficiary Telehealth Utilization amid Covid-19," 2020, https://www.hhs.gov/about/news/2020/07/28/hhs-issues-new-report-highlighting-dramatic-trends-in-medicare-beneficiary-telehealth-utilization-amid-covid-19.html.
[19] Ibid.
[20] Mike Miliard, "CMS relaxes more rules around telehealth, allowing care across state lines," 2020, https://www.healthcareitnews.com/news/cms-relaxes-more-rules-around-telehealth-allowing-care-across-state-lines.

What sometimes goes hand-in-hand with telehealth is the need for in-home testing. It helps to limit exposure from people who may have COVID-19 and in some cases lower transportation costs for hospitals that may previously been inclined to move the patient for testing purposes. Many healthcare organizations were offering this as a service, but the trend has been accelerated by the pandemic.[21]

By the Numbers

What is more staggering than the technological trends themselves is just how pervasive those trends are. More than 430 million internet-connected medical devices have already been shipped worldwide.[22] Presently, the compound annual growth rate (CAGR) of internet-connected medical devices is growing by 25%, and that is expected through at least 2023.[23] The data is not out yet, but COVID-19 is expected to accelerate some of those trends as hospitals and doctor offices are experiencing pressure to not only be remote, but often are expected to do more with less. Let's take a look at those trends. A Zingbox survey stated that there are an estimated 10 to 15 internet-connected medical devices per patient bed. By itself that is staggering and a statistic worth remembering as we dig further into the issues related to these devices.[24]

What many people do not realize is how often healthcare companies are the target of attacks. That trend is only increasing. The HIPAA Journal

[21] Anita Gupta, "Five Healthcare Trends That Have been Accelerated in 2020," 2020, https://www.forbes.com/sites/forbesbusinesscouncil/2020/07/02/five-healthcare-trends-that-have-been-accelerated-in-2020/#3895d5305d6a.

[22] Safi Oranski, "The Internet of Medical Things (IoMT) Punctuates a Century of Progress," accessed October 2019, https://www.cybermdx.com/blog/the-internet-of-medical-things-iomt-punctuates-a-century-of-progress.

[23] "IoT Medical Devices Market by Product (Blood Pressure Monitor, Glucometer, Cardiac Monitor, Pulse Oximeter, Infusion Pump), Type (Wearable, Implantable Device), Connectivity Technology (Bluetooth, Wifi), End User (Hospital)—Global Forecast to 2023," https://www.marketsandmarkets.com/Market-Reports/iot-medical-device-market-15629287.html.

[24] Heather Landi, "82% of healthcare organizations have experienced an IoT-focused cyberattack, survey finds," 2019, https://www.fiercehealthcare.com/tech/82-healthcare-organizations-have-experienced-iot-focused-cyber-attack-survey-finds.

published some fantastic statistics for the United States. For example, between 2009 and 2019 for breaches larger than 500 records, there have been more than 3,000 healthcare data breaches. Figure 1-2 shows a chart they published detailing the number of healthcare data breaches that occurred in those years.

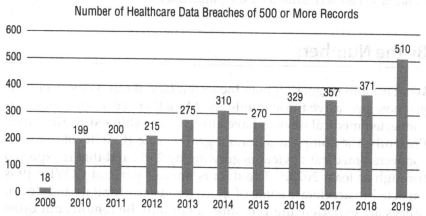

Number of Healthcare Data Breaches of 500 or More Records

Figure 1-2: Number of healthcare data breaches of 500 or more records

While 510 cases may not seem like a lot, healthcare organizations are one of the most attacked verticals. One survey demonstrated that over a two-year period, 89% of healthcare organizations suffered a data breach. Another source that echoes that information is the Verizon Data Breach Investigations report. It has one of the largest data sets available and covers global rather than local numbers. Verizon's 2020 Data Breach Investigations Report showed 521 breaches in 2019 versus only 304 breaches in the previous year.[25] So the issue with healthcare being one of the most attacked sectors is not just a local United States problem, but a global problem.

The problems are only growing worse as a result of COVID-19. Along with COVID-19 are some trends that are changing the technology landscape comprising medical care. Some key considerations are telehealth, home healthcare, and remote patient monitoring—many of which are tied to internet-connected medical devices. Each of these technologies has its own set of challenges and cybersecurity risks that correspond to those challenges. Let's briefly take a look at some of these trends.

---

[25] Verizon, "2020 Data Breach Investigations Report," 2020

Telehealth

Telehealth is essentially providing medical services remotely. It is important in this context as medical devices are often used to enable remote communication. What is interesting to note is that access to telehealth is dependent, in part, on income. The pandemic has proven the "generalizability of telehealth," the CMIO of NYU Langone Health stated, where virtual visits have skyrocketed since COVID-19 lockdown measures have been in place. Meanwhile, HHS recently awarded $20 million to increase telehealth access.[26] This, along with the pandemic, is only going to accelerate the demand for telehealth.

Home Healthcare

The growth of home healthcare is staggering. It is estimated that it will grow more than 18%.[27] Presently, there are roughly 1.4 million people employed in home healthcare services.[28] 2015 was the first year that more money was spent. The global home healthcare market size was valued at USD 281.8 billion in 2019 and is expected to grow at a compound annual growth rate of 7.9% from 2020 to 2027. Population aging around the world and increased patient preference for value-based healthcare are anticipated to fuel market growth. According to the World Health Organization (WHO), there were 703 million persons aged 65 years or over in the world in 2019. The number of older persons is projected to double to 1.5 billion by 2050. The aging population demands more patient-centric healthcare services, which in return increases the demand for healthcare workers and agencies and is anticipated to drive market growth.[29]

---

[26] Ibid.
[27] Kate Rogers, "As the US population ages, the need for home health-care workers skyrockets," https://www.cnbc.com/2018/05/31/as-the-us-population-ages-the-need-for-home-health-care-workers-skyrockets.html.
[28] John Elfein, "Home care in the U.S.—Statistics and Facts," 2020, https://www.statista.com/topics/4049/home-care-in-the-us/.
[29] "Home Healthcare Market Size, Share & Trends Analysis Report By Equipment (Therapeutic, Diagnostic), By Services (Skilled Home Healthcare Services, Unskilled Home Healthcare Services), By Region, And Segment Forecasts, 2020–2027," May 2020, https://www.grandviewresearch.com/industry-analysis/home-healthcare-industry.

Remote Patient Monitoring

Remote patient monitoring is critical for today's world. The best way to do that is with biosensors. Presently there is an 8% CAGR for biosensors, and the total market is expected to be over $29 billion by 2024.[30] The demand for sensors of various kinds will be growing. COVID-19 has already accelerated that trend.

From a numbers perspective alone, it is clear that connected medical devices are not going away. They provide too much value for patients and institutions. All that said, having more devices that are less secure than they should be is creating more opportunities for hackers. Some of the problems are due to more records being digitized as part of the Affordable Care Act, but connected medical devices are most certainly a major concern for organizations.

The Road to High Risk

The key foundation for commerce is trust—trust in the exchange of money and/or good and services. Without trust, trade becomes riskier and less likely to happen. A thousand years ago you could touch, feel, see, and work with products. Today, in the IT world, we test products, read reviews, talk to peers, and so on. We install them, ensure the functionality, and do what we can to see if they work.

What is sometimes difficult to tell is how secure the product is. I once worked with a piece of software designed to examine security requirements. It did not meet many of the requirements it was examining in other products. While this may seem very rudimentary, it is not that uncommon for vendors not to do as they ask others to do. One famous case where this happened was a company formerly known as Bit9—a company that provides security protection software. They were hacked, but they did not use their own software to protect their environment. If they had, they would not have been hacked.[31]

---

[30] "Biosensors Market outlook will register 8% CAGR to overtake $29 billion by 2024," 2018, https://markets.businessinsider.com/news/stocks/ biosensors-market-outlook-will-register-8-cagr-to-overtake- 29-billion-by-2024-1027453347#.

[31] John Leyden, "Bit9 hacked after it forgot to install ITS OWN security product: Malware signed by stolen crypto certs then flung at big-cheese clients," 2013, https://www.theregister.com/2013/02/11/bit9_hack/.

What may be surprising to some of you is that some medical devices are built with old or outdated operating systems.[32] What this means is the systems are full of weaknesses (called vulnerabilities in the security world) that can be exploited by hackers. The vulnerabilities are often so severe that the entire system can be compromised. Every shred of data related to the system can also be compromised. What is worse, that system can then be used to compromise other systems in a hospital. The fact that so many systems have severe vulnerabilities compounds the problems of security practitioners trying to protect the hospitals in the first place.

To make matters worse, in many cases the interface to the machine completely obfuscates the operating system, making it difficult to assess the underlying technology. The manufacturer can also add security on the front end of the medical devices, making it seem as though the security is high. For example, some systems will provide strong password requirements such as long password length, complexity, password rotation, and so on, making it seem as though the system is built securely. That aspect of the system may be relatively secure, but not necessarily the rest of the product.

Many of you may be thinking that this is an old issue and that operating systems are usually up to date. The hard reality is that these outdated operating systems are almost par for the course when it comes to internet-connected medical devices. Recently Palo Alto Networks put out a report demonstrating that 83% of medical imaging devices had operating systems that could not be updated.[33] This is very serious as it means those operating systems have vulnerabilities that were not previously known and they cannot be remediated. From a hacker's perspective, these internet-connected medical devices are a metaphorical gold mine—not only because they have data, but also because they are relatively easy to hack—often allowing hackers to jump from one system to another within an organization.

This very same idea can be applied to other internet-connected medical devices that do not utilize a full operating system. In those cases, the system has a very small operating system known as firmware. On a personal computer firmware can be updated very easily, but devices that are very small with firmware only may or may not be

---

[32] Heather Landi, "70% of medical devices will be running unsupported Windows operating systems by January: report," 2019, https://www.fiercehealthcare.com/tech/medical-devices-running-legacy-windows-operating-system.

[33] "Unit 42 IoT Threat Report 2020" 2020, https://unit42.paloaltonetworks.com/iot-threat-report-2020/.

updatable—cybersecurity patches cannot be applied In some cases, what is included is unalterable. The unalterable nature of the device is referred to as *hardcoded*. This is where passwords are hardcoded into some of the devices.

Processors are another avenue of attack. In January 2018, two new processor vulnerabilities, Spectre and Meltdown, hit the news and security staff across the world like a ton of bricks. They uncovered, and subsequently demonstrated, flaws in the way that motherboards were designed over the last few decades. As a result of the motherboard flaws, operating systems could be compromised in ways that previously the hardware would have provided some protection. Ultimately, if an attacker had access to a system, data could be exposed by the combination of the two vulnerabilities (of which there are three variations). For Meltdown, an attacker gains access to data they normally shouldn't see by "melting" the division of protected memory normally enforced by hardware. Spectre, on the other hand, is about making a system reveal data that it should not reveal to the attacker.[34]

Both Spectre and Meltdown are examples of what were zero-day vulnerabilities—flaws that, at the time, were out but, as they are too new, do not have remediation. Hardware (such as motherboards), operating systems, and internet-connected medical devices are all prone to zero-day vulnerabilities. They are the bane of IT and security practitioners alike. They are the kind of situation, due to the severity of the vulnerability, that requires companies perform out of band patching (also called emergency patching), which can seriously disrupt the schedule of the IT department. While some zero-day vulnerabilities are of little consequence, many are much more serious—as Spectre and Meltdown were.

But why do we have these challenges with internet-connected medical devices to begin with? An incomplete and simplistic perspective might be to say that the dollar is king, security costs money, and therefore it is not done until companies are pushed into it. The reality is far more complex than that.

If we step back in time a decade for the purposes of looking at internet-connected medical device security, there were no regulations concerning their construction—very little regulatory oversight. In theory they had to meet HIPAA requirements, but many connected medical device

---

[34]Josh Fruhlinger, "Spectre and Meltdown explained: What they are, how they work, what's at risk," 2018, https://www.csoonline.com/article/3247868/spectre-and-meltdown-explained-what-they-are-how-they-work-whats-at-risk.html.

companies did not always adhere to those—not by a longshot. Quite often these companies were not even striving to meet HIPAA requirements. The features and functions of the devices were the key capabilities they had to focus on—not security capabilities.

What makes matters worse is not every company is validating the security or making security the priority when purchasing a medical device when making a purchase. Think of it this way: If you are looking at a half-million-dollar piece of medical equipment and one company has a product that the doctors find far better than other pieces of equipment and has a better chance of saving lives, versus another product that may not save as many lives but may be a little more secure, which product do you buy? Many companies would want to purchase the product that would save more lives. It is almost common sense when weighing one concern verses another. Many hospitals would not give security a second look. Further, if you have only one or two devices that are connected, it is easy to overlook the one insecure exception in your environment. This is the way medical equipment was for decades as internet-connected medical devices first made their appearance. Keep in mind that when this started taking place, connected medical devices were not commonplace and security was not as large of a priority as it is today. Context is everything.

Another challenge that hospitals are sometimes faced with two products with poor security (or sometimes even one product with poor security). In these situations, hospitals need to choose a product and simultaneously make the hospital less secure. In those situations, you kind of have to live with the an imperfect decision of having an insecure device or decide not to help people. For most, not helping people is unthinkable for very good reasons.

Innovate or Die

Peter Drucker, considered the father of modern management techniques, popularized (or perhaps originated) the phrase "Innovate or die."[35] What he was referring to was that companies needed to stay ahead of the pace of change from a market perspective or face obsolescence. In business today that means continually changing and updating your products to ensure marketability. As a former salesperson myself, if a competitor has an innovation you lack, that could be enough to give them the competitive edge to stay in business. Innovation is here to stay.

---

[35] Adi Ignatius, "Innovation on the Fly," 2014, https://hbr.org/2014/12/innovation-on-the-fly.

Perhaps the most poignant example of this is Blockbuster Entertainment Inc., more commonly known as Blockbuster. It had a brilliant business model in the 1990s. It offered a very convenient way to rent movies, video games, and so on, but it did not innovate. Blockbuster held the philosophy that people enjoyed going to a store to rent movies. They did not anticipate that people would prefer the advantages that a modern streaming service offers people. That philosophy was its undoing, and now it is out of business. The world is full of examples where this is true. For instance, Polaroid, Compaq, Borders, Tower Records, Atari, Kodak, and Xerox were all big, recognizable names 20 years ago. But the reality is, they did not innovate with the times and thus suffered or went out of business as a result. So, too, is that true for medical device companies.

Numerous studies have been done on the companies that have survived for decades or longer. The number-one trait that all of the companies share in common is adaptability—a willingness to change with the times. What is interesting to note is that this "innovate or die" attitude has taken on another life in Silicon Valley. At this point it is well known for both its innovation and its technology disruption. Deloitte stated it best: "More than one-third of the 141 companies in the Americas, Europe, and Asia Pacific that grew to a valuation of greater than $1 billion between 2010 and 2015 were located in the Bay Area."[36] CEOs and entrepreneurs know this. While there are countless keys to success, part of the success criteria is to make companies more agile by shortening the time to market. Indeed, many companies have had to shift their overarching philosophy. Large companies used to take the time to create products that were fully ready for the market. Billions of dollars were lost this way as a result of smaller, more agile, more innovative companies creating something more quickly. The old ways of doing business simply do not apply anymore.

In short, innovation is not just a random concept that is haphazardly thrown into business. It is the basis for business models. Companies are shaped around this philosophy and quite often far more successful than they were as a result of the transformations that go along with the desire to innovate. As you can imagine, the pressure to innovate is a very strong driving force in companies today. If we look back at the CEOs who were responsible for the downturn (and sometimes demise) of companies, they were under very harsh criticism for not turning

---

[36] Maximillian Schroek, Gopal Srinivasan, and Aishwarya Sharan, "How to innovate the Silicon Valley way," 2016, https://www2.deloitte.com/us/en/insights/topics/innovation/tapping-into-silicon-valley-culture-of-innovation.html#endnote-4.

companies around or losing business due to lack of innovation. This kind of pressure leads people and thus companies to make decisions that do not always have security in mind.

This kind of pressure also affects medical device manufacturers—so much so that there is a new name for the medicine coming out of connected medical devices: Medicine 2.0. Medicine 2.0 utilizes digital diagnostic capabilities, including wireless devices, mobile health solutions, data, smartphone apps, wearable devices, and remote monitoring. Other technologies such as cloud and artificial intelligence allow for greater innovation and more rewards for both the medical industry and the patient. These technologies are only accelerating as the pace of innovation changes and grows.[37]

Imagine what kind of pressure CEOs, product marketers, etc., face when creating products. Where does security fit in in this kind of world? Is it surprising that there are as many vulnerabilities in products that we are seeing today? The sad answer is no, and this is for multiple reasons. If we sidestep to nonconnected devices for a brief minute, the Associated Press reported that since 2008, medical devices for pain have caused more than 80,000 deaths—and this is a 2018 statistic.[38] The same Associated Press article talked about how little testing there is for those pain stimulators. That article was fair in that it pointed out that there are more than 190,000 devices on the market and very rarely do they need to pull devices. Yes, occasionally things get through that are bad, but the system is working remarkably well in the FDA's estimation.[39] The central point here is that despite having processes in place, those processes are far from perfect and could use greater transparency so we as consumers can make better decisions.

To that point, Kaiser Health News (KHN) did a fantastic report in late 2019 about patient deaths related to heart devices. In this case, the report discussed more than 5,800 deaths reported about the MedTronic

---

[37] Tom Van De Belt, Lucien Engelen, JLPG, Rafael Mayoral, Sivera AA Berben, Lisette Schoonhoven "Definition of Health 2.0 and Medicine 2.0: A Systematic Review," 2010, https://www.ncbi.nlm.nih.gov/pmc/articles/PMC2956229/.
[38] https://www.statnews.com/2018/11/25/medical-devices-pain-other-conditions-more-than-80000-deaths-since-2008/#:~:text=The%20media%20partners%20found%20that,FDA%20over%20the%20last%20decade.
[39] "Medical devices for pain, other conditions have caused more than 80,000 deaths since 2008," Associated Press, November 25, 2018, https://www.statnews.com/2018/11/25/medical-devices-pain-other-conditions-more-than-80000-deaths-since-2008/#:~:text=The%20media%20partners%20found%20that,FDA%20over%20the%20last%20decade.

heart valve since 2014. FDA made it sound as though the deaths were related to the heart valve. As it turns out, the FDA was not as transparent as it could have been about the deaths. KHN reported that many of the deaths were due to how fragile the people were who were receiving the heart valve and not related to the heart valve itself. Many of the device injury reports were kept effectively hidden from the public. Even safety experts were not aware of the problems.[40] What this does point to is that we do not have enough information to make a strong judgment call about the risks pertaining to internet-connected medical devices in all cases.

There is the obvious feature and hardware side of things when it comes to connected medical devices, but the more important part from this perspective is the software that is written in and around medical devices. As the business world must evolve or die, so must software live within those paradigms. To that end, software security has often taken a back seat compared to other disciplines. There is an old joke that has evolved since 1997 about how unstable Windows is and comparing its operability to that of a car.[41] The joke is much more involved, but it does serve to illustrate the problems with software development even back then—not just from a security standpoint, but an overall operability standpoint.

Automobile engineers have to have high safety standard. People can die as a result of a car's brakes not working (for example). With software it is historically acceptable to have flaws because, generally speaking, lives are not on the line. The discipline never developed the kind of rigor typically found in automobile engineering. Software coding is a little bit more of art than science in many cases because there can be numerous ways of obtaining an objective. The end result is systems that are riddled with vulnerabilities. Windows 10, at the time of this writing has 1,111 known vulnerabilities.[42] The more complex a system is, the more likely there will be risks associated with those vulnerabilities.

---

[40] Chistina Jewett, "Reports Of Patients' Deaths Linked To Heart Devices Lurk Below the Radar," 2019, https://khn.org/news/reports-of-patients-deaths-linked-to-heart-devices-lurk-below-radar/.

[41] David Mikkelson, "General Motors Replies to Bill Gates: General Motors responds to Bill Gates," https://www.snopes.com/fact-check/car-balk/.

[42] "CVE Details The ultimate security vulnerability datasource," accessed October 2020, https://www.cvedetails.com/vulnerability-list.php?vendor_id=26&product_id=32238&version_id=&page=23&hasexp=0&opdos=0&opec=0&opov=0&opcsrf=0&opgpriv=0&opsqli=0&opxss=0&opdirt=0&opmemc=0&ophttprs=0&opbyp=0&opfileinc=0&opginf=0&cvssscoremin=0&cvssscoremax=0&year=0&month=0&cweid=0&order=1&trc=1111&sha=41e451b72c2e412c0a1cb8cb1dcfee3d16d51c44.

What is almost as concerning as the number of vulnerabilities is how we got here. In 2016, Global Newswire published the results of a Cloud-Passage study of United States' universities failing at cybersecurity. The key findings brought out by the study may be jaw dropping for the uninitiated, but not surprising for those in the cybersecurity profession. The most startling finding was the almost complete lack of security required by computer science programs for graduation. Of the top 36 Computer Science Programs (according to *U.S. News and World Report*) only one had a cybersecurity required course. According to *Business Insider*'s top 50 list, there were only three programs that required cybersecurity to graduate.[43]

When it comes to cybersecurity, quite often universities are not the place to get that education. People walk out of school barely cybersecurity literate, but eager to start building IT systems. How secure do you think those systems will be if no one educates them on how to build secure systems? While there are certainly exceptions and companies have degree programs in cybersecurity, it does show the extreme deficit about the methods for protecting organizations. People who are interested in cybersecurity either need to learn on the job, go to a very specialized school, or go get cybersecurity certifications.

From a software development perspective, organizations need to supplement the understanding of the workers to get on board. Further, the lack of cybersecurity education helps to contribute to a lack of understanding of cybersecurity within organizations. That, in turn, affects the culture of the organization and ultimately the cybersecurity posture within organizations. Only companies with strong regulatory requirements or that have gone through a breach feel that they need a team to get them up to speed. Some of the requirements of cybersecurity may even appear bizarre due to cybersecurity illiteracy.

We could stop here, but the story is really more complex than that. Todd Fitzgerald, in his book *CISO Compass*, brilliantly lays out the course of cybersecurity over the last 30 years. He points out from the 1990s to 2000 that security was seen as an IT problem—basically login security, passwords, antivirus, and the firewall. From 2000 to 2004 we started to see more regulatory security practitioners as the regulations began kicking in, so there was an emphasis on the regulatory landscape. From 2004 to

---

[43] "CloudPassage Study Finds U.S. Universities Failing in Cybersecurity Education," Cloud Passage, April 7, 2016, https://www.globenewswire.com/news-release/2016/04/07/1312702/0/en/CloudPassage-Study-Finds-U-S-Universities-Failing-in-Cybersecurity-Education.html.

2008, there was a turn toward a more risk-oriented approach to doing information security, and from 2008 to 2016 the move was more toward understanding the threats and toward understanding the cloud. After 2016, the move was to privacy and data awareness as another aspect of security evolution.[44]

Having worked in IT and security for roughly 25 years, I have seen firsthand the evolution that Todd Fitzgerald is talking about. All of these are extremely valuable insights that demonstrate the growth and change within the information security landscape. Given that company culture can take up to five years to make changes[45] (depending on the size and speed of cultural change), often businesses are well behind the curve of what they ought to be doing from a cybersecurity perspective (depending on the organization, of course). That said, appropriate momentum is required to make the appropriate changes. Obviously, for areas of resistance or where there is a lack of knowledge, such as in software development, changes can take quite a bit longer.

Another side of the equation is business perception around value. When IT was an up-and-coming phenomenon, many businesses perceived it as a cost center. They did not want to put the time and effort into supporting the men and women in that department. IT is now seen as a business enabler. Information security has had one foot in the cost center arena according to some businesses. The higher-risk and more highly regulated businesses elevated security more quickly as a business enabler—partially because it was. Various vendor risk programs required the security be heightened in order for business to commence. In heavy regulatory environments, they often had data breaches that cost them more and therefore security was given more clout to get the work done—they were not merely a cost center. They were protecting the business. They were seen as a business enabler. In these environments, despite the lack of education, they are able to form stronger cybersecurity practices—generally speaking.

Microsoft spends over a billion dollars a year on security, and some of that is devoted to patching the vulnerabilities in its operating systems.[46] Not all companies are as diligent as Microsoft, but it does

---

[44] Todd Fitzgerald, *CISO Compass: Navigating cybersecurity leadership challenges with insight from pioneers*, CRC Press 2019, page 5.

[45] Barry Phegan, "314 - How Fast Can a Culture Change," https://companyculture.com/314-how-fast-can-culture-change/.

[46] Dan Patterson, "Why Microsoft spends over $1 billion on cybersecurity each year," 2018, https://www.techrepublic.com/article/why-microsoft-spends-over-1-billion-on-cybersecurity-each-year/.

demonstrate that even security-conscious companies like Microsoft still find vulnerabilities in their code. In the IoMT world, not all companies will invest in the legacy systems to the degree Microsoft will. This can lead to vulnerabilities remaining on the systems. What is worse, many internet-connected medical devices cannot have agents installed on them.[47] On Microsoft Windows, there are hundreds if not thousands of agents that can be installed to help protect the system. That single fact alone makes protecting internet-connected medical devices more challenging—alternative strategies must often be utilized.

All of these are influences on the security of internet-connected medical devices, but they still do not tell a sufficient story. Obviously, internet-connected medical devices are influenced by the prevailing culture, but the security behind these devices has often lapsed well behind the security of other pieces of software. This, of course, does not mean there isn't software that isn't riddled with flaws, but it does mean that medical device security has often taken a back seat to security requirements if security is recognized at all. Combined with the constant drive to innovate, this only exacerbates the security challenges.

To top it all off, the manufacturers are doing what they can to limit their liability in case things go awry. In March 2019, Bethany Corbin elucidated the challenges both brilliantly and clearly the legal challenges affecting internet-connected medical devices:

"Compounding this issue of non-regulation and insecure code is the lack of a comprehensive and workable liability framework for consumers to follow if their IoMT device malfunctions or is hacked. The application of tort principles to evolving IoMT devices is imperfect, creating challenges for plaintiffs seeking damages. In particular, the numerous actors in the IoMT supply chain make it difficult to apportion liability, with no clear boundaries establishing which party is at fault for a hack or breach. Similarly, defect-free software does not exist, which complicates the application of strict products liability. Further, end-user licensing agreements contractually limit manufacturer liability for defective devices, shifting the risk of harm to consumers and eliminating manufacturer incentives to comply with cybersecurity best practices."[48]

---

[47] Greg Murphy, "No Time to Waste: Why Automation Will Shape The Future of IoMT Security," https://www.healthitoutcomes.com/doc/no-time-to-waste-why-automation-will-shape-the-future-of-iomt-security-0001.
[48] Bethany Corbin, "When 'Things' Go Wrong: Redefining Liability for the Internet of Medical Things," March 2019, https://papers.ssrn.com/sol3/papers.cfm?abstract_id=3375070.

In Summary

In the end, we have a tremendous number of factors that play into the challenges we face when it comes to protecting internet-connected medical devices. With no clear liability, there is little incentive to make secure products. The deck appears stacked against strong security in connected medical devices, and the drive to innovate further into Medicine 2.0 only compounds the issues over time. What we need to do is take a deeper dive into the technology to help us better understand the technological forces at play. What is underneath the proverbial covers is more concerning than the strategic challenges we face related to not just cybersecurity, but to the medical devices, our data, and in rare cases, our very lives.

Just because something rarely takes place does not diminish its importance. As internet-connected medical devices grow in number and complexity, so too will the vulnerabilities related to them, and ultimately this has an impact on the security of not only the devices, but also our data. To accentuate the point of continual innovation, that innovation is often on the software side of the house, and keeping up with the micro changes in each device can and does mean more security risks if proper oversight and process is not taken into account. The Silicon Valley approach of working directly with the customers to create changes almost on the fly is alluring to customers, but can also provide the fuel for more vulnerabilities in the ever-more interconnected world of internet-connected medical devices.

The Internet of Medical Things in Depth

Leaving a broken system the way it is, that's not a solution.
—Barack Obama

In order to understand the risks related to internet-connected medical devices, it is important to understand what medical devices are. That requires not only understanding the individual components that comprise internet-connected medical devices, but also how the parts fit into the larger ecosystem of devices and technology and, in some cases, ultimately services. This, in turn, has a huge impact on the security of healthcare organizations and potentially our very lives.

To accomplish this, we'll explore a bit of the evolution into internet-connected medical devices and the current challenges with the various kinds of devices and technology—including the vulnerabilities. Think of a vulnerability as a weakness in the system. Those vulnerabilities are such a pervasive part of the building blocks of internet-connected medical devices that it may seem hard to understand how to get past them from a layperson's perspective. This is such a critical chapter because it sets a central foundation that will be explored throughout this book—how we protect medical devices, our medical institutions, our data, and our lives.

What Are Medical Things?

The first device to be connected to the internet was not a medical device. Of all things, it was a toaster. This was back in 1990.[1] The only capability it had was to turn on and off over the internet. For historical contrast, it would not be until 1991 when the first web page was created. These were very early days. The idea for having devices connect to the internet is quite old—the idea was around even during the 1970s. It was often referred to as the "embedded internet" of "pervasive computing." In 1999, Kevin Ashton was giving a presentation to sell an idea he had to Proctor & Gamble.[2] He knew executives thought this internet was going to kick off so he wanted them to quickly understand what he was talking about. For the presentation he coined the phrase "internet of things." Now internet-connected devices are commonly referred to as IoT for short.

The primary consideration for an IoT device is that it is a physical object. In the consumer market we can see examples of IoT devices such as thermostats, physical security systems, and appliances. This only scratches the surface of what IoT can do. Now IoT is used in a vast array of applications. There are IoT cars, energy management systems, industrial applications, manufacturing, agriculture, environmental monitoring, military equipment, and so on. IoT is so pervasive that there are many offshoots of the technology. Medical devices are only one such offshoot. They are typically called the internet of medical things, or IoMT.

But what differentiates IoMT from IoT? Not considering the connectivity and sufficient to forward our discussion, the FDA defines a medical device as

> *"An instrument, apparatus, implement, machine, contrivance, implant, in vitro reagent, or other similar or related article, including a component part, or accessory which is:*
>
> 1. *recognized in the official National Formulary, or the United States Pharmacopoeia, or any supplement to them,*
> 2. *intended for use in the diagnosis of disease or other conditions, or in the cure, mitigation, treatment, or prevention of disease, in man or other animals, or*

---

[1] Trevor Harwood, "Internet of Things (IoT) History: A closer look at who coined the term and the background evolution into today's trending topic." November 12, 2019, https://www.postscapes.com/iot-history/.

[2] Alison DeNisco Rayome, "How the term 'Internet of Things' was invented," 2018, https://www.techrepublic.com/article/how-the-term-internet-of-things-was-invented/.

3. *intended to affect the structure or any function of the body of man or other animals, and*

which does not achieve its primary intended purposes through chemical action within or on the body of man or other animals and which does not achieve its primary intended purposes through chemical action within or on the body of man or other animals and which is not dependent upon being metabolized for the achievement of its primary intended purposes. The term "device" does not include software functions excluded pursuant to section 520(o)."[3]

But we have not touched on the connected medical devices. Many medical devices are connected, but not necessarily directly connected to the internet. In many cases the connection is through Bluetooth, a short-range wireless network that can be accessed over a few feet. In other cases, Near-Field Communication (NFC) is used, and one must be as close as 10 centimeters (roughly 2.5 inches) in order to connect.

From an internet-connected medical device perspective, there are two primary types of devices: telemedicine and data analytics. It is important to explore them as they are fundamental to future discussions.

Telemedicine

One of the most profound revolutions in Medicine 2.0 is telemedicine. It involves a range of technologies that has revolutionized how we diagnose, monitor, and treat patients today. We have only seen the beginnings of where this technology will eventually go. Right now it is limited by the types of technology we have for monitoring and communicating. Imagine one day when we have powerful nanotechnology capable of detecting, diagnosing, and treating medical issues long before they become bad enough for us to be aware of them. The potential for cost savings in the future, I believe, lies with telemedicine.

But what is telemedicine? For some, it means doctors talking to patients over a computer or an app on a cell phone. It can also include, in specific situations, diagnosis over radios. This is definitely a strong part of what telemedicine is about—and is not to be understated. With COVID-19 many people do not want to leave their homes and potentially be infected. The safest way to not be infected is to not be around COVID-19, and telemedicine allows doctors to assess and treat patients remotely.

---

[3] "How to Determine if Your Product Is a Medical Device," https://www.fda .gov/medical-devices/classify-your-medical-device/ how-determine-if-your-product-medical-device.

Telemedicine comes in two primary varieties: real time and store and forward. Real time is information that is very close to real time that is sent to devices. An example of this could be Zoom where people are talking to one another in near real time. Store and forward refers to devices that provide the information when the patient is in proximity to a device that will submit the information when possible. For example, some internet-connected medical devices are paired with Bluetooth and are only send information when the Bluetooth device is paired. It isn't always live information. For some devices, this makes much more sense.

If we kept this definition as the only definition of telemedicine, we would be missing key parts of why it is so important. Telemedicine also includes many types of monitoring tools, such as wearable devices, implanted devices, and, yes, ingestible devices. They allow doctors to detect medical problems as they come up and, more importantly, before they become emergencies. They can even be used to determine if patients are taking their medicine.

The wearable device market is all about monitoring a patient's vitals. Typically, they are worn on the wrist, but variations can be included on clothing or placed on the skin. What is great about wearables is that they do not require a significant amount of interaction other than wearing the devices. This includes, but is not limited to, heartbeat, stress levels, respiration, blood pressure, and temperature. Many of these devices use wireless technologies.

Implanted medical devices are devices that are stored within us, such as cardiac pacemakers, cardiac defibrillators, insulin pumps, and gastric stimulators. As with the wearables, many of these devices utilize wireless technology. They also cross over into medication management because they can help release medicine based on what they are sensing.

Ingestible IoT is critical for diagnosing and treating certain kinds of problems. It involves swallowing a pill with a camera or sensors. Even tiny X-rays can be used with ingestible devices. The information is then relayed wirelessly to nearby devices for analysis.

Data Analytics

Technically data analytics are not IoMT devices themselves, but they are tied into many IoMT systems. There are two types of technology that data analytics can rely on—machine learning and artificial intelligence. Think of machine learning as a stepping stone to artificial intelligence. Quite often machine learning can be used to sense trends more quickly than a human and, more often than not, reasonably accurately. With exceptions, machine learning is typically being used in most cases.

What is important about data analytics is how it is rapidly changing the playing field in medicine. The stream of data from IoMT devices is helping the medical community to identify not only problems but solutions at a faster pace than ever before. From a scientific perspective, it allows the medical community to use more fact-based cases to study, which will only improve the overall process.

Data analytics is also valuable from a population perspective. If a medication is causing problems in a population or for a particular pharmacy, data analytics is probably the best place to make that discovery. Another example is a medicine that may not be as effective for a particular case of a specific disease. This makes diverse populations like NYC especially attractive because we have a range of ethnic diversities, which may provide more insights related to diseases than focusing on a single demographic.

For many patients, especially the elderly, medication management is extremely important. It helps patients take the right amount of medication at the right time. And yes, there can be a connected component to this. Other devices, such as ingestibles, can actually monitor if the patient is really taking the medication or not.

The term *stationary medical devices* refers to the range of medical equipment that stays in the hospital setting. This can include everything from MRI systems to X-ray machines. Even beds are connected to provide additional information related to the status of a patient.

Asset management refers to the tracking and monitoring of high-value devices within hospitals. While this can be related to IoMT devices, it can also be related to tracking other valuable equipment such as wheelchairs.

Obviously, a tremendous number of IoMT devices have proliferated over the last few years. All of them bring value to hospitals and other organizations or they would not be there. In general, the IoMT is greatly reducing the costs of medical care today and allowing people to live better, more fulfilling lives. What is not always recognized are the risks that these modern technologies bring. For that, it is helpful to look at the history of IoMT and put IoMT technologies in context.

Historical IoMT Challenges

We have all heard the phrase that history repeats itself. Unfortunately, that is true for the security of IoT/IoMT as well. While not true for all companies and there has been a great deal of recent innovation related to IoT/IoMT security, historically this has not been the case. Historically speaking, companies do not want to invest more into the product than they have to. It is an additional cost and hurts the overall bottom line. Since cost is a factor when making business decisions, going the extra mile is not always a wise business decision. Combine with that the slow approval rates by the FDA, and it is no wonder that security is not as high as it could be.

Those in the software development space or the security space may be familiar with something called the Open Source Web Application Security Project (OWASP). It helps developers and security practitioners with secure programming practices. In 2018 OWASP released the Top 10 internet of things (IoT) vulnerability list.[4] It is one of the best aggregated lists of problems with IoT (and thus IoMT) devices. As we will explore, the IoT vulnerability list is an egregious list of challenges. From a security practitioner's perspective, it is appalling to design a system this way. The problems cited here are so severe, it is worth exploring all of them because they all apply to the historical challenges of IoMT. They also hint at the cultural challenges surrounding the IoT market, which, from a security standpoint, is very different from other IT markets such as Microsoft, which takes security very seriously.

Number one on the list is "Weak, Guessable, or Hardcoded Passwords."[5] Security practitioners have known for more than 20 years the importance of good password hygiene. Leaving the default password in place means that almost anyone with access to the network can own the device. Weak or easily guessable passwords are also just as unforgivable. Every year the top passwords used are published and they do not vary a great deal. Unsurprisingly, weak passwords tend to be the most hacked. This means a hacker can gain control of that data in many instances.

Second on the list is "Insecure Network Services."[6] This refers to vulnerabilities that could be exploited over a network that allow the system to be compromised. Not surprisingly, in some cases this refers to components that are not required for functionality of the device.

Third on the list is "Insecure Ecosystem Interfaces."[7] The ecosystem refers to all of the interconnections that device may have to other devices that could allow the device to be compromised. This includes various wireless communication, cloud connections, no authentication (no user-

---

[4] OWASP Internet of Things Project 2018 https://wiki.owasp.org/index.php/OWASP_Internet_of_Things_Project.
[5] Ibid.
[6] Ibid.
[7] Ibid.

name/password), no encryption in the communication, and lack of input and/or output filtering. Lack of authentication means that anyone with access to the interface can gain access to the information. Lack of encryption means that the system is vulnerable to a man-in-the-middle attack. This is someone who hasn't authenticated to the device, but may be inline from the communication. Essentially the information is in plain text and can be pulled. If it isn't clear, poor interface security can lead to data breaches, stolen passwords, etc.

The fourth item on the list is "Lack of Secure Update Mechanism."[8] Many IoT devices simply cannot be updated. In some cases this ties into hardcoded passwords, while in others it is the operating system or firmware that cannot be updated. This means that any vulnerabilities found cannot be remediated. Alternative methods must be used to protect the device.

If there was one item that causes a cascade of other items, it would be the fifth item, the "Use of Insecure or Outdated Components."[9] Having up-to-date components is critical as those components are foundational for everything else. Think of it this way: a percentage of you have thought about upgrading your computer, but were prevented from doing so because the hardware could not handle the upgraded operating system. Without the proper hardware, the operating system may get to a point where patching the system is simply not possible. Even worse, outdated components may have known vulnerabilities in it that can be compromised by an attacker.

We will get into some of the intricacies of privacy in Chapter 6, but "Insufficient Privacy Protection,"[10] the sixth item on the list, is almost an epidemic of its own. Based on everything identified so far, not only are there privacy gaps, but in many cases, there are compliance gaps. This particular deficit also points to the data being used improperly, such as storing on devices or with poor encryption or even no encryption in many cases.

"Insecure Data Transfer and Storage"[11] is also a serious problem with IoT devices. The range of issues on this seventh item include lack of encryption of the data at rest, in transit, or in use. Almost all of the compliance regulations require encrypting the data. Of course, that depends on the type of information. Not all information is regulated, so the type

---

[8] Ibid.
[9] Ibid.
[10] Ibid.
[11] Ibid.

and amount of information collected will influence the importance and the risks related to the data.

The eighth item on the list may not as intuitable as some of the others for the less technically inclined. It details the "Lack of Device Management."[12] What this means is that there is no centralized oversight of the IoT devices. This is important as the only way to discover a problem is to be at the specific IoT device. You have no way of knowing in a centralized fashion if data is leaving the device or not (at least through the existing technology). Also, if there is an issue on a thousand devices (for example), instead of making a change centrally and then pushing that change throughout the organization, each device must be connected to individually. Simple tasks can become monumental efforts. An extra console can make all the difference in the world.

"Insecure Default Settings" is number nine on the list.[13] In many cases this is much worse than it sounds. If an operating system can change the settings on the device, the risks can be reduced with due care. What they are also talking about is locking operators out from the system so they cannot make changes. In many cases, this is very prudent because an operator could prevent key functionality on the system thus rendering the device nonfunctional. Most manufacturers do not want to support a device if changes are made. This is even true for some software, so it is not just an IoT issue. This is often tied to outdated components or the ability to update the core operating system.

The final item on the list may also not be immediately intuitable as a problem for some of you. Number 10 is "Lack of Physical Hardening."[14] There is an old expression in security, "If you have physical access to a device, you own it." Not providing physical security for the devices is particularly concerning—especially if brought over to the medical world where outsiders have access to some of the medical devices when seeing patients.

It is important to keep in mind that not all of these items will be applicable to connected medical devices, but given the roots of medical devices within IoT, many of these items are quite common. In 2018, the FDA put out new regulation regarding the security of IoMT. While that was a large step forward, hospitals can hold onto devices for many years— often longer than they were intended to. This means that many of the previously approved devices may have one or more of these problems.

---

[12] Ibid.
[13] Ibid.
[14] Ibid.

But let us take a practical example of how these weaknesses in IoT can have disastrous and unforeseen consequences. In 2016, Paras Jha, an undergraduate at Rutgers University, wanted to see how DDOS attacks could be used for profit, so he attacked Rutgers so that the University would hire him. Eventually the DDOS tools used by Jha were enhanced and augmented by himself and a few friends. That code was posted online. Someone else decided to use the code against Dyn, an infrastructure company. This was on October 12, 2016. The resultant attack was a massive distributed denial of service (DDOS) attack that took out a large portion of the internet on the Eastern seaboard of the United States. A DDOS attack is caused when hundreds or thousands of IoT devices are compromised and then used to point internet traffic at one or more sources. In this case the hackers used the malware that, once it took over devices, then removed other pieces of malware that may be infecting the device so they could claim the device for themselves. All it took was to look for internet-exposed IoT devices to pull off the attack, along with a little ingenuity. In this case, the code had 61 usernames and passwords, which allowed the attackers to compromise devices such as cameras, home routers, and baby monitors. All of the devices were using a stripped-down version of the Linux operating systems, which the malware was looking for.[15] These were just a few kids who had no intention of causing the extreme problems they did.

While this story is not directly related to IoMT, it is indirectly related and serves as a strong cautionary tale. The security of these random internet-connected devices is very important. Lack of security can cause severe problems. The reality is governments and organized crime took note of what was going on. IoT was hitting center stage, and variants of Mirai were created after the fact—just looking for vulnerable devices to compromise.

Whether the devices had hardcoded passwords or it was just poor management on the part of the individual IoT device owners is more than an immaterial distinction. If the manufacturers had hardcoded passwords, it means that if the system is on the open internet, it can be compromised by looking up the default password. The two most obvious ways to protect the device is to not have it directly exposed on the open internet or to limit the inbound traffic on the internet that can

---

[15] Josh Fruhlinger, "The Mirai botnet explained: How teen scammers and CCTV cameras almost brough down the internet," 2018, https://www.csoonline.com/article/3258748/the-mirai-botnet-explained-how-teen-scammers-and-cctv-cameras-almost-brought-down-the-internet.html.

reach the device. While there are a few other options, it does illustrate the challenge of trying to protect devices with known vulnerabilities.

Let us take a look at a more recent case to validate this point. On January 9, 2017, the FDA released a statement saying that patients with a St. Jude Medical implantable cardiac device (along with the corresponding transmitter) were vulnerable, which could affect how the medical devices work.[16] The FDA went on to say that the Merlin@home Transmitter could ultimately be used to provide inappropriate shocks, cause rapid battery depletion, and so on. A device without battery life at a critical time could have potentially deadly consequences.

It may seem that 2017 was not that long ago, but from a technology perspective it was. Since then, the FDA has enacted new rules to help protect medical devices. Understanding that challenge, though, requires an understanding of the technology—the subject of the next section.

IoMT Technology

Security and technology go hand in hand. To understand the security risks within the IoMT, it really helps to understand the technology. Because this book is aimed at a general audience and not a technical one, we are only going to go deep enough to explain what the general issues are from a security standpoint. Please keep in mind much of what is discussed here is not true across the entire spectrum of medical devices. Each piece of technology has its own specific applicability.

Part of the reason it is so important to define what medical devices are is that it helps to determine what kinds of technology are built into the devices. Just as there is no one-size-fits-all in the medical device world, that is true for IoMT as well. Any generalizations made here are not meant to be applicable across the whole spectrum of IoMTs.

Electronic Boards

In a traditional computer there exists something called a motherboard. Without going into too many details, it is the central circuitry that connects

---

[16] "Cybersecurity Vulnerabilities Identified in St. Jude Medical's Implantable Cardiac Devices and Merlin@home Transmitter: FDA Safety Communication," https://www.fda.gov/medical-devices/safety-communications/cybersecurity-vulnerabilities-identified-st-jude-medicals-implantable-cardiac-devices-and-merlinhome.

different aspects of the system such as memory, the processor(s), input and output functions, the hard drive, monitor, and so on. What is important to consider from an IoMT perspective is that for some medical devices, many of the aspects of a traditional computer are baked into the motherboard. The end result is that memory, processing power, communications, and so on are severely limited. Often the "operating system" (firmware for the technophiles) is extremely limited and in some cases is not possible to upgrade or patch.

Operating Systems

Operating systems are another aspect of many connected medical devices. In many cases these are the same operating systems you may have at home. The first chapter covered medical imaging devices running on Windows XP. Another report from 802secure stated that 83% of the systems are running on outdated operating systems—a 56% jump from the previous year as a result of Windows 7 not being supported any longer.[17] In some cases these systems can be and are updated, but in other cases, the manufacturer will not support upgrades, making things a bit more challenging in hospitals.

Sometimes the issues of old operating systems are beyond the control of the manufacturers. The FDA can take as much as 5 to 6 years to approve a particular device.[18] Many companies are on a 3-year cycle for upgrading hardware. Imagine the quandary device manufacturers are in. Quite often the devices are released to the public with known vulnerabilities. The manufacturers can't change operating systems mid-stream. To make matters worse, many medical devices have a 15- to 20-year life span.[19] As of this writing, Windows XP has 741 known vulnerabilities[20]— many of which cannot be patched because it is not supported. This is a huge challenge because sometimes the hardware cannot support new operating systems. The fact that many IoMT systems are kept for 15 to 20 years creates other challenges. It is simply impossible for manufac-

---

[17] "Securing the Internet of Medical Things (IoMT)," https://802secure.com/wp-content/themes/802secure/pdf/AIRSHIELD-Health-Data-Sheet.pdf.

[18] "Clearwater Medical Device Security and CIO Insomnia," https://clearwatercompliance.com/blog/medical-device-security-and-cio-insomnia/.

[19] Ibid.

[20] "CVE Detail," https://www.cvedetails.com/product/739/Microsoft-Windows-Xp.html?vendor_id=26.

turers, developers, and operating systems to keep patching systems for 15 plus years. Inadvertently, it becomes an intersection where all of these problems create an environment that is essentially a hacker's paradise.

Software Development

Secure software development is arguably one of the more important controls in information security—especially if data is accessed through that software. If you have a poorly written application, it can mean the difference between securing the data and not securing the data. The challenge with software development is that there can be ten ways, all legitimate, of accomplishing the same control. In many other parts of information technology, there is a button to press and you are done. From a historical perspective, there are some cultural challenges.

Typically, developers use something called the software development lifecycle (SDLC). The SDLC includes methods of eliminating the various problems. These include peer review, unit testing, line testing, and a host of other techniques. What is missing from the SDLC processes of less mature organizations (from a security standpoint) is security. Depending on when and where you went to school, security may or may not have been a consideration. Oftentimes, it is up to organizations to train developers about security.

Training developers on security can be a little like herding cats. Doing it right means you have to have several things in place. First, you need a set of guidelines and security standards for the team to follow. Just right-sizing the amount of information to provide the developers can be a daunting task for organizations. Providing too much information means it will not be retained right away. Not providing enough means other challenges for the organizations.

Another aspect of a good coding environment is tooling. There are fantastic tools on the market that can detect problems before the product goes into production, and using them in the right way is one way to reduce the risks to the organization. However, the tools do have blind spots when it comes to human logic flaws. It is not something these kinds of applications are good at, and thus penetration tests are critical to the final product being secure. A penetration test is a process where both vulnerabilities and human logic flaws are discovered. While tools are used, there is a human aspect to the assessment process.

Sadly, not all companies have the time or resources to have a mature secure SDLC that includes all of the right tools being used in the right way. In cybersecurity there is a phrase called "Separation of Duties"

(SoD). In this specific context, it is important to have some SoD between the software developers and the cybersecurity team signing off that the software is ready for production. If a software developer checks the software, they may or may not adhere to the requirements depending on the person or context. They may or may not ensure that what goes onto the market does meet FDA security requirements.

Software development has shifted considerably over the years. What is common now is an iterative approach to software development known as scrum. Many years ago, software was only created in versions. The first version was 1.0. Bug fixes could take it to 1.01. while minor revisions could take the software to 1.1. Larger revisions would go to 2.0. While versioning is still common and highly practiced, when it comes to the cloud aspects of development, an iterative model is much more common. Iterative means the product continually improves as part of the Software-as-a-Service. It is also a good business practice to ensure you continually evolve to meet the client's needs. The challenge here is for that development to be continually secure—assuming the software was secure to begin with. It takes time to perform the aforementioned penetration tests. Given that updates can now occur multiple times a day, it is a challenge for security to keep up.

Wireless

There are multiple types of wireless connections for medical devices. The full range of wireless connectivity includes Wi-Fi, near-field communications (NFC), cellular, Bluetooth, and occasionally RFID. All have their strengths and weaknesses—especially when you consider the potential 20-year life span.

Wi-Fi is particularly attractive for many of the remote monitoring capabilities built into connected medical devices. There is an easy bridge to the internet, which means the system can be monitored in the cloud (more on the cloud in a while). From there, hospitals, doctors, and patients can be alerted in a moment's notice if there are any issues. As a result of COVID-19, the wireless technologies are gaining in popularity—especially as they relate to telemedicine. They are also important for some hospitals that have rooms that block cellular service (as a byproduct of blocking other systems).

Over Wi-Fi's comparatively long history there have been a great number of improvements, not only from the functional standpoint, but also with regard to security. The precursor to Wi-Fi, Wavenet, was created back in 1991—just after the dawn of the internet. Wireless signals were not encrypted back then. It would not be until 1997 that Wire Equivalent Privacy (WEP) was created and included with Wi-Fi devices. It had a 10- or 26-digit key written in hexadecimal, but with modern technology WEP can be hacked in under a second. What replaced WEP is Wi-Fi Protected Access or WPA. This was back in 2003. Now WPA has had several different iterations—WPA, WPA2, and WPA3. WPA3 was most recently included in modern Wi-Fi devices in 2018. The upgrades in encryption are substantial between the versions, but each one was replaced partially because vulnerabilities were discovered in the system.

Vulnerabilities are not the only problem with Wi-Fi. Configuration is also a huge problem. Many systems are configured to be encrypted. This is important because anyone in range can sniff the traffic over that connection. Having performed many Wi-Fi assessments myself, I know it is a very common problem. Interestingly enough I was just reading about a case where the FBI warned against using hotel Wi-Fi for work purposes because of the often-lax security standards in Wi-Fi configurations.[21] Not every company gets Wi-Fi security right. Combine this with hospitals using IoMT systems for extended periods of times, and old insecure protocols in Wi-Fi are required to support older devices.

But let us switch to cellular systems. Right now, we are seeing the shift from 4G cellular technology to 5G technology. For many devices switching from one technology to another is not a huge challenge—often, but not always, it is a feature that can be plugged into a motherboard that can be easily replaced. But, as you may have guessed, cellular technologies are not without their vulnerabilities that can be easily exploited. One of the black market accessible devices are "Stingrays," which are also known as International Mobile Subscriber Identity "(IMSI) catchers."[22] They are capable of interfering with cellular communications. From a hospital's perspective this is extraordinarily dangerous because some of their systems are dependent on cellular communications. In security shorthand, this is an attack on availability.

Another weakness in cellular technology is something referred to as SS7 and the IP version of the protocol known as SIGTRAN—protocols designed more than a decade ago. They were designed without consider-

---

[21] Matthew Humphries, "FBI Warns Against Using Hotel Wi-Fi for Work: The FBI says hotels in cities across the US have lax security allowing for easy exploitation by malicious actors," 2020, https://www.entrepreneur.com/article/357524.
[22] Jefferson B. Sessions II, 2018, https://www.wyden.senate.gov/imo/media/doc/08212018%20RW%20Stingray%20Jamming%20Letter%20to%20DOJ.pdf.

ations to modern security. No one had envisioned the widespread use of wireless technology. The current 4G protocol is based on Diameter. Diameter, without getting too technical, is a protocol that enables validation of technology, and sometimes users, over a network. Now it is built on the internet protocol, but is essentially only marginally better. But what is worse, in early 2019, a new flaw was discovered that allows attackers to intercept calls and track phone locations. This is true for both 4G and 5G cellular service,[23] despite the newer protection in 5G.[24]

Several more pages could be devoted to exploring the intricacies of vulnerabilities in cellular service, but the point here is that cellular technologies also have vulnerabilities as a key aspect of the technology. But let us turn our attention to short-distance wireless communication—with exceptions, this typically means Bluetooth. Bluetooth development was initiated in 1989 by Ericsson Mobile in Sweden. The purpose of Bluetooth was essentially for wireless headphones. Of course, the uses for Bluetooth have expanded well beyond that (yes, including medical devices) to the point where it is almost ubiquitous around the world. What is unique about Bluetooth compared to other technologies is that it is easy to trick users into allowing a connection to a device. This process is so common that it has a name—BlueSnarfing. This brings the fallible human element to the security of systems in the environment. But what is more alarming is the sheer number of vulnerabilities that have appeared over the years. At the moment of writing this, in 2020 alone there have been 49 vulnerabilities found in Bluetooth. Many of the vulnerabilities allow for access to the full system. Four of them are from the applications designed to help with COVID.[25]

If you extend the timeline back to 2002 when the MITRE corporation was publicly tracking the vulnerabilities, at the time of this writing, there were 388 vulnerabilities. As fantastic as MITRE is, this is far from a complete list. For example, on March 3, 2020, the FDA released a warning about a set of vulnerabilities known as "SweynTooth." SweynTooth affected certain medical devices that utilized Bluetooth Low Energy—in particular, pacemakers, glucose monitors, ultrasound devices, electrocardiograms,

---

[23] Zack Whittaker, "New flaws in 4G, 5G allow attackers to intercept calls and track phone locations," 2019, https://techcrunch.com/2019/02/24/new-4g-5g-security-flaws/.

[24] Wikipedia, https://en.wikipedia.org/wiki/Bluetooth, accessed October 24, 2020.

[25] "Common Vulnerabilities Exposures," https://cve.mitre.org/cgi-bin/cvekey.cgi?keyword=Bluetooth, accessed October 24, 2020.

and monitors. This was not listed by MITRE.[26] In a worst-case scenario the vulnerability can stop a device from working, or allow an attacker to access the device functionality, which is usually available only to authorized users.[27] While the attack would have to be within a few feet, the *Homeland* scenario of stopping a pacemaker does not seem so farfetched.

The SweynTooth family of vulnerabilities was linked in part to manufacturers of microchips. Think of a microchip as a tiny part of a motherboard. This means that the fault may not be with the makers of the motherboards, but with some of companies that help with subcomponents of the motherboards. The challenges from a security standpoint are widespread to say the least.

NFC has a very short range—roughly 4 inches. As a result, it has a very unique place within the arena of connected medical devices. Some of the applications of NFC include logical access to medical information, Intelligent ID bracelets, tagging of medications, physical access, and so on.[28] The tagged ID bracelets and other such items do not store medical information. That reduces the risk considerably, which is a good thing because there is no authentication within NFC. The risks concerning NFC generally are around two devices in active mode—where information can be transferred. For many uses, NFC is typically in passive mode for tagging purposes. While it is a huge help for hospitals, from a connected medical device perspective, the risks tend to be lower, but not zero. For example, in 2019, Android devices had an NFC vulnerability that exposed the devices to malware attacks and, worse, privilege escalation (which means anyone can do almost anything to the device).[29] In most settings this is not a huge risk, but if you had a device that uses NFC, that could be a risk to all the other systems the device was connected to. In some environments, this includes protected health information.

---

[26] "FDA News Release FDA Informs Patients, Providers and Manufacturers About Potential Cybersecurity Vulnerabilities in Certain Medical Devices with Bluetooth Low Energy," March 3, 2020, https://www.fda.gov/news-events/press-announcements/fda-informs-patients-providers-and-manufacturers-about-potential-cybersecurity-vulnerabilities-0.

[27] Ibid.

[28] Cristina Ardila, "Six Ways NFC Helps Healthcare," 2015, https://www.nxp.com/company/blog/six-ways-nfc-helps-healthcare:BL-6-WAYS-NFC-HELPS-HEALTHCARE.

[29] Zak Doffman, "New Google Android Threat: NFC Exposes Devices To Malware Attack—Update Settings Now," 2019, https://www.forbes.com/sites/zakdoffman/2019/11/02/new-android-threat-contactless-payment-technology-open-to-attackchange-your-settings/#4ed6ccf45cde.

Wired Connections

Wired networks have a very different security concerns than wireless networks, generally speaking. People can use devices to snoop wireless traffic, pretend to be an access point you would want to connect to in a local coffee shop, and so on. Wired networks, from a healthcare perspective, are generally where there is an aggregation of devices—where all the IoMT devices are located. Wireless networks are also where some of the other more breached systems are located. There are a host of problems related to wired networks, which will be discussed in Chapter 10, "Network Infrastructure and IoMT."

The Cloud

Twenty years ago, most companies had their own electronic infrastructure to store, process, and transmit information. They had independent servers that had a one-to-one relationship to the operating system. Later, virtualized operating systems hit the scene, so many servers could be on one system. Now, due to business advantages, many companies utilize cloud services for the same purpose. In the cloud, systems are divided virtually and logically in cloud environments. The economics of scale within the cloud make a great deal of sense for many companies due to a principle known as elasticity. This means that systems can spin up and down both servers and can add and/or remove compute power to meet immediate demands. While traditional systems have virtualization technology, what most virtualization technology accomplishes is the ease of scalability. Traditional systems have to purchase the computing power, storage, and memory maximum that are required. With the cloud, these maximums do not need to be purchased. In the end, for companies who need this kind of elasticity, the cloud makes perfect sense. Cloud has proven a lifesaver for companies that have had to shut down or reduce their footprint due to COVID-19. They don't have expensive equipment to power, thus saving money that is not possible with traditional infrastructure. They do not have to pay for processing power—only storage for keeping their virtualized systems powered down, which is a huge cost savings.

For the IoMT, the cloud is a very critical component because for some companies the growing ubiquity means that companies will need to grow as their devices grow. While there are a range of technologies that aid or support connectivity, the cloud is one of the key technologies. That being said, cloud technologies come with their own types of unique risks. Mature companies have the issues related to those risks mostly accounted for, but smaller companies are not always as adept at understanding or compensating for those risks. For example, where companies had traditional physical security to keep track of, a cloud provider takes full responsibility for that security.

Some of the differences that take some getting used to for many companies are cloud native capabilities. For example, years ago, traditional systems used a database. Think of a database as a giant electronic repository of data. It is more complex than that, but it is sufficient for this discussion. Today, a separate database does not need to be purchased. Many cloud systems have databases built into the infrastructure. We refer to those as cloud native systems. The challenge for companies is that there is a learning curve when it comes to cloud native systems. Let's take the example of the S3 bucket, which is a cloud native database within Amazon Web Services (AWS). (I almost wish I had kept track of the number of organizations—both government and corporate—that have been hacked as a result of a misconfigured S3 bucket.) It is a very common occurrence despite the fact that AWS has increased the security and brought to the attention of others the dangers related to it and has educational information on how to configure the S3 bucket securely. One of the proverbial sins of IT is to make sure that a system works, but not to make sure that the system is secure. If everyone on the internet can access the system, it is probably working from an IT perspective—often the administrator not realizing they just opened the database to hackers as well. This is not just a problem of small companies; some of the major breaches that have hit the news are related to S3 bucket security. Examples include such prominent names as Uber, Accenture, and even the United States Department of Defense.[30] While there is a much deeper dive that can be had related to this specific topic, suffice it to say that cloud native technology has its challenges, and not all companies are equally up to those challenges.

The reason this is important to consider is that companies often store the information related to the connected medical devices in those buckets—often without the knowledge of the end users of those systems. All a physician cares about is ensuring their system works properly when they need it to. They are operating under the assumption the host company is doing the security properly.

---

[30] Marc Laliberte, "How data breaches forced Amazon to update S3 bucket security," 2019, https://www.helpnetsecurity.com/2019/09/23/s3-bucket-security/.

Many of you may be thinking that the problem has to be resolved soon. The reality is the problem does not appear to be going away. In August 2020, Truffle Security reported that they uncovered thousands of leaky S3 buckets in AWS that are accessible to anyone on the internet without authentication.[31] To make matters worse, they believe that these open buckets are "wormable." This means that software could be written so that one bucket leads to another, magnifying the impact of a leak. With all of these leaks, it is only a matter of time before ransomware based on misconfigured S3 buckets will become a new norm. Already the proof of concept has been created.[32]

While AWS is the focus of this discussion, most of the major cloud providers have their own versions of the AWS S3 buckets. Since AWS is the largest player in the market (and one of the most mature of the cloud players), it is used by many and thus these issues are more prevalent. As the other cloud providers become more prevalent, these issues will pop up. There are numerous articles about some of their competitors.

A few of the more astute readers have probably noted that this chapter has not touched on the most obvious aspect of databases—encryption. A foundational requirement in information security is to encrypt data. HyTrust performed a survey of companies moving to the cloud. The survey uncovered that 25% of healthcare organizations are not encrypting data in the cloud.[33] What has not been specified is if this is related to cloud native databases or installed, non-native databases. Either way, it is a very serious issue and points to lack of due diligence and/or due care in organizations.

Another cloud native technology that is a challenge for some businesses is the portal to the clouds themselves. Think of that portal as an administrative gateway that provides full access to one or more virtual data centers. That access includes all cloud native infrastructure, and now, quite often, virtual computers used by everyday corporate employees.

[31] Truffle Bot, "An API Worm In The Making: Thousands of Secrets Found In Open S3 Buckets," 2020, `https://trufflesecurity.com/blog/an-s3-bucket-worm-in-the-making-thousands-of-secrets-found-in-open-s3-buckets`.

[32] Spencer Gietzen, "S3 Ransomware Part 1: Attack Vector," `https://rhinosecuritylabs.com/aws/s3-ransomware-part-1-attack-vector/`.

[33] HyTrust, "HyTrust Cloud Survey Finds 25% of Healthcare Organizations Are Putting Patient Data at Risk in the Public Cloud," February 15, 2017, `https://www.hytrust.com/news-item/hytrust-cloud-survey-finds-quarter-healthcare-orgs-putting-patient-data-risk/`.

So far, though, I have not touched on a branch of the cloud known as Software-as-a-Service (SaaS). Instead of needing to build your own tools in the cloud, services are available to do many of the common actions that hospitals and doctors' offices would otherwise need to create on their own. While sometimes there is a significant customization effort, these tools can provide companies with huge cost savings. Many of these companies also provide the compliance and security necessary to secure the data. Of course, these third-party vendors are far from perfect. Atrium Health had to notify 2.65 million individuals of a data breach as a result of AccuDoc being breached.[34] So, due diligence related to the vendors is a must just as with any technology.

Mobile Devices and Applications

The use of mobile applications in medicine is becoming more common with each passing year. They cover everything from information and time management, access to records, communication and consulting, patient management and monitoring, to aids for clinical decision-making. They are helping to lead the charge for better decision-making and improved patient outcomes. With digitalization of records, healthcare professionals can access the information from anywhere. For some this is a marvelous miracle. For devices that are heavily controlled by corporations, the risks are relatively low. The challenge comes in with consumer technology. We do not necessarily have the most up-to-date versions of the software. While some people buy the latest technology, keep up to date with patching, and have antivirus installed on their devices, others do not. There is also a tremendous number of risks from downloading applications with malicious software in them. Review 42 identified that one in 36 phones had a high-risk application in them.[35] If you tie that back to phones that are not patched or protected, this is a very large volume of phones at high risk.

---

[34] Marianne Kolbasuk McGee, "Attack on Billing Vendor Results in Massive Breach: Atrium Health Says Attack on Accudoc Affected 2.65 Million Individuals," 2018, https://www.bankinfosecurity.com/attack-on-billing-vendor-results-in-massive-breach-a-11740.

[35] Nick G., "35 Outrageous Hacking Statistics & Predictions [2020 Update]," accessed October 24, 2020, https://review42.com/hacking-statistics/#:~:text=The%20cost%20of%20a%20data,high-risk%20apps%20in%202018.

Let's take a look at this from another perspective. *Science News* had an article where a research team from the University of Sydney, the University of Toronto, and the University of California studied how top-rated medicine tracking mobile apps shared data. They looked at the top 24 apps on the Android platform within the United States, United Kingdom, Canada, and Australia. They were looking for potential data leaks beyond the apps themselves. They found that 19 out of 24 of the apps shared data outside of the apps. A total of 55 unique entities were receiving the data. Those unique entities were owned by 46 parent companies. The entities they analyzed could share the information with 216 fourth parties, including multinational technology companies.[36] What they did not state in the article was whether those 216 parties had limitations about the data that is shared. Nonetheless, this is fairly concerning as it does shed light on how many companies do business this way from one app.

Clinal Monitors

Clinical monitors are the lynchpin that helps to coordinate a wide range of IoMT devices so that medical information regarding a patient is all together in one location. They also make sure that the records are fed directly into Electronic Health Record (EHR) systems. The data can then be reviewed by specialists at a later point in time. Almost predictably at this point, vulnerabilities have been found in clinical monitors, too. In September 2020 DataBreachToday reported about several vulnerabilities in a Philips monitor.[37] While the problems may be the equivalent of speaking a foreign language to some of you, the mitigations step should give a better idea about how bad these vulnerabilities are. Paraphrasing, they recommend that the device essentially be quarantined (from a network perspective) until it is patched. They also want the device to be physically blocked off to prevent unauthorized login attempts and only allow access on a must-have basis.[38] The list is more extensive (and more technical as I am trying to save my non-technical audience), but

---

[36] "Unprecedented privacy risk with popular health apps: Clinicians and consumers warned of privacy risks," University of Sydney, 2019, https://www.science-daily.com/releases/2019/03/190321092207.htm.

[37] Marianne Kolbasuk McGee, "Patient Monitoring Software Vulnerabilities Identified Philips and DHS Issue Advisories; Mitigation Tips Offered," 2020, https://www.databreachtoday.com/patient-monitoring-software-vulnerabilities-identified-a-14991.

[38] Ibid.

the mitigation steps are non-trivial in many environments. Some hospitals have the equivalent of a flat network, which means the network is essentially wide open, and trying to block the devices is time-consuming from a network standpoint, but also from a physical standpoint. If a large manufacturer like Philips is making these kinds of mistakes, it is even more difficult for the smaller companies.

Websites

Part of the connected world is a need for instant access to data—especially when it comes to hospitals. The more up-to-date the information, the more valuable that information is. There are numerous ways of collecting that information, but quite often with IoMT, that information's repository is an EHR system. That means the mobile devices, which are quite often connected via cellular technology, will need a way to access the data from the internet. Websites are a common tool to collect that information—whether it is directly through the EHR or through an independent website. Websites have all the flaws that we have previously mentioned and tend to be dependent on hardware or the cloud, an operating system, and software development.

Putting the Pieces Together

Just like a car, the more parts there are in the system, the more things can break. Similarly, in the electronic world, each piece of the system adds complexity and more room for vulnerabilities. Not only can they break, but they may have unforeseen vulnerabilities. Since one or more of the systems identified in Figure 2-1 are part of the IoT ecosystem, they all can have potential issues. When considering the security of a hospital, this is a daunting and growing challenge.

Current IoMT Challenges

A few might argue that recent legislation may have solved the problems related to vulnerabilities found within connected medical devices. While improvements have been made, there are still enormous challenges related to securing these devices. Legacy systems pose tremendous risks for organizations. With IoMT devices providing more value, especially in the time of COVID-19, the problems are only going to grow over time.

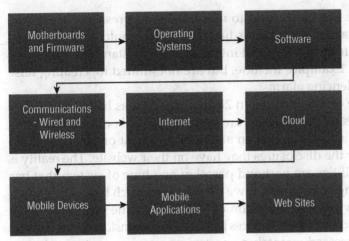

Figure 2-1: The interconnection of IoMT technologies

On January 23, 2020, the FDA released a warning on GE Healthcare's Central Stations and Telemetry Servers—essentially medical equipment that monitors patients.[39] Just the day before on January 22, 2020, GE posted the list of devices that are much broader. They listed six vulnerabilities that can allow an attacker to:

"Make changes at the operating system level of the device with effects such as rendering the device unusable, otherwise interfere with the function of the device, and/or

Make certain changes to alarm settings on connected patient monitors, and/or

Utilize services used for remote viewing and control of multiple devices on the network to access the clinical user interface and make changes to device settings and alarm limits, which could result in missed or unnecessary alarms or silencing of some alarms."[40]

---

[39] Kate Fazzini, "FDA issues cybersecurity warning on GE medical equipment that monitors patients," 2020, https://www.cnbc.com/2020/01/23/fda-issues-cybersecurity-warning-on-ge-medical-equipment-that-monitors-patients.html.

[40] GE Healthcare Product Security Portal, accessed October 12, 2020, https://www.gehealthcare.com/security.

In this case machines used to monitor blood pressure, heart rate, temperature, and patient status had a flaw that could allow a person to tamper with the devices and interfere with the standard operations of the device. Examples include, but are not limited to, creating false alarms and silencing alarms.

At the time of this writing, in 2020 alone, GE has had eight critical vulnerabilities released. These are easily explorable on their website, so I will not list each one. I can also look at a host of other competitors and show the disclosures they have on their website. The reality is that vulnerabilities are part and parcel of any type of system that has a programming component. If we expand the search beyond internet-connected devices into the realm of just devices, the problem is even greater. Connected medical devices just have extra considerations because they can be accessed remotely as part of a greater ecosystem, whereas before they were a disconnected box.

Some of this stems from the continuous software development process. IoMT manufacturers are continually making improvements and upgrades to their devices—even adding new features. If a device is certified at a specific point in time, even if it is perfectly secure, there is no guarantee that the device will be secure after one or more updates. Over a few years the original software can vary greatly—especially if you consider a life span that may be up to 15 years.

Another reality facing manufacturers is stiff competition. The timing of the release of a device (often any product) is absolutely critical. Security is a known way of slowing down the release of a product because it takes time and money to make sure that things are evaluated in a mature way—not to mention the resolution time to remediate any findings security assessments may find. If you are a CEO and are dealing with the pains of the market versus the pains around a device, sometimes a cost benefit analysis means things may not be perfect—especially if patches can fix the problems later. From an advertising perspective, sometimes the negative press is also seen as a positive—especially for non–life critical systems.

In Summary

All this said, as we have seen with Spectre and Meltdown in the previous chapter, vulnerabilities exist that nobody would have predicted. Even if a company is extremely diligent with its security, vulnerabilities can be found. They are inevitable even in the best of situations. That does not mean we should not strive for better. Too often, IoMT manufacturers use the excuse of ever-present vulnerabilities to not focus on the security of their products as much as they should. Again, this does not apply to every company, but unfortunately it applies to too many companies. As hospitals adopt IoMT technology in greater quantities, there will be a tipping point for security to become of greater importance than it currently is from a manufacturer's perspective.

In the end, both lives and data are important to protect. So far, we have been focusing on the technology. The data that comes out of that technology is also extremely important. The cost of a breach is heavily linked to the amount of data. All of these IoMT vulnerabilities inevitably lead to a loss of data. IoMT is causing a data explosion, and thus the risks for hospitals are greater than they ever have been—not just from IoMT devices, but also from the data they produce. We'll explore the data side of the equation in the next chapter.

It Is a Data-Centric World

The price of light is less than the cost of darkness.
—Arthur C. Nielsen, Market Researcher & Founder of ACNielsen

In the last few years, we have seen an explosion of data unlike anything in history. Most of that data is in electronic format, meaning that it is more accessible than ever before. On one level it has provided us with an opportunity to not only advance our scientific (and medical) understanding, but it has allowed us to apply new technologies such as artificial intelligence to further our understanding faster and more thoroughly.

That data has a dark side and a cost, however, as the data is dispersed in more directions than most people are aware of. With modern technology and data analysis, it is becoming easier to link people to data that is supposedly anonymous. There are tremendous challenges that we as a country need to make some decisions about. This chapter elucidates the second leg of IoMT devices: the data that they produce. It is ultimately why the IoMT ecosystem needs to be protected.

The Volume of Health Data

The United States has one of the largest per-capita expenditures on healthcare of any modern nation. We have been looking for solutions to reduce those overall costs. The causes of the expenditures are up for debate, but some of the prevailing issues cited include everything from administrative overhead to heavy use of both emergency room visits and acute care utilization. Obviously for the latter, IoMT has the ability to play a part in reducing the overall cost. One study cited by T-Mobile stated that the end result of combining wireless and IoMT devices created a 40% reduction in acute care utilization and a 65% reduction in emergency room utilization. To top things off, IoMT also resulted in a 30% increase in workflow efficiency.[1]

Think about this from both a hospital and a patient perspective. Trends could indicate a worsening of conditions early on and allow the hospital and patients to respond more quickly. This is a tremendous win across the board. IoMT technology can help in many other ways. Remember the NFC communications in the previous chapter? Just putting an NFC bracelet on a patient and an NFC tag on medicines has resulted in faster validation, fewer incidents of people getting the wrong medicine, and an overall improvement in the system.[2] To get this to work, simply check the tag on the patient, and when they need medicine, the medicine is matched against the NFC tag to validate that the patient is receiving the correct medicine. It is a very effective method to reduce problems related to medication errors. Some estimates are between 55% and 86% reduction in errors.[3] All of these small changes help to improve many aspects of today's medical treatments.

With so many success stories occurring as a result of improvements, it is no wonder that all the devices that support Medicine 2.0 are proliferating so quickly. COVID-19 is only accelerating the pace of change. This is all part of the beginning stages of Medicine 2.0, which stands on the proverbial back of Web 2.0 technology—basically technology that includes more audio and video content than Web 1.0. We now have more hard drives and more ways of connecting to the internet than ever before. I would also argue that the cloud principle of elasticity has been a huge boon to collecting and storing information. In the past, companies had to spend a tremendous amount of money to continuously expand their

---

[1] "Using IoMT to serve medically high-risk populations. How Catalytic Health Partners uses IoMT solutions to provide cost-effective, quality care," https://www.t-mobile.com/business/resources/articles/catalytic-health-partners.

[2] "Using RFID technology to reduce medication errors," https://hospitalnews.com/using-rfid-technology-to-reduce-medication-errors/.

[3] Nir Menachemi and Taleah H. Collum, "Benefits and drawbacks of electronic health records systems," 2011, https://www.ncbi.nlm.nih.gov/pmc/articles/PMC3270933/.

infrastructure. The cloud allows companies to get out of the hardware business and focus on the technology that is truly important to them.

If you recall, we stated the average hospital has between 10 and 15 medical devices per patient. While not all of them are producing continuous information, they are providing more and more detailed information at often close to real-time speeds. All that data begins to add up to volumes of information. A December 2019 report by the World Economic Forum said the average amount of data a hospital produces is 50 petabytes (PB) per year.[4] While data was collected prior to Medicine 2.0, the volume of data has exploded exponentially—mostly due to the advent of IoMT. Lifewire put together some fantastic statistics to help understand the sheer volume of information. One petabyte is equal to roughly 1.5 million CD-ROM discs, which is equal to 4,000 digital photos taken per day over the course of your entire life.[5]

Also, to help put things in perspective, since 2016, there has been an 878% growth in the amount of data that has been collected electronically. Some of this is due to the Affordable Care Act, but a large amount of it is due to the proliferation of IoMT devices. Health data is here to stay and is not going away anytime soon.

Projecting into the future, the proverbial holy grail of medicine would be to get a full 360-degree view of a person—to understand what is going on with them on a constant basis. The more data you have, the better and stronger recommendations that may be given. We have a long way to go before we get there, but the technological seeds are in place to cause data to grow exponentially—far more than the amount of data we collect now.

Data *Is* That Important

No matter your perspective on the Affordable Care Act (ACA), it has hastened the push toward Electronic Health Records (EHRs) that both technology and the HITECH Act began. It represents another step toward a more paperless office. The overarching goals are about transforming the medical care through the sharing and analysis of information. There are several benefits to doing so, but the outcome is more data in more locations.

---

[4] "4 ways data is improving healthcare," 2019, https://www.weforum.org/agenda/2019/12/four-ways-data-is-improving-healthcare/.

[5] Tim Fisher, "Terabyte, Gigabytes, & Petabytes: How Big Are They? An understandable guide to everything from Bytes to Yottabytes," 2020, https://www.lifewire.com/terabytes-gigabytes-amp-petabytes-how-big-are-they-4125169.

Providing insurance to millions of Americans who did not have it before is a tremendous help—especially during a pandemic. Aggregating the information from insurance companies, hospitals, doctor's offices, and so on, can help leaders identify key neighborhoods where the problem is worse and provide appropriate responses. New York City, for example, is starting to experiment with closing areas that are harder hit from COVID.[6] Whether or not that plan is successful, it demonstrates the power of what data can be used for. It also aids in community outreach so we can respond more locally to local problems. This would not be possible without solid actionable data being at least semi-centralized.

From a hospital perspective, that information is very valuable. Thirty years ago, if a patient came into a hospital unconscious, there was no information about that patient. Today, depending on the sharing capabilities of a region, doctors have the ability to look up the medical history of a patient or even lab tests they have had in the past. This prevents the waste of performing the tests again and provides healthcare professionals with invaluable information on how to treat patients more quickly based on their background. That extra information can help save both lives and money.

But from a pandemic perspective, it can help hospitals predict where the influx of patients will be coming from so they can better plan to handle those patients. Information is absolutely critical. Without it, hospitals can be overwhelmed. Even with that information, hospitals can be overwhelmed, but at least they are better prepared to save lives.

The ACA also has provisions for fighting fraud from potentially dishonest providers. Being specifically focused on the data, participating organizations can have their data accessed to search for fraudulent activity. Centralized data does have specific value as part of an overall fraud reduction strategy.[7]

The ACA also has provisions for Accountable Care Organizations (ACOs). The primary function of ACOs is to create cost savings by encouraging doctors, hospitals, and other health providers to coordinate patient

---

[6] Matt Troutman, "See If Your NYC Neighborhood Falls in A Coronovirus Closure Zone: Maps show the borders of a new color-coded, tiered closure system that takes effect Thursday in Brooklyn and Queens," 2020, https://patch.com/new-york/new-york-city/see-if-your-nyc-neighborhood-falls-coronavirus-closure-zone.

[7] D. P. Paul III, S. Clemente, R., McGrady, R. Repass, & A. Coustasse, "Medicare and the ACA: Shifting the paradigm of fraud detection." Presentation at the Academy of Business Research Fall 2016 Conference, Atlantic City, NJ, September, 2016, https://mds.marshall.edu/cgi/viewcontent.cgi?referer=https://www.google.com/&httpsredir=1&article=1171&context=mgmt_faculty.

care more efficiently. In order to do that, they need data from the members who are part of the network of services that the ACO is part of. So again, the drivers are there to have data in more locations.

In the final analysis we certainly have improvements to make, but we are making very larges strides as a society to cut back on individual medical expenses through the use of IoMT and better communication networks. Our care is becoming more personalized as we gather data on patients on a regular basis. We are responding to medical issues before they become major problems. The access we have to medical records is saving us from having to redo the same tests time and again. We are reducing our error rates, which is a boon for hospitals and patients alike.

This Is Data Aggregation?

Almost ironically, the need to aggregate data is also a cause of some of the dispersion of data. Every company needs data in order to operate effectively. The more centralized that information, the better. Years ago, the information was by hand and needed to be pulled out manually—a time-consuming and painful process by today's standards. Assessments on that data were time-consuming and difficult. Now, with modern technology, they are much easier. But each system needs the data for different purposes. The insurance company needs to get all the requisition codes to analyze the data in a different way. A hospital needs to aggregate data from a host of different systems so that it has a more complete record. In the end, it is not about one aggregation, but many.

Many IoMT devices do not keep the data local to the hospital they are operating in. They send data to the cloud. This is not by accident. It has tremendous advantages for both the hospital and the device provider. Previously, a physical server needed to be installed and supported within the organization in order to maintain medical records. This created an extra burden for the IT staff and the hospital to support. Many things could go wrong—servers could go down, connectivity could be blocked, etc. There is also a maintenance overhead that comes with that extra device. The manufacturers of IoMT devices that depend on servers would need to support a patching process, provide tech support when the software components would go down, etc. This equals a lot of overhead that hospitals and manufacturers would like to avoid. Having a cloud service is a win-win for the providers because it reduces the technical overhead for IoMT and then provides an additional service that the manufacturer can charge for continually. Years ago, companies would sometimes forgo support to save time and money—a loss of revenue. It also helps the manufacturers because they can have more data to analyze and make their product better.

EHR systems are used to aggregate and access health records by hospitals, doctors, and other health providers. They are critical for the purpose of having centralized data. They also are moving to the cloud with many of the same advantages that are afforded to the IoMT cloud providers with similar benefits to the providers. The cloud, in short, helps to get companies out of the IT game (to an extent), allowing them to focus on what they do best—helping people.

Health insurance companies also need many of the same records that hospitals and doctor's offices require. They have to analyze the data and pay out claims, and they too are utilizing the cloud for many of the same reasons as other companies. Again, aggregation means diffusion of data.

With Health Information Exchanges (HIEs) we start to get into connections that not everyone is aware of. HIEs aggregate data within a Health Information Network. The goal of HIEs is to facilitate a faster, safer, and more efficient transfer of data than the previous way of having to walk or fax information over from one place to another. While typically they do not exchange information outside of their networks, they are known to connect to state or federal bodies to exchange information—yet another place where data interconnects.

There are additional grants built into the America Recovery and Reinvestment Act (ARRA) of 2009 for building Regional Health Information Organizations (RHIOs). The primary goal of RHIOs is to share health information within a region while following both state and local guidelines. Part of the overarching goal of RHIOs is to allow for the interconnection of medical information to a specific region. In some cases, they even share information with multiple regions.

The Center for Medicaid and Medicare Services (CMS) has the tremendous responsibility of overseeing patient data for several medically related federal programs. They do not necessarily collect the data themselves, though. Many of their programs are contracted out to third-party companies. When you connect into CMS web sites, these sites are often built on corporate networks.

All of these institutions that have medical information are the tip of the iceberg for where and how medical information is aggregated, stored, and exchanged. There are claims clearinghouses, labs, other types of information exchanges, data warehouses, other government entities, research institutions, service providers, biopharmaceutical agencies, aggregators, and so on. The potential location for data almost never stays within a single organization. It becomes part of an extremely rich interconnected ecosystem of partners.

So far, we have been exploring data strictly from a HIPAA perspective, but there is also data that looks like HIPAA data, but in reality, it is not.

Non-HIPAA Health Data?

Over the last decade, a number of new devices and applications have hit the market. These include everything from wearable devices that track physiological data to health and fitness applications designed to make you healthier. What is interesting is that many fitness devices are eerily similar to IoMT devices that collect many of the same types of data as IoMT—in many cases, using the same types of technology. By all considerations, many of the devices are collecting HIPAA-like data, but the data they collect is not considered HIPAA data because the data created is not by a covered entity. A covered entity, defined in the HIPAA rules, is a health plan, healthcare clearinghouse, or health provider. Covered entities are beholden to HIPAA and have strong privacy and cybersecurity requirements. Data from health devices, despite the similarity to health data, does not have the same privacy or cybersecurity requirements. Data from health and fitness applications oftentimes has a great deal of additional information about you such as where you are, where you have been, personal information such as your address, and so on. These "free" applications mean you give up information about yourself, which is healthcare-like information.

A challenge with many of the health applications on the market is that some of them are providing health advice without sufficient science behind them to back up the claims. Within iTune and Google Play stores, there are more than a hundred thousand health applications. There have been numerous fines against many of these companies, but given the relative ease of designing apps and getting downloads, it becomes an almost impossible task of keeping track of them all and determining which are legitimate and which are not. Making an unsubstantiated claim may ultimately harm some people. The FDA has made recommendations for companies or individuals who develop these applications, but not everyone follows those recommendations.

There are also a host of companies that focus on your family tree based on some personal information and your genetic information. Today, that information can tell a tremendous amount about you. While not all genetic tests are equal, generally speaking genetic testing can tell if you have a genetic predisposition for specific diseases. The FDA prevents these companies from doing any kind of diagnostics, however.[8] What these companies do is reference key information against publicly available databases—some of which have incorrect information. In the end, from a disease standpoint, the tests only have a 40% efficacy rate.[9]

Like fitness devices and applications, genetic testing that is direct to consumers is not covered by HIPAA. In many cases, it is the same as HIPAA data, but because it is not coming from doctor or hospital, it isn't afforded the same protections. The data walks like a duck. It quacks like a duck. It is a duck, but it does not have the same security considerations as the other ducks because it did not come from a doctor or hospital.

It should be pointed out that just because the data is not HIPAA data, it does not mean that the data is not sensitive. That additional information like name, address, and phone number is sensitive information. It is considered personally identifiable information (PII). PII is essentially information that can help identify someone including Social Security numbers. In the United States, PII must be protected, but the protection requirements are much less stringent for PII than it is for Protected Health Information (PHI). PHI is the data that is protected under HIPAA. It includes PII, but also the information required under covered entities. In the cases of fitness devices, genetic ancestry testing (not performed under a covered entity) the data is PII but also has health data that is not governed by the HIPAA law. Oftentimes, that means that the data is less secure.

But the story of this non-HIPAA medical data does not end here.

Data Brokers

In today's data-centric world, data is the new gold. Perhaps nowhere is that truer than with data brokers. In the simplest terms, data brokers source and gather data and then resell the most important parts. Today, some extremely large and well-known companies, including Oracle, McKinsey, Accenture, and Experian, act as data brokers. It is a multi billion-dollar-a-year industry that is not just growing rapidly from a business perspective, but ballooning along with all the sources of data.

---

[8] Stephany Tandy-Connor, Jenna Guiltinan MS, Kate Krempely MS, Holly LaDuca MA, Patrick Reineke, Stephanie Gutierrez, Phillip Gray PhD, Brigette Tippin David PhD, "False-positive results released by direct-to-consumer genetic tests highlight the importance of clinical confirmation testing for appropriate patient care," 2018, https://www.nature.com/articles/gim201838.
[9] Ibid.

From a health perspective, a large percentage of the data that data brokers have is from hospitals, doctor's offices, ACOs, and so on. That data must be anonymized prior to sale. In fact, Health and Human Services (HHS) has a 32-page document stipulating the requirements around de-anonymized information.[10] Quite often, though, the byproduct of the anonymization process is that age, gender, partial ZIP codes, and doctors' names are still in the data.[11] It becomes relatively easy in most cases to match that data with other large data sources. In fact, that is a challenge for healthcare adjacent organizations that work with the data. They can and do send out unmatched data against alternate sources in order to accurately identify individuals—all in the name of helping people. Many of these legitimate companies do not permanently save that information. That is not to say that data brokers are illegal; it is just that they have found a way to profit off a loophole in privacy regulation given more modern capabilities.

We, as individuals, in most states, do not have the right to prevent that data from going to data brokers—or to delete it once it is part of that data ecosystem. That means our data is often shared without our knowledge with an array of different brokers that can make use of the information in literally untold ways. In some cases the data really does move science forward, but in other cases it is used for advertising purposes. Each piece of data is valuable in different ways to different organizations.

We are just beginning to learn about that market, but Patientory estimates that it is a multi billion-dollar-a-year market for healthcare data.[12] Putting together the full list of your doctor visits, blood tests, prescriptions, IoMT, and so on, is extraordinarily valuable. But so far we have been talking about data from covered entities that are being used. Data brokers also pull data from health applications, fitness watches, and genetic testing. Tie these data sources together and it is a cornucopia of valuable data. In the end, data brokers can gather thousands of data points on any given person. They quietly sell your personal information without any of us being the wiser.

---

[10] Bradley Malin PHD, "Guidance Regarding Methods for De-identification of Protected Health Information in Accordance with the Health Insurance Portability and Accountability Act (HIPAA) Privacy Rule," 2012, https://www.hhs.gov/sites/default/files/ocr/privacy/hipaa/understanding/coveredentities/De-identification/hhs_deid_guidance.pdf?language=es.
[11] Patientory Inc., "Data Brokers Have Access to your Health Information, Do You?" November 16, 2018 https://medium.com/@patientory/data-brokers-have-access-to-your-health-information-do-you-562b0584e17e.
[12] Ibid.

If we sidestep the conversation about HIPAA data and look more keenly at some of the uses of other kinds of data, the story takes an interesting turn. A tremendous amount of available data relates to location data from a variety of sources. Some of the sources include loyalty cards, public records, social media posts, cell phone data, browser behaviors, and so on in order to get as complete a view as possible about consumers— about you and me. [13]

There are some concerns about the accuracy of the data, however. *Harvard Business Review* did a test by gathering data from multiple data providers to assess how accurate it was. The results left much to be desired. For example, identifying if someone was male or not only had a 42.5% accuracy. Age was a little better at 77% accuracy.[14] But what does this mean if inaccurate information is mixed in with personal details such as name, address, and phone number? On the innocent side of things, you will gain advertisement you may or may not be interested in. On the opposite side of things, false information can prevent you from getting a job, or worse.

To address this, the Federal Trade Commission (FTC) is looking into studying the harm that can befall consumers as a result of bad data. Some of the harms they have noted include predatory pricing and racial profiling. Many key companies change their prices depending on the location of the individuals or their racial and ethnic backgrounds.[15] In another case the FTC cites, Google was allowing illegal pharmacies to target users in the search engines—for which they paid a $500 million civil forfeiture.[16] The FTC even goes so far as to say big data helped to facilitate the subprime mortgage crisis in the mid-2000s.[17] Years later, there is relatively little oversight of big data despite these not so insignificant problems.

Still, advertisers love to know this information so they can send targeted advertising. That seems innocent enough if that is all that is being done with the data. Mobilewalla, a Singapore-based search portal for applications

---

[13] Catherine Tucker and Nico Neumann, "Buying Consumer Data? Tread Carefully," 2020, https://hbr.org/2020/05/buying-consumer-data-tread-carefully.

[14] Ibid.

[15] Nathan Newman, "How Big Data Enables Economic Harm to Consumers, Especially to Low-Income and Other Vulnerable Sectors of the Population," https://www.ftc.gov/system/files/documents/public_comments/2014/08/00015-92370.pdf.

[16] Ibid.

[17] Ibid.

that target mobile devices, decided to publish age, sex, and ethnicity data related to the George Floyd protests. For many, this was a wake-up call for how much data is leaking out of our mobile phones.[18] It should also be a wake-up call that information about American citizens can be bought and sold all over the world. Why does a Singapore company have that much data on United States citizens? Why bother hacking organizations if any country can buy any information on any citizen? Internet trolls can also use this kind of information to target individuals. They know who you are and what your preferences are and can use that information to manipulate public opinion. This was a big concern in the 2016 election, no matter what side of the political fence you straddled.

From a legal perspective, unless the data broker uses the data from credit, employment, insurance, or housing, there is no requirement to keep the data private. They can even sell information about health conditions—so long as the data is either anonymized or not from a covered entity.[19] This means that there are robust amounts of data with very few protections.

What makes data brokers more interesting is that today we have more data than at any time in history. The digitization of information makes it far easier to stream data all over the planet in a comparatively short period of time. Sifting through that data is also far easier, which means corporations, governments, and people have that information. We truly are in the era of big data.

Big Data

Big data has been around since at least 1937, on a project that Franklin Roosevelt's administration had in relation to the Social Security Act, whose goal was to keep track of 26 million Americans. IBM developed the punch card to keep track of the process.[20] It wouldn't be until 2005 when the

---

[18] Zak Doffman, "Black Lives Matter: U.S. Protesters Tracked by Secretive Phone Location Technology," 2020, https://www.forbes.com/sites/zakdoffman/2020/06/26/secretive-phone-tracking-company-publishes-location-data-on-black-lives-matter-protesters/#7dcab0984a1e.
[19] Louise Matsakis, "The WIRED Guide to Your Personal Data (and Who Is Using It): Information about you, what you buy, where you go, even where you look is the oil that fuels the digital economy," 2019, https://www.wired.com/story/wired-guide-personal-data-collection/.
[20] Mark van Rijmenam, "A Short History of Big Data," 2013, https://datafloq.com/read/big-data-history/239#:~:text=In%202005%20Roger%20Mougalas%20from,using%20traditional%20business%20intelligence%20tools.

term "big data" would be coined by Roger Mougalas.[21] Big data is exactly what you might think it is—very large sets of data. From a hyperconnected perspective, it ties into many different data sets. The more data from more sources, as long as it is accurate, the better discoveries that can be made as a result of the assessment. It is generally accepted that there are four Vs that go along with big data—volume, velocity, variety, and veracity. All are critically important to the accuracy of information and helping advertisers more accurately target individuals.

Volume is really critical to big data because the more information you have, the better chance you have of having a particular *piece* of data. Think about it from a COVID-19 perspective. If you had only two people and those two people died as a result of COVID-19, you might come to the erroneous conclusion that COVID-19 was 100% fatal. While that example is absurd, having a large volume of data helps to weed out the statistical improbabilities that a small volume of data might indicate. The larger the data set, the more reliable that data tends to be.

Velocity, generally speaking, centers around the analysis of streaming data. The more sources of information—the more sensors that are on a person (patient or not), the better overall picture the data brokers or hospitals concerning the person or patient. The more real time the data is, the more useful that data can be to an organization because near-real-time judgment calls can be made. The store-and-forward technique discussed in the previous chapter means that decision making has a lag and may not be as relevant depending on the circumstances. When we talk about the instantaneity of the world, this is what people are talking about.

Variety is also key from a big data perspective. Having a single type of data source is good, but having more data sources is even better. Let us use COVID-19 data as an example. If all we had was the data on young children, our view on the disease would be different. We know that it disproportionately affects the elderly in terms of severity. The larger the variety of sources, the better analysis we have overall.

Veracity pertains to the accuracy of data. If our data set was very diverse when analyzing COVID-19, but it was wildly inaccurate to the point where it looked like everyone was affected the way the elderly are, we probably would be taking very different actions. Having accurate data really matters. If any one of the four Vs fails, we are provided with less than optimal information.

Today we have data scientists who work with these large volumes of data to extract patterns and knowledge. The buzzword for what they

---

[21] Ibid.

do is called "data mining." While technically inaccurate, it is the most common and easiest way to explain to a general audience what data scientists do. In reality, data mining is an interdisciplinary field that combines both statistics and computer science. While there are a host of other processes that go into what they do, sifting through that data to create accurate data models and trends is crucial. Visualization of that data is the ultimate goal because they need to communicate to others what trends they are discovering.

Big data has a tremendous number of advantages for things other than healthcare data. Cost savings alone is a very strong motivator. It is used to identify better ways of doing business. Quick, actionable information is very critical to the heart of many businesses. From a marketing perspective, it can help to understand market conditions and the sentiment of people online. Toward this end, companies can better target marketing strategies to help boost customer acquisition and retention. All of these can be used to fuel better product innovations.[22] These are just the beginning, however. Almost every industry is reaping the rewards of big data. In 2017, *Forbes* identified that 53% of companies are adopting big data analytics.[23]

Healthcare tends to be a little less mature in its data analysis techniques, but richer in its data sources, especially when considering IoMT devices.[24] Now many of those data-rich healthcare companies are eager to utilize that data, not only to improve their own practices and knowledge, but to sell. In fact, all of the data sources that IoMT brings to the table have seen an explosive 878% growth since 2016.[25] With 80% of healthcare

---

[22] "Big Data - Definition, Importance, Examples & Tools," https://www.rd-alliance.org/group/big-data-ig-data-development-ig/wiki/big-data-definition-importance-examples-tools#:~:text=The%20use%20of%20big%20data%20allows%20businesses%20to%20observe%20various,is%20important%20to%20trigger%20loyalty.&text=Big%20data%20analytics%20can%20help%20change%20all%20business%20operations.

[23] Louis Columbus, "53% Of Companies Are Adopting Big Data Analytics," 2017, https://www.forbes.com/sites/louiscolumbus/2017/12/24/53-of-companies-are-adopting-big-data-analytics/#2f2c78eb39a1.

[24] Jessica Kent, "Nearly 80% of Healthcare Execs Investing More in Big Data, AI Healthcare data executives are upping their investments in big data analytics and artificial intelligence, but many are still struggling to overcome organizational resistance," 2019, https://healthitanalytics.com/news/nearly-80-of-healthcare-execs-investing-more-in-big-data-ai.

[25] Fred Donovan, "Organizations See 878% Health Data Growth Rate Since 2016," Healthcare organizations have seen an explosive health data growth rate of 878 percent since 2016, according statistics compiled by Dell EMC. 2019, https://hitinfrastructure.com/news/organizations-see-878-health-data-growth-rate-since-2016.

executives investing in big data, big data is just not going away without additional influence. In fact, there is a hefty supply of big data—some of which has been in place for decades.

QuintilesIMS, a company dedicated to improving patient outcomes through the analysis of data, was created in the 1950s and now collects data on most prescription sales in the United States and many other countries.[26] Health insurance companies are also involved in selling this data. Blue Health Intelligence, part of Blue Cross Blue Shield, has data on at least 165 million people dating back to 2005 and helps to supply QuintilesIMS. Big data also pulls data from IoMT, EHRs, providers, patient registries, private players, government health plan claims, and pharmacy claims.[27]

Today, anonymized health data is being bought, sold, and used by large corporations to get more information and improve their products and/or services. What is concerning about the data brokers is that they are able to add disparate pieces of information to the anonymized data collection that allow big data companies to determine an individual's identity.[28] Anonymizing the data in the fashion that HIPAA requires is simply insufficient in today's world.

What is a concerning is that there are no federal laws against re-identification of information.[29] From a HIPAA standpoint, once it is anonymized, it is no longer HIPAA data. If the data is de-anonymized, it has the same structure as HIPAA data, but it is no longer has the HIPAA compliance requirements—even if that data has all the same elements. For many this is a concerning loophole. Many organizations, even if they legally anonymize the data, are, in effect, giving out HIPAA data. They follow the letter of the law, but not the spirit of the law. The law was intended to keep people's data private, but with modern data mining techniques that data is no longer protected. What is worse, that data may be bought, sold, and traded without consent or even anyone's knowledge that this is going on.

---

[26] Adam Tanner, "Strengthening Protection of Patient Medical Data," 2017, https://tcf.org/content/report/strengthening-protection-patient-medical-data/.

[27] Ibid.

[28] Adam Tanner, "How Data Brokers Make Money Off Your Medical Records: Data brokers legally buy, sell and trade health information, but the practice risks undermining public confidence," 2016, https://www.scientificamerican.com/article/how-data-brokers-make-money-off-your-medical-records/.

[29] Natasha Singer, "When 2+2 Equals a Privacy Question," 2009, https://www.nytimes.com/2009/10/18/business/18stream.html?_r=1<br%20></a>.

Brokers now sell very detailed information about population segments, including name, address, phone number, email address, and such information as people with cancer, erectile disfunction, bladder control, STDs, etc. Not all brokers provide information that is this specific, but it does allow for targeted advertising campaigns.[30]

It will be interesting to see how this plays out as more and more people become aware of the roles of data brokers. Many of these data brokers were unknown until Vermont created a law to govern them in 2018.[31] Since then, we have started to discover many of the companies that are in the data broker market. By March of 2019, 121 companies were identified—obviously not all of them are interested in HIPAA data. In terms of being aware of where your data is, it is much more challenging than ever before because that data could literally be anywhere on planet Earth.

If only anonymized data were the only concern. Kevin O'Reilly, a news reporter for the American Medical Association, reported about Project Nightingale, which puts patient data from the 2,600 hospitals that are part of Ascension health into the hands of Google. Google's intent is to use artificial intelligence on the data. In fact, prior to that it spent $2.1 billion to acquire healthcare data on its users.[32] Of course, data provided in this form is HIPAA data, and the requirements for HIPAA must be followed. From a privacy standpoint, providing that data is done without informed consent, people do not have control of their own data.[33] Given some of the flagrant violations of data usage by Facebook and other technical giants, there is understandably some concerns related to that data.

In the previous section we talked about applications that have medical that are not validated by science or contain false information. Given that volume is important, the more sources of data presented, the better. If one of those applications sends erroneous data, the data

[30] Adam Tanner, "Strengthening Protection of Patient Medical Data," 2017, https://tcf.org/content/report/strengthening-protection-patient-medical-data/.

[31] Steven Melendez, "A landmark Vermont law nudges over 120 data brokers out of the shadows," 2019, https://www.fastcompany.com/90302036/over-120-data-brokers-inch-out-of-the-shadows-under-landmark-vermont-law.

[32] Kevin B. O'Reilly, "Google-Ascension deal comes as concerns rise on the use of health data," 2019, https://www.ama-assn.org/practice-management/digital/google-ascension-deal-comes-concerns-rise-use-health-data.

[33] Ibid.

stream may be polluted. Remember that volume, velocity, and variety are extremely important from a sales standpoint. Veracity, to an extent, can be validated by stating that the data is top notch. Undoubtably, when it comes to the buying data, some companies will do a better job validating the data prior to purchase. Given the volume of potential data sources, this can be a daunting task for many organizations.

Another challenge is that oftentimes this means sharing data globally, which means data can literally be anywhere. Health data can physically be located in any country. Although frowned upon, there is no law requiring U.S. health data to remain in the United States. Oftentimes, depending on the platform, that is exactly what happens. Some data brokers, not all, send data throughout the planet to ensure that, in case of an emergency, it is backed up. Unless a thorough investigation is performed about the platform and someone thinks to ask that question, the hospital or doctor's office may be blissfully unaware that the data is being spread throughout the world.

In the end, big data is about sharing of data and aggregating the right data sets in the right way. That data may or may not be HIPAA data, but may have all the markers of HIPAA data. The data may be collected from applications and shared in ways that we, as consumers, may not be aware of. It also holds the promise of expanding our scientific under-standing and taking us into future directions we have only begun to imagine today. Big data is not about the data itself. There are goals and objectives from many different angles that make it important. There are also tools that data scientists use to sort through the volumes of data.

Data Mining Automation

Analyzing the volume of data that comes out of big data is not a minor undertaking. As the volume of data increases and we become more and more subtle in terms of our analysis of data, often it is worthwhile to get some extra help to analyze that data. Unsurprisingly, there are numerous ways to help with that analysis. Most people immediately start to think of artificial intelligence—partially popularized by IBM's Watson that beat out other contestants on *Jeopardy* in 2011 and partially by science fiction. While certainly artificial intelligence is used, often the term is overused by marketing teams. Some of the subcomponents of artificial intelligence are more than sufficient to meet the data analytics needs of many companies. For example, many tools use machine learning or deep learning for analytics purposes. Each method has its own pros and cons, and each may bring value depending on the context. Nonetheless, while there are many other tools for working with data, the range of tools that data scientists use to correlate data and discern patterns offer vast improvements over the activity that people perform on their own. Figure 3-1 demonstrates the relationship between the different technologies relating to data science and artificial intelligence. For purposes of simplicity, let's use the term *artificial intelligence* broadly to talk about the full range of available tools, although it is not technically accurate.

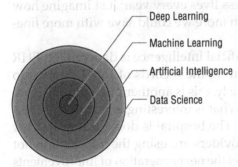

Figure 3-1: Relationship of data science to enablement technologies

One thing to keep in mind is that artificial intelligence and many of the related tools are in their infancy and require tremendous amount of maturation to meet their full potential. Even in the healthcare market, the full potential has yet to be reached. McKinsey and company identified three stages of artificial intelligence uses that are helpful to highlight the context. The first phase is that we are striving to work on repetitive and largely administrative tasks to reduce the existing workload. We are beginning to see this for specializations that work with images as well. The second phase is to use artificial intelligence in home care—often related to remote monitoring. In this phase artificial intelligence will be utilized more often as an aspect of the connected devices themselves. Phase three will be focused more on being embedded within the clinical processes.[34] Being a cautious technological optimist, I am sure there will be further applications of artificial intelligence in the future, especially when it is tied to robotics.

---

[34] Angela Spatharo, Solveigh Hieronimus, & Jonathan Jenkins, "Transforming healthcare with AI: The Impact on the workforce and organizations," 2020, https://www
.mckinsey.com/industries/healthcare-systems-and-services/
our-insights/transforming-healthcare-with-ai#:~:text=It%20
can%20increase%20productivity%20and,patient%20care%20and%20
reducing%20burnout.

It is important to look more deeply at these phases described by McKinsey. Having artificial intelligence injected into telemedicine has tremendous potential to push medicine into a more proactive mode than ever before. If we took the technology within health applications and tied them into augmented forms of monitoring devices that tie into artificial intelligence systems, we could begin to detect potential medical issues (or diseases) early prior to onset of symptoms. The proactive measures of some of the simpler forms of artificial intelligence are already saving us millions of dollars and countless lives every year; just imagine how many more people and how much more we could save with more fine-grained medical information.

Another area of interest for artificial intelligence is data mining EHR records, which does include mining the records of IoMT devices to look for predictors of risk. Obviously, this is another proactive measure that companies are focusing on. What is interesting is that this process is valuable from multiple angles. The hospital is doing it to help their patients, and the IoMT device providers are using the information not only to help patients, but also to fuel the next generation of improvements in the devices. The more data you have, the more you know what you need to go after from a data perspective. That information can be used to focus product innovation. Quite often, this ties back to the Silicon Valley business model, which works with hospitals and other health practitioners to get feedback from them about improvements that need to be made. This, in turn, will increase the amount of data, which is a small part of the reason we will continue to see more data in the years to come.

In Summary

We have been on a short exploration of how big data fits into the big picture of both hospitals and IoMT devices. We have explored how big data fits into the overall Medicine 2.0 as data is part of the advancement of not only medical science, but also for protecting patients that utilize IoMT. As our IoMT devices become more sophisticated and capable of even deeper readings than ever before, this will only catapult our understanding of medicine even further. That shift will help us be more preventative and thus save lives and also further reduce our healthcare expenditures.

On the data science side of things, whether you are talking about deep learning, machine learning, or artificial intelligence, these practices help the data scientists to aggregate, correlate, and present key findings more quickly. They are a critical tool to help sort through vast quantities of data. They help to make data science much easier and the role of data scientists more important for the companies that rely on big data whether they are working on population health, advertising, or myriad other disciplines—including information security.

The utilization of this data is a brilliant and clearly fantastic use of resources on many fronts. But, there is clearly room for improvement as privacy rights, from many people's perspective, are being violated. We clearly need a better approach going forward not only from an IoMT perspective, but also from a data perspective.

IoMT and Health Regulation

Supply always comes on the heels of demand.
—Robert Collier

IoMT manufacturers are still not entirely on board with securing IoMT devices. There are clear rules with HIPAA regarding how things should be secured. From a manufacturer's perspective, it is the hospital that faces the HIPAA fines, not the manufacturer. If most companies are not meeting security requirements and it is the innovation of the health technology and not the security that gives the competitive edge, security will always lose out.

This chapter explores how the industry has made some positive steps forward in securing the medical devices despite the manufacturing challenges. Maybe it can be an indicator of go-forward approaches in the future.

Health Regulation Basics

At the time, the Health Insurance Portability and Accountability Act (HIPAA) of 1996 was landmark legislation for protecting health data. It was far from complete, however, as additions were made to the various rules in 2003 (Privacy Rule), 2005 (Security Rule), 2006 (Enforcement Rule), and 2013 (Final Omnibus Rule). That and the HITECH Act of

2009 comprise many of the key aspects of the legislation, but these are not the only considerations.

HIPAA, at the time, was a big shock for many healthcare providers. This kind of legislation was very different from anything that had come out prior. It involved a new breed of legal specialists to interpret the requirements and make sure the healthcare providers were following the new law. As each new rule came out, the requirements became stricter. It took a while for organizations to adapt to the new regulations.

The enforcement arm of HIPAA is through the Office of Civil Rights (OCR). HIPAA had requirements, but the fines for HIPAA violations were relatively low—only up to $25,000. OCR also developed specifics for organizations to follow above and beyond the HIPAA requirements, such as risk assessments. While the fines were a bit of a concern before 2009, it wouldn't be until the Health Information Technology for Economic and Clinical Health (HITECH) Act came out in 2009 that HIPAA really grew teeth. With the HITECH Act, the minimum penalty was based on the assessment of negligence. Now the maximum is $50,000 per violation with a cap of $1.5 million per year.

The HITECH Act was signed into law by President Obama in 2009. The central goal of the bill was to promote and expand the adoption and use of Health Information Technology (HIT). It also closed a few glaring loopholes in HIPAA and used tougher penalties for compliance failures as incentive to follow HIPAA requirements. Additionally, it requires notifications be sent to individuals if their information is compromised. The HITECH Act is also important because business associates that have access to data now have to comply with HIPAA. Yes, you read that right: business associates that had access to data were not required in any way to be compliant with HIPAA unless the parent organization built it into a legal agreement.

Given that HIPAA and HITECH are laws, they hold a unique place from a corporate perspective compared to other forms of compliance. There is no certification process that companies can go through to declare compliance. They can have an assessment performed to validate compliance, but there is no HIPAA certification for covered entities. This differs greatly from other compliance standards such as credit card compliance (PCI-DSS), ISO 27001, or other security frameworks. At best, a letter of attestation can be achieved, but there are no universally compliant formal audit standards. The closest standard to HIPAA is HITRUST. In fact, HITRUST was born out of HIPAA compliance, and many organizations and regulatory bodies consider passing a HITRUST audit roughly equivalent to being HIPAA compliant.

While numerous security requirements are important in our story about IoMT related to HIPAA, one of the key considerations is around covered entities. The HIPAA Privacy Rule defines a covered entity as follows:

"Covered entities are defined in the HIPAA rules as (1) health plans, (2) health care clearinghouses, and (3) health care providers who electronically transmit any health information in connection with transactions for which HHS has adopted standards. Generally, these transactions concern billing and payment for services or insurance coverage. For example, hospitals, academic medical centers, physicians, and other health care providers who electronically transmit claims transaction information directly or through an intermediary to a health plan are covered entities. Covered entities can be institutions, organizations, or persons.

Researchers are covered entities if they are also health care providers who electronically transmit health information in connection with any trans-action for which HHS has adopted a standard. For example, physicians who conduct clinical studies or administer experimental therapeutics to participants during the course of a study must comply with the Privacy Rule if they meet the HIPAA definition of a covered entity."[1]

From an IoMT perspective, device manufacturers were claiming that manufacturing companies are not covered entities—even if they collect medical like data for testing purposes. Just as fitness devices and many health applications do not capture PHI (only PHI-like data), the same is true for IoMT. For all intents and purposes the data can be given the same consideration as PII (if it includes name and address). The updated fines in HITECH also do not apply. The reality is, the IoMT manufacturers that make the claims that they are not covered entities may or may not be right. The key differentials are that if the IoMT manufacturer has a service related to the covered entity or is collecting data on behalf of a covered entity, then the manufacturer must comply with HIPAA. This is yet another tug of war that hospitals were dealing with as the technologies started to mature. While many manufacturers were on board with the HIPAA requirements because services are an intelligent sales approach for many organizations, there were always stragglers

---

[1] "To Whom Does the Privacy Rule Apply and Whom Will It Affect," U.S. Department of Health and Human Services National Institutes of Health, https://privacyruleand-research.nih.gov/pr_06.asp#:~:text=Covered%20entities%20are%20defined%20in,which%20HHS%20has%20adopted%20standards.

or newfound companies that could stay in business while providing products that could not meet minimal HIPAA requirements. In short there was often no guarantee of perfect security in the medical devices from a HIPAA perspective.

Some of the weaknesses within the IoMT are due to heritage and cultural issues. As previously discussed, the IoT world is full of gaping vulnerabilities. For the most part, there are no specific requirements to follow—especially for home systems. For example, as a result of poor camera security, 50,000 homes have been hacked with the footage posted online.[2] Apparently lifetime access for cameras is only $150. Some of the cameras caught people in compromising positions and later posted the videos online.[3] The IoT security gaps are almost a pandemic on their own. For manufacturers that produce both IoT and IoMT, there may be little difference between an internet-connected camera and an internet-connected clinical monitor—especially for the smaller manufacturers that may not have a refined legal team to help them sort out the requirement differences.

Another enabler of lax IoMT standards for years has been the "black box" defense. It is how security practitioners have dealt with the unfortunate findings from the weaknesses of IoMT devices. The security team uses the defense that the auditors cannot dictate what medical equipment is to purchase for their organization. Given that so many hospitals are stuck between insecure devices and insecure devices, what are the alternatives? Close the hospitals? That is clearly not a rational alternative for any society. Sure, there are technologies in place to reduce the risk, but they are a Band-Aid over the problem. As a result, any deficiencies that an insecure medical device brings cannot be used against the covered entity for using insecure IoMT devices. The devices literally are an untouchable black box. Unfortunately, this defense has only enabled IoMT manufacturers to get away with poor standards—even in the federal space, which is well known for having stricter standards than other organizations. Maybe the FDA would have a better approach as they have had a long history of pulling medical devices from the market.

The one provision in HIPAA that can be used to document the risks related to IoMT is the risk assessment. HIPAA requires that companies

---

[2] Amer Owaida, "50,000 home cameras reportedly hacked, footage posted online. Some footage has already appeared on adult sites with cybercriminals offering lifetime access to the entire loot for US$150," 2020, https://www.welivesecurity.com/2020/10/14/50000-home-cameras-reportedly-hacked-footage-posted-online/.
[3] Ibid.

do risk assessments that take into account the confidentiality, integrity, and availability of the system. These three concepts are fundamental within HIPAA-compliant risk assessments. IoMT devices, especially en masse, represent a risk to all three. The risk assessment process is so important that OCR also has a requirement for risk assessments and helps to ensure the work that is done properly aligns to HIPAA. Of course, this takes someone with a thorough understanding of IoMT devices and their corresponding weaknesses to properly identify the risks. This can take a significant investment in time and resources to really see the big picture related to IoMT challenges and then accurately translate those into a mature risk assessment process. Translating the outcomes of these risk assessments is another challenge altogether—one that we will pick up in Chapter 17.

What hospitals are often left with, especially after budgetary considerations, is a choice of one insecure device or another. Features and functions often overrule security considerations if security is given a seat at the table. The number of IoMT devices started growing rather rapidly over the last few years. This meant that there were more and more vulnerabilities within the hospital network with no real recourse except to work with more and more unique technologies to help detect, but often not protect, against the advanced threats hitting hospitals. The vulnerabilities keep piling up as more and more IoMT devices were being purchased. Things were starting to seem hopeless for hospitals. Then the United States Department of Veterans Affairs made a bold step to change the way manufactures were approaching security within IoMT devices as we will explore later in this chapter.

In the end, though, HIPAA is a powerful piece of legislation for protecting our data, but has insufficiently addressed the security of IoMT devices. From a data perspective it has only offered a dated method to protect our data from data brokers. Clearly, we need other forces that can help improve the security and privacy relate to IoMT devices and the corresponding clouds, and the data brokers that protect our data. To continue the story, we'll turn to the Food and Drug Administration.

FDA to the Rescue?

The United States Food and Drug Administration (FDA) is a federal agency within the Department of Health and Human Services. It has the awesome responsibility of protecting public health. It covers everything from tobacco to drugs, vaccines, biopharmaceuticals, animal feed, and of course medical devices.[4] While this is not a complete list, it does begin to demonstrate how widespread the FDA's responsibilities are. Like any agency, or any company, it has budgets or limitations to work with to prevent them from being able to protect the American people and hospitals from the poor security found in medical devices. That being said, the FDA can pull devices off the market whose poor cybersecurity may affect human life or, as is most often the case, require urgent correction to the cybersecurity vulnerabilities. Usually this means that the device manufacturer will have to create a patch to correct the vulnerabilities.

For historical context, medical devices were not part of the original purview of the FDA. An amendment to the Food, Drug, and Cosmetic Act added medical devices to their purview in 1976. That amendment included a premarket approval process for devices that have valid scientific evidence that the device is safe and effective. Congress also included an alternative pathway to getting devices on the market known as the 510(k) provision. The 510(k) provision to allow a less burdensome route for new devices that were on the market that were substantially similar to what was on the market in 1976. They allowed new companies to have small improvements without going through the extensive premarket approval process.[5] The reality is the FDA simply did not have the resources to review all the new devices that were entering the market. It felt it needed greater oversight of the process, but things went in the opposite direction.

Congress passed the Medical Device User Fee and Modernization Act of 2002 (MDUFMA). This called for reducing the burden of approach for device regulation. As a result, this 510(k) pathway was the predominant method of allowing new devices on the market. Unfortunately, this allows a large number of devices to enter the market that are unvalidated from a security perspective unless there is a safety concern.[6] The FDA responds to the problems, in many cases, well after the release of the product.

What is interesting is that these reviews are primarily safety oriented. Insofar as cybersecurity is concerned, it is a big enough problem

---

[4]Food and Drug Administration, Wikipedia, https://en.wikipedia.org/wiki/Food_and_Drug_Administration, accessed October 24, 2020.
[5]Diana Zuckerman, Paul Brown, & Steven Nissen, "Medical Device Recalls and the FDA Approval Process," 2011, https://jamanetwork.com/journals/jamainternalmedicine/fullarticle/227466.
[6]Ibid.

if human life is at stake, but not for many of the comparatively minor cybersecurity issues. Of course, companies are compelled to follow HIPAA, but enforcement and oversight are severely lacking. It is really helpful from a free market perspective, and it is good that the FDA recalls devices for cybersecurity issues if they are large enough to be of risk to the patient, but not in many other cases. The FDA wants secure devices, but it is left challenged to validate their security.

The FDA has a fact sheet concerning its role surrounding medical device cybersecurity. It is very enlightening and concerning at the same time. It does clearly specify that medical device manufacturers must comply with federal regulations. The facts as the FDA lays them out specify "Medical device manufacturers must comply with federal regulations. Part of those regulations, called quality system regulations (QSRs), requires that medical device manufacturers address risks, including cybersecurity risk. The pre- and post- market cybersecurity guidance's provide recommendations for meeting QSRs."[7] What is interesting to note is that there are no formal processes or regulations concerning how those QSRs are met. They have guidance. Guidelines are not mandates, so it provides manufacturers with some leeway for how they approach the problems. Guidelines are not without reason, however. The approach can be different based on many different factors as the technologies are rapidly changing. There is no such thing as a one-size-fits-all approach when it comes to protecting systems. For example, you could have an in-depth software testing program and then utilize a deficient web encryption protocol on the final product that wasn't part of the original testing.

The second chapter of this book mentions that when it comes to IoMT, each piece of the ecosystem needs to be examined holistically as part of the others. Once more, each part needs to be reevaluated on a periodic basis. What may seem like a small decision from a business standpoint may have large ramifications from a security standpoint depending on how astute the people making the decisions are. Let's use the deficient web encryption protocol example mentioned earlier. Let's expand the example to state that no sensitive data is sent nor does it include any kind of authentication—such as a login to a system. If business leaders decided to add the name of a person onto the data, that data may become HIPAA data when a few fields are added. A simple IT process change can change everything from a privacy and security perspective. The details really do matter.

---

[7]U.S. Food and Drug Administration FDA Fact Sheet, "THE FDA's ROLE IN MEDICAL DEVICE CYBERSECURITY," https://www.fda.gov/media/123052/download.

The FDA also recognizes that there are some systems that cannot be updated or patched. In these cases, healthcare organizations need to work with manufacturers to see that deficiency or vulnerability is remediated.[8] To anyone outside of IT this may seem reasonable, but the reality is, depending on the context, this may or may not be possible. Usually the manufacturer can provide the fix for the vulnerability or not, and that is the end of the story. Special considerations often become prohibitively expensive if it is possible to remediate a vulnerability. Take the recent situation with Windows 7 expiring under the covers of IoMT devices. It is a hefty price tag for the manufacturer to upgrade—if it is possible for them. With each Windows upgrade, the system has to have the appropriate hardware to support it. If the hardware doesn't support an upgrade, the only option is to upgrade the entire system to the latest model. Given how expensive some of the medical systems are, this is sometimes not realistic due to the competing needs of the organization. Companies have to make do—sometimes for years.

The most concerning thing that the FDA does from this same fact sheet is to have companies self-validate the security of the IoMT devices they are manufacturing. Yes, there are some companies that have top-of-the-line security built into the products, but other companies may not be so stringent. For example, there is something called static analysis security testing (SAST). SAST evaluates the base code of a product for security vulnerabilities. It is critical for strong software hygiene. There are some fantastic SAST products on the market. There are also some mediocre products on the market. A poor SAST product is an indicator that the end product will probably not be as secure as it would have been otherwise.

There are companies that perform detailed security testing–related to IoMT, but it may be prohibitively expensive depending on the context. With the example provided earlier about the poor encryption and no authentication capabilities, continual evaluation becomes critical to ensure security. Take a look at Windows. The 1,111 vulnerabilities in Windows 10 noted in Chapter 1 are not just from new software. They are often new vulnerabilities found with existing software. Continuous monitoring is absolutely critical to a secure system.

One result is that hospitals do not really know how secure a manufacturer's equipment is. Nor is the FDA currently designed to keep up to date with all of these devices—or with continual monitoring to keep organizations safe—especially if you consider that hospitals can

---

[8] Ibid.

keep devices for years past the end of life—past the time when there are no more security patches for a product. The reality is, vulnerable IoMT devices are usually in use well after they are released in many cases.

While things may seem bleak for the security of IoMT devices, the story does not end here. The FDA would find an unlikely bedfellow with the United States Department of Veterans Affairs (VA). It was all inspired out of 2015 when the healthcare crisis came to a head. The statistics they cite are staggering to say the least. There were 258 large breaches of health information, which resulted in over 113 million records being lost. This was an 897% increase over 2014 numbers. 98.1% of the incidents were the result of hacking attacks.[9] The now famous Anthem attack occurred in 2015, which totaled roughly 78 million records stolen by cybercriminals. UCLA also lost 4.5 million different healthcare records.[10] While this was a wake-up call for hospitals that had become complacent with poor security, it was also a wake-up call for the VA. The events of 2015 inspired them to do something about the problems related to the poor state of IoMT security.

The Veterans Affairs and UL 2900

For context, the VA is the second largest department within the U.S. It helps to protect the 17.4 million veterans who served within the United States military and provides care at 1,255 healthcare facilities including 170 medical centers.[11] It is larger than any healthcare organization in the U.S. When the VA has a concern, manufacturers listen. It has a tremendous amount of buying power.

To that end, in 2016, the VA, in conjunction with UL, a global safety science leader, developed a Cooperative Research and Development Agreement (CRADA). A CRADA is an agreement between a government agency and a company or university for the purpose of research and development. The goal, in this case, was to create a stronger safety standard for medical device cybersecurity not only for the VA, but across

---

[9] RedSpin Breach Report 2015: Protected Health Information (PHI), February 2016.
[10] Sara Heath, "Majority of 2015 Data Breaches Due to IT Hacking," 2016, https://healthitsecurity.com/news/
majority-of-2015-healthcare-data-breaches-due-to-it-hacking.
[11] US Department of Veterans Affairs Veterans Health Administration, https://www
.va.gov/health/aboutvha.asp#:~:text=The%20Veterans%20Health%20
Administration%20(VHA,Veterans%20enrolled%20in%20the%20VA, accessed
October 24, 2020.

the whole United States healthcare system.[12] They wanted to cover such challenges such as in-home care, coordinating connected technologies for emergency situations, allowing FIPS 140-2-compliant cryptographic modules with minimal impact on the system, and acceleration of the utilization of leading connected medical devices.[13]

The requirements that the VA had in place are quite rigid. The FIPS 140-2 cryptographic modules are a federal standard for ensuring cryptographic integrity. It is a huge step above non-validated cryptographic modules that are sometimes built insecurely. For example, two systems can use AES-256 encryption, but a system without the NIST validation of FIPS 140-2-compliant algorithms has a greater chance of being less secure. The VA had 174 security requirements for the UL 2900 standards. As a test, the VA had a penetration test (an authorized hack) against a UL 2900 certified device to validate its security.[14]

The UL 2900 standard was actually much broader than IoMT devices, however. It covered all IoT devices. There are actually a few parts to UL 2900. UL 2900-1 applies software security for network-connected products. UL 2900-2-1 applies to healthcare and wellness systems. UL 2900-2-1 was recognized by the FDA in June of 2018 for premarket submissions and post-market management. UL 2900-2-2 applies to industrial control systems. UL 2900-2-3 applies to IoT signaling systems. UL also has a Cybersecurity Assurance Program (CAP) for validating devices.[15] In that service they test the controls related to the IoMT device to validate the requirements.

From a cybersecurity perspective, this is a huge leap forward for IoMT security. If you are a hospital looking at products, the UL 2900 certification is critical from a cybersecurity perspective and a huge boon for getting through the FDA approval process and a great way to reduce hospital risk—especially systems with NIST-validated, FIPS 140-2-compliant cryptographic modules. Expectedly, not all manufacturers can afford to

[12] Steve Alder, "Adoption of Standards Improves Cybersecurity of Internet of Medical Things (IoMT) Devices," 2019, https://www.hipaajournal.com/adoption-of-standards-improves-cybersecurity-of-internet-of-medical-things-iomt-devices/.
[13] Anura Fernando and Marc Wine, "How the VA and UL Created an Orchestrated Approach to Healthcare Cybersecurity Assurance," 2020, https://www.openhealthnews.com/story/2020-01-03/how-va-and-ul-created-orchestrated-approach-healthcare-cybersecurity-assurance.
[14] Ibid.
[15] Synopsis UL 2900, https://www.synopsys.com/glossary/what-is-ul-2900.html, accessed October 23, 2020.

see the cryptographic modules are validated as that can be an extensive process on its own—let alone combined with the UL 2900 program.

Not all manufacturers use UL 2900 when producing devices, though. It is also somewhat new being that it was released in 2018. It also does not help with non-medical IoT devices that may be mixed in the environment, such as beds. In 2018, Deloitte reported that 48% of the medical devices are IoMT, but expected that number to grow to 68% in 5 years.[16] As previously discussed, COVID-19 is hastening the adoption of IoMT devices. That being said, despite the efforts of the FDA, the VA, and UL, there is still a great deal of work that needs to be done—especially in hospitals with legacy IoMT devices. Unless the healthcare institutions change their spending habits to only go for devices that are secure such as what the VA has done, IoMT devices will continue to have a large number of flaws.

In Summary

Getting IoMT manufacturers to be compliant with even basic security practices continues to be an ongoing struggle, but with the help of the VA, a tremendous amount of progress has been made. For some, that progress is not enough, but some manufacturers voluntarily do what they can to increase the security of their products and/or are moving to UL 2900. Companies that understand the risks within their organizations and are willing to pay for the extra layers of security are a step ahead in the security game. Of course, for some product types, secure solutions may not exist.

The other tug of war is between UL 2900 certification and innovation. As discussed in Chapter 1, manufacturers that work with hospitals will be more adaptable to the needs of the hospital—creating new products and furthering innovation. That innovation can happen more quickly than the UL 2900 certification process, which means that there can be a slippery slope away from security products that leads to demand for products from the medical side of the house that may be less secure, but better able to protect human life.

---

[16] Karen Taylor, Amen Sanghera, Mark Steedman, & Matthew Thaxter, "Medtech and the Internet of Medical Things: How connected medical devices are transforming health care," 2018, https://www2.deloitte.com/content/dam/Deloitte/global/Documents/Life-Sciences-Health-Care/gx-lshc-medtech-iomt-brochure.pdf.

But the regulatory arena is only one part of the story. On the other side of that coin are the privacy frameworks, which also come from a legal standpoint and are interrelated to HIPAA and HITECH, but also extend to the data side of the proverbial coin and are starting to make a dent in how both data and IoMT devices are treated. Before we do that, however, we'll be taking a deeper dive into breaches, how they happen, and the impact on hospitals so that a better picture of the problems can be ascertained.

blished that healthcare is the most breached sec

Once More into the Breach

*Facts are stubborn things; and whatever may be our wishes, our inclinations, or the
dictates of our passion, they cannot alter the state of facts and evidence.*

—John Adams, *The Portable John Adams*

People tend to learn by analogy, by telling stories. They think about how events might affect them personally or affect other people. Those stories are critical to starting down the road to creating change. Yet facts and statistics are what should be driving behavior. Whether we're talking about a cost/benefit analysis or the likelihood and impact of a risk assessment, it is the facts that should drive our behavior regardless of how we contextualize them. With this in mind, learning both the stories and the facts is critical, and one of the reasons that security professionals should study cybersecurity breaches and why they happen. Once you have convinced people of the why, only the how remains.

Understanding what happens in company breaches can help us to understand not only the stories, but also the facts. This chapter is about exploring breaches, how they happen, what some of the key elements are, and how IoMT plays a pivotal role in them—and not a positive role. First we'll explore the statistics, then go into some common actions taken by hackers when breaching systems, and finally tie it all together by looking at some common locations where data is stored and how IoMT vulnerabilities can ultimately lead to data theft.

Grim Statistics

We have already established that healthcare is the most breached sector via the 2020 Verizon Data Breach Investigation Report. The numbers are downright staggering. The National Institutes of Health (NIH) did an assessment of those numbers and found that from 2015 to 2019, 76.59% of the breaches were in healthcare.[1] That is not a typo. Healthcare data is valuable, and hackers are often lazy. Anyone with more than ten years of experience in cybersecurity will tell you hackers tend to go after low-hanging fruit. They go after the easy targets. The concern here isn't just the number or the percentage of breaches, it is also the number of records. Figure 5-1 shows how severe that trend is within the United States.

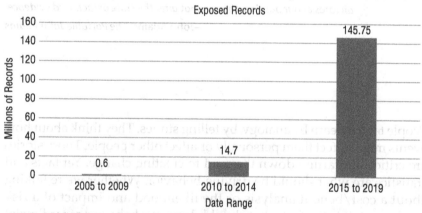

Figure 5-1: Number of exposed records 2005 to 2019

Source: Adil Hussain Seh, Mohammad Zarour, Mamdouh Alenezi, Amal Krishna Sarkar, Alka Agrawal, Rajeev Kumar, and Raees Ahmed Khan," Healthcare Data Breaches Insights and Implications," 2020, https://www.ncbi.nlm.nih.gov/pmc/articles/PMC7349636/.

If you recall from the first chapter, there has been an uptick in the number of breaches, but that uptick in the number of breaches does not fully account for the dramatic uptick in the amount of data compromised in those breaches. This is due in part to the increased amount of data required by the HITECH Act and the Affordable Care Act. It is also due

---

[1] Adil Hussain Seh, Mohammad Zarour, Mamdouh Alenezi, Amal Krishna Sarkar, Alka Agrawal, Rajeev Kumar, and Raees Ahmed Khan, "Healthcare Data Breaches Insights and Implications," 2020, https://www.ncbi.nlm.nih.gov/pmc/articles/PMC7349636/.

to the number of records sent through IoMT devices to EHR and other systems. The more data that exists, the more data cybercriminals can compromise. As a result of the breadth and impact of breaches, 2015 was a turning point for the VA, as it was for many in healthcare.

As if all of this is not bad enough, the breach costs in healthcare are high compared to other sectors. Take a look at NIH-provided data from 2015 to 2019 in Figure 5-2. The costs are more than double per record in healthcare than any other sector.

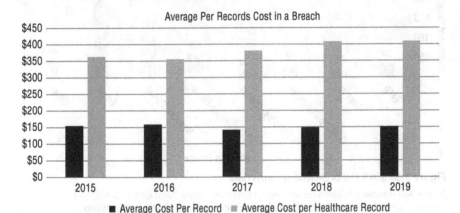

Figure 5-2: Average per record cost in a breach

Source: Adil Hussain Seh, Mohammad Zarour, Mamdouh Alenezi, Amal Krishna Sarkar, Alka Agrawal, Rajeev Kumar, and Raees Ahmed Khan, "Healthcare Data Breaches Insights and Implications," 2020, https://www.ncbi.nlm.nih.gov/pmc/articles/PMC7349636/.

Again, these are very sobering statistics for healthcare practices. The healthcare sector also has the highest industry average breach cost at a whopping $713 million according to IBM. This trend has been true for at least a decade—it's not just an anomaly.[2] The NIH did a study to discover why the number of hospitals have been breached in recent years. From the perspective of a proportion of records exposed, the vast majority (92.59%) were from hacking/incident response, which looked at data from 2015 to 2019. Many of these incidents were related to IoMT, but also all the technology that surrounds IoMT and other IT systems including smart phones, applications, etc., as part of the full ecosystem of vulnerable devices.[3]

---

[2] IBM Cost of a Data Breach Report, 2020, page 11.
[3] Adil Hussain Seh, Mohammad Zarour, Mamdouh Alenezi, Amal Krishna Sarkar, Alka Agrawal, Rajeev Kumar, and Raees Ahmed Khan, "Healthcare Data Breaches: Insights and Implications," 2020, https://www.ncbi.nlm.nih.gov/pmc/articles/PMC7349636/.

If we step beyond looking purely at medical devices and look at the broader cybersecurity challenges that health institutions face, the problems of lost data are larger than just medical devices, as shown in Figure 5-3.

Email and paper breaches, while clearly the top vector for data breaches, are largely due to human error—people sending information to the

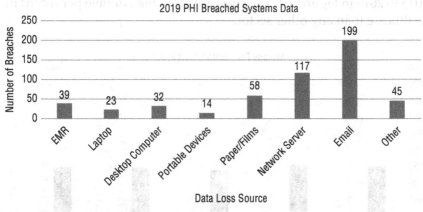

Figure 5-3: 2019 PHI breached systems data

Source: Adil Hussain Seh, Mohammad Zarour, Mamdouh Alenezi, Amal Krishna Sarkar, Alka Agrawal, Rajeev Kumar, and Raees Ahmed Khan, "Healthcare Data Breaches: Insights and Implications," 2020, https://www.ncbi.nlm.nih.gov/pmc/articles/PMC7349636/.

wrong location or other unintended disclosures. These are very important to consider from the data security/privacy side of the story we are telling because it demonstrates that more due care is required when preparing and/or sending information. There are cybersecurity implications that can also play into these sources of data loss—clearly something that healthcare institutions need to take into account. They should be a concern for everyone in America.

But from an IoMT perspective, that is not the most interesting story to tell. Most of the other devices in Figure 5-3 can play a part in the overarching healthcare ecosystem—one that IoMT is part of. The compromise of one device leads to the compromise of other devices. How that takes place is important to understanding the complete picture related to IoMT devices and ultimately to understanding why and how breaches take place.

Breach Anatomy

If breaches were only simple phenomena, security would have been solved a long time ago, and we would not have the problems we are facing today. Instead, we have a world of ever-increasing complexities and thus ever-increasing vulnerabilities, as talked about in Chapter 2. Breaking down how systems are compromised starts to put the challenges of having vulnerable IoMT systems into perspective and better explains why they are such a problem for hospital security and ultimately our data.

Because this is not a how-to book on hacking IoMT, we are only going to look at the high-level issues without going too deep—only enough to explain why insecure devices are so perilous from a data perspective. Our first step on this journey is to look at something called the *kill chain*. A kill chain was originally a military concept that Lockheed Martin adapted to describe the steps that attackers take in order to compromise individual systems.[4] Today, cybersecurity professionals of all types use it to describe how attacks take place. Figure 5-4 outlines and paraphrases the basic steps.

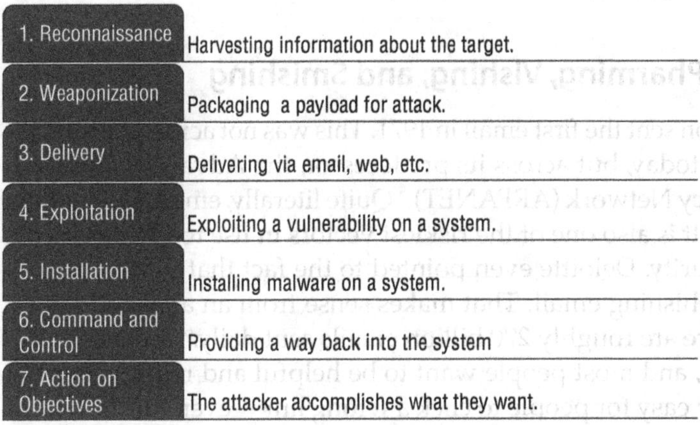

1. Reconnaissance	Harvesting information about the target.
2. Weaponization	Packaging a payload for attack.
3. Delivery	Delivering via email, web, etc.
4. Exploitation	Exploiting a vulnerability on a system.
5. Installation	Installing malware on a system.
6. Command and Control	Providing a way back into the system
7. Action on Objectives	The attacker accomplishes what they want.

Figure 5-4: The cyber kill chain in a nutshell

Source: The Cyber Kill Chain, https://www.lockheedmartin.com/en-us/capabilities/cyber/cyber-kill-chain.html.

---

[4]Cyber Kill Chain, https://www.lockheedmartin.com/en-us/capabilities/cyber/cyber-kill-chain.html.

Of course, there are variations of kill chains to fit a wide variety of attack circumstances, but it does give a general overview of some of the key actions and objectives. For IoMT devices that have no operating system, obviously implanting malware is not always an option. Then again, some devices with smaller operating systems have been compromised in various ways. While there are some limitations to what an attacker can do to a system (IoMT or not), in many cases what an attacker can do is limited by the vulnerability and their imagination.

From our story's perspective, it is not important to understand every single detail of the kill chain. That said, it is important to understand "command and control" and "actions on objectives." Command and control is a type of malware that not only allows access back into the system, but also allows the attacker to perform further objectives within that specific system. Attackers do not want to just attack the system they have access to. They also want to attack other systems to gain access to data or systems that might help them obtain their objectives. Sometimes those objectives are best met by blending social engineering with technical attacks on systems. Social engineering is about finding ways to use human behavior to trick the intended victim into doing something harmful to the system.

Phishing, Pharming, Vishing, and Smishing

Ray Tomlinson sent the first email in 1971. This was not across the internet as we know today, but across its predecessor, the Advanced Research Project Agency Network (ARPANET).[5] Quite literally, email is older than the internet. It is also one of the riskiest vectors in use today despite its relative maturity. Deloitte even pointed to the fact that 91% of attacks begin with phishing email. That makes sense from an attacker's point of view. There are roughly 270 billion emails sent daily.[6] It is a communication tool, and most people want to be helpful and reply via email. It is also very easy for people to click a wrong link—even for the best of us that tend to be conscientious.

Today, most people are aware that email is not the most trustworthy application in terms of trusting the location. The Nigerian Prince scam, so prevalent a decade ago, is more of a reminder today of what phishing

---

[5]Evan Andrews, "Who Invented the Internet," 2019, https://www.history.com/news/who-invented-the-internet.

[6]Radicati Email Statistics Report, 2017–2021, 2017, https://www.radicati.com/wp/wp-content/uploads/2017/01/Email-Statistics-Report-2017-2021-Executive-Summary.pdf.

scams used to be. Today, phishing is often used by malevolent nation-state actors and organized crime not only as a way to compromise computers, but as a gateway into networks.

Phishing techniques have also advanced quite considerably in the last ten years. Spear phishing is now a common technique. It consists of using someone's name to make the attack more personal. The victim is more likely to click the link because it is directed at them. Another common tactic is for criminal organizations to pretend like they are a friend of yours. In many cases, they create an email address that looks like it is from someone you know, but when you look at the underlying address, it is different—in many cases, they can spoof that address to make it seem as though it came from your contact. A more advanced form of phishing is known as *whaling*. It is essentially phishing, but against a C-level executive. The value here can be increased access, or sometimes companies fall for financial transfers. Imagine an email from a CEO telling a CFO to transfer funds to a fraudulent account. Those fraudulent attempts happen all the time. Security professionals today just assume this is part of the background noise of the internet.

Another is a technique called *pharming*. Pharming utilizes fake websites that often accompany a phishing email, but can stand on their own. These websites might be hard to spot substitutions in the names of the companies such as replacing an "l" (lowercase L) with a "1" so the reader may not realize they are going to a fraudulent site. These few techniques are really just the tip of the iceberg. There are hundreds of tricks and techniques that people use to fool others. There are secure email gateways (SEGs) to help companies stop these kinds of attacks, but even using those products is insufficient. Security Magazine estimates there are at least 3.4 billion fake emails sent every day.[7] Even the secure email gateways, however great they are, are not perfect, and many of those phishing emails make their way to the intended targets.

But phishing and pharming are far from the only avenue of attack. Many attackers are brazen enough to call the intended victim. This is referred to as *vishing* (voice phishing). In these cases, they may pull information from LinkedIn, the company website, or other sources to pretend to be an insider and then use the name of that insider to talk

---

[7] "More Than Three Billion Fake Emails Are Sent Worldwide Every Day," *Security Magazine*, www.securitymagazine.com/articles/90345-more-than-three-billion-fake-emails-are-sent-worldwide-every-day#:~:text=At%20least%203.4%20billion%20fake,Spring%202019%20Email%20Fraud%20Landscape.

to the intended victim. In some cases, they will have pharming sites set up and ask users for their username and passwords. Wary users will not easily fall for this kind of attack, but some users may.

Finally, there is *smishing* (SMS phishing). Smishing is about links sent to your phone via text message. Unsurprisingly, clicking these links can mean your phone, watch, or other SMS device can be infected with malware. Given how important mobile devices are for IoMT security and thus hospitals, smishing is a serious concern.

Phishing, pharming, vishing, and smishing fall under the general category of social engineering—they just use technology as the path to obtain their goals. They are extremely critical to the security of IoMT. Quite often, the compromised device is the foothold into that organization. In the case of mobile devices, they may now be embedded into the data collection process—very dangerous. From a computer perspective, the foothold can be very concerning. As mentioned previously, if the environment has a flat network, that foothold may be one hop away from compromising IoMT devices. The fact that IoMT devices have so many vulnerabilities often means they are easy for hackers to compromise. Once they are on the device, those devices can provide access to EHR systems. This is where that interconnection capability is both a positive and a negative trait. It also demonstrates the weaknesses of interconnected environments. The more devices are interconnected, the easier it is to compromise those devices.

Web Browsing

Part of the purpose of the internet is to read, watch, and explore content that might interest us. Hackers have taken advantage of that natural inclination in order to trick us into going to a domain. Unfortunately, as previously discussed, criminals will feed on our fears and concerns—even related to a pandemic. Palo Alto Networks did a study of coronavirus-related domains that were popping up between February and March of 2020. Some of their findings are very concerning. They noted a 656% increase in the average daily COVID-19–themed domains that popped up. They also saw a 569% growth in malicious domain registrations that included malware and phishing, and a 788% growth in domains that included scams, coin mining, etc. In the end, they had 116,357 newly registered COVID-19 domains, with over 40,000 of those domains in the high-risk category.[8] Even in times like these, we have to keep our

---

[8] Janos Szurdi, Zhanhao Chen, Oleksii Starov, Adrian McCabe, and Ruian Duan, "Studying How Cybercriminals Prey on the COVID-19 Pandemic," 2020, https://unit42.paloaltonetworks.com/how-cybercriminals-prey-on-the-covid-19-pandemic/.

collective suspicions up and be very careful about where we go on the internet. Combine these with phishing attacks and it is easy to see how even the best systems might miss a few dangerous sites—especially if more than half seem to be legitimate.

Sometimes, even going to seemingly legitimate websites can be very dangerous. Most well-known websites use publicly available advertisers to supply their ads. The legitimate website is not aware of the advertisements that cycle through its site. In some cases, the links to sites may be one of those malicious websites that can put malware on your computer. This is referred to as *malvertising* (malicious advertising). What is worse is that sometimes the advertising system used by the vendor adds malware to a legitimate website. All it takes in some cases is for the end user to move the mouse over the advertisement to get their system infected. You can be a reasonably good internet user, think you are only going to reputable websites and striving to do the right thing, and then get your system infected with malware.

If someone is browsing the internet from within a hospital or on a mobile device that then connects to IoMT devices, that, in turn, can allow in criminals who do essentially whatever they want from within a network. The internet is far from a safe and social place to be. Threat actors can set up malicious websites very easily for only a few dollars. What they get back is often worth far more. What and where we browse is a critical part of keeping our networks and our data safe.

Black-Hat Hacking

Not all attacks involve social engineering—tricking someone into doing something that would cause harm. Some of them involve hacking. Essentially it involves taking advantage of existing vulnerabilities in systems in order to compromise that system. There are good hackers that hack systems in order to inform organizations of vulnerabilities. These are known as white-hat hackers. The key distinction between white-hat hackers and other hat hackers is permission. They are authorized to attack an organization and stay within the boundaries of that authorization. There are also gray-hat hackers that are not authorized to hack into systems, but do so anyway. Usually they do not exploit the vulnerability or they report the vulnerability so the company can do something about it. Finally, there are black-hat hackers. These are the unauthorized individuals who exploit the vulnerabilities they discover for personal or organizational gain to the detriment of the victim. With previously noted exceptions, these are the ones that attack hospitals in the middle of a pandemic.

What is common to all of these hackers, no matter what hat they wear, is that they use vulnerabilities to gain access to systems. There are a lot of methods and tools both freely available and on the market that organizations can use to detect these vulnerabilities. Other times simple commands can be used to pull data from a website. Another kind of hacking uses stolen usernames and passwords to gain access to a system.

A key difference about hacking is the types of systems that the attackers have access to. If they use phishing to gain access to the initial system, they then have to move laterally within an environment to gain access to other targets. If they attack a server, they may be a single hop away from a server with data—or worse, by hacking a server exposed to the open internet, they have access to the data on that server. Either way, hacking is one of the most common actions used in breaches and is something that organizations need to be very wary of. Most of the breach stories that hit the news are as a result of black-hat hacking.

Speaking of hitting the news and hacking, as I write this chapter, the FBI, DHS, and the HHS warns of a fresh round of ransomware attacks hitting hospitals as being imminent.[9] The timing couldn't be worse as there is currently a heavy spike in COVID-19 cases—over 500,000 new cases a week.[10] Long before this book is printed, there may be more unfortunate deaths at the crossroads of the pandemic and ransomware. To make matters worse, half of the ransomware attacks now involve theft of data prior to the ransom.[11]

IoMT Hacking

As we have described from multiple perspectives, IoMT devices are full of vulnerabilities that hackers have a field day with. I have repeatedly said that IoMT has a great number of vulnerabilities. What has been implied has been compared to other technologies. For example, most of us have a phone or a computer at home. Unless the system is old, those systems can be patched and updated—reducing the vulnerabilities. The

---

[9] "FBI warns of 'imminent' ransomware attacks on hospital systems," CBS News, 2020, https://www.cbsnews.com/news/fbi-warns-ransomware-attack-us-healthcare-system-hospitals/.

[10] Helen Sullivan, "Global coronavirus report US added nearly 500,000 cases in a week; Europe faces more lockdowns," 2020, https://www.theguardian.com/. world/2020/oct/28/global-coronavirus-report-us-adds-nearly-500000-cases-in-a-week-europe-faces-more-lockdowns.

[11] Steve Alder, "Half of Ransomware Attacks Now Involve the Theft of Data Prior to Encryption," 2020, https://www.hipaajournal.com/half-of-ransomware-attacks-now-involve-the-theft-of-data-prior-to-encryption/.

same thing goes for servers and a host of other systems. As mentioned in Chapter 2, often IoMT devices are partially built on an operating system. One would think that those operating systems would be updated. Contrary to what you might think from a cybersecurity perspective, the manufacturer will void the warranty if the system is updated because they do not want to support a device through upgrades or changes of any kind. Remember those 1,111 vulnerabilities for Windows 10? Guess what? Those are now "magically" turned into IoMT vulnerabilities. Quite often the manufacturer will not support industry-standard security software on those systems either. In many cases, not only are they unpatched, but they are unprotected.

Let us look at this situation from the attacker's perspective. On the one hand are computers that are patched and protected sitting out on the network. On the other hand, there are a bunch of unpatched, unprotected systems. Wouldn't that be a great place to establish a permanent watering hole? What? There are hundreds of these systems? All the better. Thus, IoMT stands out from the background simply from that perspective alone. They make, ripe, juicy targets for attackers, and because they are often not protected, the attacker is almost assured of having a permanent connection into the environment. From there, they can reach out to other systems to accomplish other objectives. In short, IoMT vulnerabilities affect the security of the whole organization.

Breach Locations

Obviously black-hat hackers are not just interested in the data on specific IoMT devices. That is small compared to the total data in an organization. They want to gather as much data as possible, which means they need to go where the data is. Generally speaking, the majority of data is sitting in servers and EHR systems. Indeed, both servers and EHR systems are in the top five locations where data is stolen according 2019 statistics.[12]

In Summary

Understanding what is happening in breaches, both from a hacking perspective and from an aggregate perspective, is critically important to

---

[12] Adil Hussain Seh, Mohammad Zarour, Mamdouh Alenezi, Amal Krishna Sarkar, Alka Agrawal, Rajeev Kumar, and Raees Ahmed Khan, "Healthcare Data Breaches Insights and Implications," 2020, https://www.ncbi.nlm.nih.gov/pmc/articles/PMC7349636/.

understanding the challenges that insecure IoMT devices bring to both hospitals and the corresponding data. It also serves to illustrate just how damaging having insecure IoMT devices are on a network and the critical need to develop alternate strategies to protecting today's hospitals and our data from hackers.

The number of attacks is clearly going up. The number of insecure devices is clearly going up. The impact of the attacks is just starting to affect human life. The ransom demands are increasing. The fines are going up. Something clearly needs to change as the current situation is becoming more and more untenable. This upward trend cannot continue indefinitely.

6

Say Nothing of Privacy

Historically, privacy was almost implicit, because it was hard to find and gather information. But in the digital world, whether it's digital cameras or satellites or just what you click on, we need to have more explicit rules—not just for governments, but for private companies.

—Bill Gates

Privacy, in some form or another, has existed for eons. There are even arguments that the desire for privacy may be innate to humans—even if survival, technology, and culture have influenced the thinking around it. In hunter-gatherer societies, it was frowned upon for children to watch parents making love—even if it was done in front of them.[1] Internal walls in buildings were not common until the 1500s, which meant that most activities were done in public. Families often slept in the same bed—often in a room with a fire. Children were exposed to the intimate activities of adults. Of course, this influenced definitions of privacy. Beds for one person were not around until the 1700s. As technology grew, we slowly moved toward separated rooms where people could have more privacy.

---

[1] Greg Ferenstein, "The Birth And Death Of Privacy: 3,000 Years of History Told Through 46 Images," 2015, https://medium.com/the-ferenstein-wire/the-birth-and-death-of-privacy-3-000-years-of-history-in-50-images-614c26059e.

97

People and societies have used many different techniques to protect and maintain privacy throughout history—a key component of privacy is cryptography. The ancient Greeks, for example, came up with a cipher device around 400 B.C.E., called a scytale, as a means to protect communication between military commanders.[2] As depicted in Figure 6-1, the scytale consisted of a baton where the paper was wrapped around it. The message was written around the baton and unreadable except when wrapped around another baton of equal size.[3]

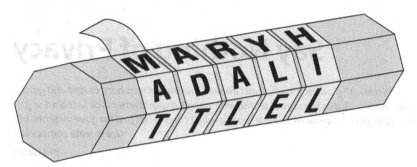

Figure 6-1: Example of a scytale

Encryption has been used throughout history for a range of functions, including protecting privacy in a wide variety of ways. It has helped to protect trade secrets, communication between royalty, as amusement, and so on. Encryption is emblematic of the need for privacy, but the encryption technology that protects IoMT and other systems does not always reflect the desire for privacy. This chapter explores the evolution of privacy in the United States, why privacy is important, and the relationship between privacy and technology.

Why Privacy Matters

In Chapter 3 we explored a bit about data and took it in the direction of compliance in Chapter 4. That protected health information (PHI) also has a great deal of personally identifiable information (PII) in it. PII has names, addresses, phone numbers, etc. Aside from the medical insurance fraud covered in Chapter 1, it also can be used for identity theft—some of that theft is a result of healthcare breaches. The proportions are higher

---

[2] The definition of cipher by the editors of Encyclopedia Britannica, https://www .britannica.com/topic/cipher.

[3] Ibid.

than you might expect. In 2019 the Federal Trade Commission reported over 650,000 cases of identity theft.[4] The cost to the American public was $16.9 billion dollars and impacted just over 5% of the population.[5] Just imagine how much higher those numbers would be if all of our sensitive information were completely public.

Figure 6-2 paints a very grim picture regarding the various kinds of identity theft going on. This does not include fraud, phishing, extortion, or other kinds of racketeering going on as a result of identity theft. What is currently supposed to be largely an advertising issue for big data has turned into real-world impacts that affect all of us. That same advertising information is also useful for nefarious purposes. Knowing something about your intended victim means that you can get them to click a link, purchase products that do not exist, and so on. Many of these crimes are a result of a violation of privacy. Medical insurance identity theft really is only the tip of the proverbial iceberg.

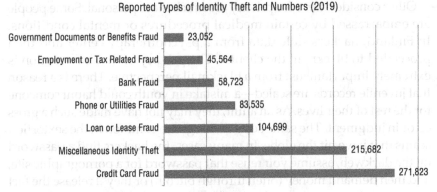

Figure 6-2: Top 7 reported types of identity theft and numbers (2019)

Source: Federal Trade Commission Consumer Sentinel Network, 2020, https://www.ftc.gov/system/files/documents/reports/consumer-sentinel-network-data-book-2019/consumer_sentinel_network_data_book_2019.pdf

Keeping data private is essential to a healthy economy. Companies spend billions on cybersecurity products every year in the hopes that they will not be hacked—essentially to maintain compliance and ensure trust from their patrons. Without privacy, people's lives can be ruined or otherwise harmed. Victims of domestic violence, for example, often want

---

[4] Federal Trade Commission Consumer Sentinel Network, 2020, https://www.ftc.gov/system/files/documents/reports/consumer-sentinel-network-data-book-2019/consumer_sentinel_network_data_book_2019.pdf.

[5] Gayle Sato, "The Unexpected Costs of Identity Theft," 2020, https://www.experian.com/blogs/ask-experian/what-are-unexpected-costs-of-identity-theft/.

to get away from their tormenters. Companies like Spokeo or MyLife contain very detailed information about people, so no matter where the victim moves, it is very easy for the abuser to find that information and pick up where they left off. Oftentimes, these applications do not have an easy or convenient way to remove the information.[6] Personal privacy matters in ways that do not always relate to an exact dollar value.

Let's look at this from the perspective of some companies. If they are spending billions to develop a product and a cybercriminal hacks in and steals the source code for the product, it can put a company out of business. It can stifle innovation if everything a company owns is known ahead of time.

This same idea also applies to the military. Arguably one of the most famous cases surrounds the story of Winston Churchill letting Coventry be bombed by the Germans in order to hide the fact that the English had broken the Enigma code.[7] Privacy, from a military perspective, can be worth sacrificing lives.

Other considerations for privacy are much more personal. Some people are embarrassed by certain medical procedures or mental conditions. In Finland, hackers stole data from a psychotherapy center and then proceeded to blackmail the clients.[8] The privacy of that information is extremely important just from a blackmail perspective. There is a reason that juvenile records are sealed—a mistake in youth could haunt someone for the rest of their lives. As an adult, they may not have made such a gross error in judgment. The same sorts of things are common in the sextortion scams that have hit the globe. In many cases, the hackers find a password on the darkweb, assume you reuse that password for a pornographic site, and then demand money (often through bitcoin) or they'll release the fact that you utilize a pornographic site.[9] While there are several variations of these kinds of crimes, what is important is that these crimes are partially enabled as a result of personal information being stolen.

---

[6] Yuri Nagano, "New State Law Pits Privacy Against Free Speech, Public Records and Data Brokers," 2019, https://www.sfpublicpress.org/new-state-law-pits-privacy-against-free-speech-public-records-and-data-brokers/.
[7] Peter J. McIver, "Churchill Let Coventry Burn To Protect His Secret Intelligence," https://winstonchurchill.org/resources/myths/churchill-let-coventry-burn/.
[8] "Finland shocked by therapy center hacking, client blackmail," News Break, https://www.newsbreak.com/news/2089427684576/finland-shocked-by-therapy-center-hacking-client-blackmail.
[9] Luis Lubeck, "Sextortion scammers still shilling with stolen passwords," 2020, https://www.welivesecurity.com/2020/04/30/new-sextortion-scam-claims-know-your-password/.

In short, whether talking about personal medical records or passwords, privacy affects us on a very personal level and is a critical foundation of our society. From a small-business perspective, it can be truly devastating. Roughly 10% of small businesses go out of business because of a data breach, and 25% of small businesses have to file for bankruptcy because of breaches.[10] So no matter which side of the metaphorical coin you are looking at—personal or business—privacy is worth protecting, even if cybersecurity is a large part of what protects that privacy.

Privacy History in the United States

Elements of privacy regulation have been around since the early days of the United States. For example, in 1782, Congress passed a law that made it illegal for mail to be opened by anyone other than the intended recipient. In 1880, there was a mandate on the privacy of telegraphs.[11] Both of these are advocating for the privacy of communication—the assumption being that harm is done by intercepting that communication. Benjamin Franklin, for example, had his employees swear an oath not to open his mail.[12] On September 25, 1789, the Fourth Amendment passed, guaranteeing the right to be protected against unreasonable search and seizures. It covers two of the seven central classes of privacy—privacy of territory and privacy of body.[13]

Over the decades since, we have refined our definitions. It wasn't until the 1970s that some of the stronger privacy legislation began to accelerate and we would see some changes as a result. This is clearly demonstrated in Figure 6-3. The first of these is the Fair Credit Reporting Act of 1970, which protects the information of credit information. This goes back to the data integrity requirement for big data. The data has to be accurate. In 1974 we saw the Privacy Act. It puts limits on how personal information can be used by the federal government.[14] In 1978 came the

---

[10] Silviu STAHIE, "Data Breaches Force 10% of Small Company Victims Out of Business," 2019, https://securityboulevard.com/2019/10/data-breaches-force-10-of-small-company-victims-out-of-business/.
[11] Daniel Solove, "A Brief History of Information Privacy Law," 2006, https://scholarship.law.gwu.edu/cgi/viewcontent.cgi?article=2076&context=faculty_publications.
[12] Ibid.
[13] National Constitution Center, https://constitutioncenter.org/interactive-constitution/amendment/amendment-iv.
[14] The United States Department of Justice Privacy Act of 1974, https://www.justice.gov/opcl/privacy-act-1974#:~:text=The%20Privacy%20Act%20of%201974,of%20records%20by%20federal%20agencies.

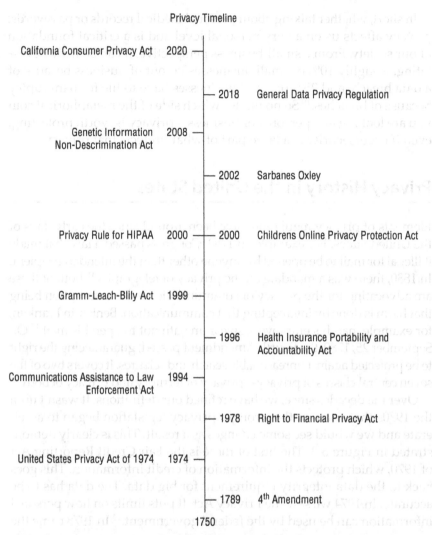

Privacy Timeline

California Consumer Privacy Act   2020

2018   General Data Privacy Regulation

Genetic Information   2008
Non-Descrimination Act

2002   Sarbanes Oxley

Privacy Rule for HIPAA   2000   —   2000   Childrens Online Privacy Protection Act

Gramm-Leach-Blily Act   1999

1996   Health Insurance Portability and
Accountability Act

Communications Assistance to Law   1994
Enforcement Act

1978   Right to Financial Privacy Act

United States Privacy Act of 1974   1974

1789   4th Amendment

1750

Figure 6-3: Some key privacy laws affecting the United States

Right to Financial Privacy Act, which required that the government must follow specific procedures in order to obtain information. In short, the 1970s were all about increasing privacy protection.

The 1980s were greatly affected by the rise of the internet. Legislation then was largely concerned with protecting electronic communication and sharing of electronic information. The Cable Communications Policy Act of 1984 was aimed at deregulating the cable industry, but it did include provisions for protecting subscriber privacy—such as not disclosing personal information without obtaining authorization. In 1986 the Electronic Communications Privacy Act protected communications while they are being made, while in transit, or stored on computers.[15] Last, but certainly not least, is the Video Privacy Protection Act (1988), which protects against the disclosure of rental records of video information.

The 1990s Turning Point

The 1990s were a time of massive improvements in the protection of American privacy. This included everything from the Children's Online Privacy Protection Act to the Gramm-Leach Bliley Act (GLBA), the Americans with Disabilities Act, and of course HIPAA. This is where privacy and security started to merge, because so much of privacy is dependent on technology. Scytales are no longer in use, but there have been a whole host of cryptographic technologies that protect the privacy of data today. In fact, many of these laws were put into place as a result of privacy violations and recognitions of harms that were done.

The 1990s also introduced a bill that is still controversial today—the Communications Assistance to Law Enforcement Act (CALEA). A few years back Apple made a choice not to unlock a terrorist's iPhone during an investigation, which violates CALEA. Apple responded strongly to the CALEA requirements because, in their own words, "First the government would have us write an entirely new operating system for their use. They are asking Apple to remove security features and add a new ability to the operating system to attack iPhone encryption, allowing a passcode to be input electronically."[16] Apple felt that adding a simple passcode would severely weaken the security of the iPhone. As Apple points out, password crackers could be used against the iPhone, and soon everyone would have access to everything on it. Plus, how do you give passwords out to all law enforcement without that information slipping out somehow? It becomes virtually impossible. Ultimately, that change would severely weaken the iPhone's security and privacy. For Apple, whether or not you agree with them, that privacy is worth putting up a fight with the United States government.

From a security standpoint, though, both HIPAA and GLBA are particularly interesting for their security requirements. GLBA breaks out the physical, technical, and administrative-level controls so it begins that

---

[15] Justice Information Sharing Electronic Communications Privacy Act of 1986 (ECPA), https://it.ojp.gov/PrivacyLiberty/authorities/statutes/1285.

[16] "Answers to your questions about Apple and security," Apple, https://www.apple.com/customer-letter/answers/.

differentiation process in terms of security. HIPAA bases the information on the protection of confidentiality, integrity, and availability—known as the CIA Triad. That triad is a foundation for information security controls today. As HIPAA expanded to include security requirements, they were becoming more mature from a framework perspective. In the end, the 1990s were a time of tremendous shift in terms of privacy regulations.

HIPAA Privacy Rules

HIPAA is not just compliance to follow, nor is it just a legal framework. There are also HIPAA privacy requirements that make it worthy of discussion from a privacy standpoint. The goal of the HIPAA privacy rules is to protect the confidentiality of patient healthcare information. Protected healthcare consists of eighteen Individually Identifiable Health Information (IIHI) that could be used to identify a patient. The data set is expanded under the HIPAA Privacy Rule to include things like drivers' licenses, license plate numbers, serial numbers, URLs, IP addresses, and so on. From a privacy standpoint it expands to include images than contain the IIHI. Disclosure is also a large part of the privacy rule. IIHI information can only be disclosed if the patient authorizes the disclosure. Those disclosures require that the covered entity that receives the data must use the minimum necessary information to accomplish the intended purpose.[17]

All this said, within the United States, HIPAA is one of the broadest and most detail-oriented privacy and security frameworks. Critics feel that there are too many loopholes in HIPAA that allow sharing of information without patient consent. This is one of the reasons that data can be provided to so many organizations. HIPAA, in a way, is caught in the modernization crossfire between the needs of big data helping society and the need to keep data safe. In the United States, we still have not found the perfect balance, and given that technology evolves so rapidly, we may be always a step behind.

HIPAA and Pandemic Privacy

The HIPAA Privacy Rule has several provisions that relate to public health that are particularly suited to pandemics. HIPAA, for example, recognizes the need for public health authorities to be aware of certain

---

[17] Health and Human Services Summary of the HIPAA Privacy Rule, https://www.hhs.gov/hipaa/for-professionals/privacy/laws-regulations/index.html.

conditions (such as COVID-19), which means covered entities can disclose PHI without authorization. Those disclosures can only be to health authorities or foreign government agencies in collaboration with the health authority. Information can also be disclosed to persons at risk as a result of the person being infected. Healthcare providers may also share the information to lessen a serious or imminent threat (such as COVID-19). In all cases, that information sharing should be the minimum necessary to accomplish the preceding goals.

HIPAA has not gone far enough in terms of working with the COVID-19 pandemic, so emergency measures have been put in place that modify the way the Office of Civil Rights (OCR) penalizes covered entities for violations. Telehealth is a good example. OCR has made a conscious decision to allow some video communication applications without risk of penalties for the companies not meeting all of the HIPAA requirements so long as the applications are not public facing (Facebook Live, Twitch, and TikTok). The Health and Human Services (HHS) website recommends that covered entities use video services that are in HIPAA compliance and will enter into Business Associates Agreements (BAAs). HHS also lists some of the services that are acceptable telehealth services such as Microsoft Skype, Teams, and Zoom for Healthcare. These services do meet HIPAA compliance sufficiently and will enter into a HIPAA BAA.[18]

A number of other changes to HIPAA became effective as of March 15, 2020. HHS put out a COVID-19 & HIPAA Bulletin to detail those changes, but the key point is that OCR would not enforce sanctions against hospitals for not complying with the following provisions of the HIPAA privacy rule:

- the requirements to obtain a patient's agreement to speak with family members or friends involved in the patient's care. See 45 CFR 164.510(b).

- the requirement to honor a request to opt out of the facility directory. See 45 CFR 164.510(a).

- the requirement to distribute a notice of privacy practices. See 45 CFR 164.520.

---

[18] Health and Human Services Notification of Enforcement Discretion for Telehealth Remote Communications During the COVID-19 Nationwide Public Health Emergency, https://www.hhs.gov/hipaa/for-professionals/special-topics/emergency-preparedness/notification-enforcement-discretion-telehealth/index.html.

- ▪ the patient's right to request privacy restrictions. See 45 CFR 164.522(a).

- ▪ the patient's right to request confidential communications. See 45 CFR 164.522(b).[19]

These are not the only pandemic-related changes. There are other recommendations that are outside the scope of HIPAA (in most cases) that have also been an influenced by the pandemic.

Contact Tracing

Contact tracing is another important way of staying safe. It involves keeping track of who you have been around and then informing people if you pick up COVID-19. If you are unfortunate enough to experience COVID-19 symptoms, you should get tested, self-isolate, and inform others you have been in contact with. Where contact tracing gets interesting are some of the new applications that are out. Some states, such as New York, have released a contact-tracing application to alert users when they have been around someone with COVID-19.

The challenge with these apps is that several of them are available on the market, and they require adoption in order to maximize utility. The large number of available apps brings confusion about which ones should be used. With disparate apps, it means reduced effectiveness of the products overall.

Privacy is obviously a big concern for anyone who uses these apps. North Dakota, for example, has a contact-tracing app that was reviewed for privacy. In theory, the North Dakota app should not share location data, but in fact, it was sharing that data with Foursquare. Foursquare was then selling the information to advertisers.[20] Privacy gaps, which are remarkably common, do push some people away from making better use of these kinds of apps.

Further, it was found that the data in the app wasn't as anonymous as it was thought to be. The app used an anonymous code in conjunction

---

[19] Health and Human Services COVID-19 & HIPAA Bulletin Limited Waiver of HIPAA Sanctions and Penalties During a Nationwide Public Health Emergency, 2020, https://www.hhs.gov/sites/default/files/hipaa-and-covid-19-limited-hipaa-waiver-bulletin-508.pdf.

[20] Pierre Valade, "Jumbo Privacy Review: North Dakota's Contact Tracing App," 2020, https://blog.jumboprivacy.com/jumbo-privacy-review-north-dakota-s-contact-tracing-app.html.

with an advertising identifier. The advertising identifier is the same across all the applications on your phone, which means aggregating that information back to data brokers could easily reveal who you are. The information was transmitted to Foursquare and Bugfender, which not only received the anonymous code, it received information like the name used by the owner of the phone.[21]

Privacy gaps are only one of the reasons for low utilization of contact-tracing apps, but they have diminished the overall value of such programs.

Corporate Temperature Screenings

As a result of COVID-19, many corporations have instituted a policy where they temperature screen employees prior to them gaining access to a facility. If they have a temperature, it is an indicator they may have COVID-19, and they will not be allowed access as a means of protecting the other employees. Like the fitness watches discussed in Chapter 3, unless the testing or information is from a covered entity, it is not considered PHI. That being said, the data collected may still be sensitive and the requirements may be different depending on the privacy laws of the state you live in. CCPA, for example, requires a disclosure about the information collected, why it is there, and how that information will be used. Employees may further request that the information be deleted. If the data is compromised, informing the attorney general may be applicable.

A Step Backward

The 2000s were a big step backward in terms of privacy. Most of that was due to the aftermath of the tragic events of September 11, 2001. With the Uniting and Strengthening America by Providing the Appropriate Tools Required to Intercept and Obstruct Terrorism Act—the USA PATRIOT Act—many agencies within the United States were given broad new powers to find terrorists. These included such powers as the ability to search business records and the ability of the NSA to collect phone records and go through the browser history of citizens. It also allows the searching of foreign intelligence information from both foreign and United States citizens—whereas United States citizens were formerly exempt.

---

[21] Ibid.

The New Breed of Privacy Regulations

The General Data Protection Regulation (GDPR) hit the scene like a brick in 2018. It is a comprehensive privacy bill that came out of the European Union that dramatically changed the nature of how privacy bills are put together and how they were thought of. Companies around the world, and in the United States, were struggling to understand what the repercussions of the bill would be. One of the defining characteristics was that it was not about geographic boarders, but about the citizens. This meant that the law technically applied everywhere a European citizen was located—even in the United States. The challenge that enforcement of GDPR has is related to where the company is located. If the company is in Europe, European has legal authority to enforce their law. They do not have the authority to enforce GDPR in the United States without the cooperation of a United States Attorneys General. While impact of the regulation was quite strong in Europe, that impact is much less strong in the United States as most Attorneys Generals will not enforce European laws here.

From a United States perspective, this would change business operating in the EU (and some degree the United States) and recognize strong rights that people have under this umbrella regulation. But probably what is more important is the influence that GDPR had on the legal thinking within the United States. California would be the state to lead the privacy charge within the United States, as you will soon read.

California Consumer Privacy Act

Following along a similar path as GDPR, the California Consumer Privacy Act (CCPA) went into effect on January 1, 2020, but its enforcement was postponed for six months.[22]

The scope of CCPA applies to residents of California, but the law can apply to companies that have data related to California residents that meet any of the following criteria:

- The business has an annual revenue of over $25 million.

- The business buys, sells, or receives the personal information of 50,000 or more California residents, households, or devices.

---

[22] Alikhani Kayvan, "California's CCPA Triggers A Tsunami of State-Level Data Privacy Laws," 2020, https://www.forbes.com/sites/forbestechcouncil/2020/02/20/californias-ccpa-triggers-a-tsunami-of-state-level-data-privacy-laws/?sh=21373cd16cad.

- Fifty percent or more of the annual income of the business is derived from selling personal information of California residents. The only exceptions to this are non-profit organizations or government agencies.

Under the CCPA, personal information is defined as any information that could be reasonably linked to you or your household. This is in stark contrast to the federal definition of personal information that is generally related to a person's name, address, phone number, and so on. The federal definition does not include your phones location (which can generally be linked to a specific home), purchase habits, and an assortment of other information related to you or your household. Under the CCPA, the definition is more broad and less specific, which makes it a bit better than the federal guidelines for protecting data—especially for protecting the privacy of your data.

The CCPA also expands the rights that California residents have. California residents, by right, can ask businesses for information that companies have about themselves. In turn, companies have to disclose that information to California residents. California residents can also choose to have the companies delete any information they may have. You also have the right to be notified prior to providing your information. Business cannot make you waive your rights nor discriminate against you as a result of exercising your rights under California law. This may not seem like much from a layperson's perspective, but these are very powerful rights—rights that most citizens in the rest of the country do not have. This means that a California resident can ask a data broker to remove their data, and they have to comply.

California has another law that requires data brokers to register with the California Attorney General. From there, the California government has the data broker's information, links, and email addresses related to the data brokers. That information is easily downloadable in a CSV format. At the time of this writing, there are more than 400 data brokers listed in the file. Of course, the challenge is knowing where your data is out of the list of 400 data brokers and then removing that data.

CCPA, AB-713, and HIPAA

When CCPA was first released, the de-identified data from HIPAA was still considered Personal Information from a CCPA perspective.[23] That

---

[23] Pepper Troutman, "CCPA Amendment Further Harmonizes with HIPAA and Provides Additional Exemptions," 2020, https://www.jdsupra.com/legalnews/ccpa-amendment-further-harmonizes-with-97666/.

has huge data privacy implications because it meant that de-identified HIPAA data could not be used in accordance with HIPAA. On September 28, 2020, AB-713, a modification of CCPA, went into effect so that de-identified PHI could be used in accordance with HIPAA and other legal requirements despite the fact that the data was PII from a California perspective.[24]

What is interesting is that AB-713 didn't stop there. It also included a clause about the re-identification of PHI. If you remember in Chapter 3, there were no national laws against the re-identification of PHI and the subsequent sale of that information. CCPA changes that, even if it is only on a state level. Under AB-713, re-identified data is no longer exempt from CCPA unless that re-identification is for use with a covered entity, or is for public health activities, for research, or specific testing purposes where the data is returned or destroyed.[25]

AB-713 goes further than this, though, in that it has strong contractual requirements for the sale or license of de-identified data, which began January 1, 2021. Those contractual requirements must include a statement about the fact that re-identified data is being sold or licensed, that re-identification is prohibited, and that the data may not be sold, unless the same (or stricter) prohibitions are included.[26]

From a data protection standpoint, these are massive changes and the first steps for protecting people's data from the harms of data brokers. While this covers California citizens' data, it does start to make a dent in the national arena—especially if that data is aggregated. While exceptions can be made for multi-state data, not every company is willing to make that exception. California is the most populated state in the country and many companies have chosen to comply with the California law across the country even if the company is not located in California.[27] Its economy is the fifth largest in the world.[28] Of course, many companies do not choose to make the California law universal—sometimes as a cost-cutting measure. The advantage that Californians have is that, being the United States, other attorneys general in the United States are more likely to take CCPA seriously if there are violations.

---

[24] Ibid.

[25] Ibid.

[26] Ibid.

[27] Marian White, "The 10 Largest States by Population," 2020, https://www.moving.com/tips/the-10-largest-states-by-population/.

[28] Alikhani Kayvan, "California's CCPA Triggers A Tsunami of State-Level Data Privacy Laws," 2020, https://www.forbes.com/sites/forbestechcouncil/2020/02/20/californias-ccpa-triggers-a-tsunami-of-state-level-data-privacy-laws/?sh=21373cd16cad.

Another consideration is that any company that does business in California, so long as it fits within the CCPA applicability criteria, will have to comply with the CCPA criteria as part of the contracts. With strong contractual requirements like this, most applicable businesses are going to push to meet CCPA requirements.

New York SHIELD Act

California is not the only state with bills that significantly transform the privacy and security landscape. New York signed into law the Stop Hacks and Improve Electronic Data Security Act, also known as the SHIELD Act. The central tenets of the SHIELD Act include expanding the scope of what a data breach entails. For example, biometric information, email addresses, passwords, or security questions and answers are not subject to data breach notification. The definition of data breaches now includes any unauthorized access to private information.

The SHIELD Act applies to any New York resident and not just companies that conduct business there. Like CCPA, this has tremendous ramifications for companies across the globe because doing business that affects New Yorkers means updating the definition of a breach—at least for New Yorkers.

Nevada Senate Bill 220

Senate Bill 220 is somewhat similar to the CCPA in that it requires that any operators of websites and online services (excluding healthcare, financial institutions covered by the Gramm-Leech Bliley Act, and certain motor vehicle manufacturers) provide opt-out requirements on the sale of their covered information if that information is for monetary consideration. There are some exceptions for data transfers to third parties, including companies that process data for the operator, who have a direct product or service business relationship with the consumer, or is consistent with a reasonable expectation of privacy that the consumer would have based on the context of the information.[29]

---

[29] "Nevada Enacts New Online Privacy Law Requiring Opt-Out Rights for Data Sales," InfoLawGroup, 2019, https://www.infolawgroup.com/insights/2019/6/4/nevada-enacts-new-online-privacy-law-requiring-opt-out-rights-for-data-sales#:~:text=While%20businesses%20scramble%20to%20prepare,be%20effective%20October%201%2C%202019.

Nevada's Senate Bill 220 is not at comprehensive as the CCPA in that the law does not include the right of access to data, nor deletion or non-discrimination related to the exercise of rights related to the bill.

Excluding healthcare data clears up some of the entanglements that the CCPA had with healthcare data, but Senate Bill 220 does not have the advantage of being able to handle re-identified healthcare information. That data can be sold if it comes from Nevada residents. Still, Nevada's opt-out clause provides a way for Nevada residents to opt out of having their data sold.

Maine: An Act to Protect the Privacy of Online Consumer Information

Maine's law to protect consumer information went into effect July 1, 2020. The law prohibits providers of broadband internet access from using, disclosing, selling, or permitting access to that information unless the customer explicitly gives consent. It also prohibits pressure tactics from the providers for customers not consenting to that agreement.[30] While not as impactful as the CCPA or the SHIELD Act, it does represent the importance of privacy and is yet another step toward creating a holistic privacy strategy—even if we have a long way to go.

States Striving for Privacy

Between 2018 and 2020, there have been more than 40 privacy bills introduced on the state level. While many of them have failed to become law, it does point to the fact that many states see a clear need to have privacy legislation. Part of the reason so many states are working toward stronger privacy laws is the privacy laws are not as strong as they could be at the federal level. This creates challenges for multi-state businesses as they strive to keep track of the quickly changing state regulations.

There has been some talk of a national privacy standard to protect data. Other than HIPAA and GLBA, which are industry specific, there

---

[30]"Governor Mills Signs Internet Privacy Legislation," State of Maine Office of Governor Janet T. Mills, 2019, https://www.maine.gov/governor/mills/news/governor-mills-signs-internet-privacy-legislation-2019-06-06#:~:text=consumer%20privacy%20online."-,LD%20946%20"An%20Act%20To%20Protect%20the%20Privacy%20of%20Online,%2C%20disclosure%2C%20sale%20or%20access.

are no GDPR or CCPA-like standards in the works. It would help us to alleviate many of the privacy violations we are facing today. In Chapter 3 we mentioned that today, foreign governments can buy data of United States citizens and potentially use it for nefarious purposes. It is clearly a gap in the protection of our citizens.

International Privacy Regulations

We have already covered a number of regulations, but far from all of them. GDPR has helped to spawn privacy regulations throughout the world. Here is a list of just a few, but experts recognize that more are on the way:

- Brazilian Data Protection Law
- India Personal Data Protection Bill
- Chile Privacy Bill Initiative
- New Zealand Privacy Bill

As a result, the way we do business is changing at a very rapid pace. The privacy landscape we are dealing with now will not be the landscape we are dealing with 10 years from now. Things will have become much more complicated.

Still, these are not the only players in the international privacy arena. Take something like credit card compliance. They have a regulation referred to as Payment Card Industry Data Security Standard (PCI DSS or PCI for short). PCI is a set of cybersecurity regulations regarding the use of credit cards. What is interesting about PCI is that it truly is an international standard because credit cards are a global standard by design. It is not originally from a law within a country, but from the collaboration of credit card companies that have experienced too much legal damage as a result of hacking.

Credit card information also accompanies personal information in many instances—especially for items that are sold through a website or an app and need to be shipped to a customer address. PCI is largely designed to protect credit card data, and not all companies use the same strategy when it comes to meeting PCI compliance. For example, many companies farm out the credit card processing to other companies to avoid having to meet all of the PCI regulations. In this sense, personal information may not be protected. Many hospitals have to meet PCI and HIPAA requirements simultaneously.

Technical and Operational Privacy Considerations

From a non-technical perspective, it may seem that a great deal of the privacy discussion is in the legal realm and does not have much of an impact from a technical or operational perspective. Nothing could be further from the truth—especially for multi-state and/or multi-country businesses. Keeping track of the types of data and the requirements related to that data can be a massive undertaking for data brokers, and without extremely thoughtful processes in place, it can create large legal problems for organizations. The way things are going, in the future there could easily be over a hundred distinct requirements related to data depending on the type of data, the location, and so on. Complexity is an invitation for mistakes to be made.

The more technically minded may think that it is easy to tag data, and they would be right. But trying to tag a hundred different types of data and remembering what all the different restrictions are with each type is not an easy task. Take the CCPA requirement for re-identified data. All it takes is a faulty tag for data to be changed from CCPA not being scope to suddenly be in scope for a specific data set. Yes, protections can be created to search for these kinds of issues, but it takes another layer of data/technical governance to monitor for them.

Once an issue is identified, the cleanup work may be more difficult than many may assume. If the data broker is interconnected to several other data brokers, information transferred may include data that should not have been sent. That may require technical intervention of standardized processes and the cooperation of the downstream entities in order to clean up the problem. Given that many of the data brokers have strong interconnections to other brokers for specific purposes, a simple technical glitch can quickly have downstream effects that are extremely difficult to rectify.

In Chapter 3, we discussed how many of the data brokers contain inaccurate information. One polluted source of information can quickly amplify across an environment. Creating a strong data governance model is absolutely critical, and that model has to be tightly interconnected with IT operations to be truly effective. In most organizations, changes to IT systems or data are performed through a centralized change management process. Change management is a process for governing changes within an organization. There are several models, but for data brokers, a team of data governance specialists have to be part of the overall decision to make changes.

Non-IT Considerations

Operations are not just an IT issue. Creating contracts, validating the contracts, and documenting what the interconnection agreements are should not be a one-time process. Every mature process has a system of checks and balances to ensure that companies are protecting themselves through the legal agreements. This means working with lawyers to ensure the contracts meet the legal requirements on a continual basis. For large data brokers it means keeping up to date with all of the privacy laws in all the states and/or countries they are operating in. This is no small challenge, and companies often rely on privacy software just to keep up with the variety of privacy changes. Continual reviews are also part of good data governance.

Impact Assessments

Two items that we have not discussed are Privacy Impact Assessments (PIA) and Data Privacy Impact Assessments (DPIA), which are also part of strong privacy programs and are required as part of many privacy frameworks. There is also some general confusion about the distinction between the two because of how frameworks label them. A PIA, generally speaking, is about designing privacy processes from the beginning or when new businesses are (about to be hopefully) acquired. Another phrase that is appropriate is privacy by design. The purpose of the process is to ensure that as new systems are in the design phase, privacy is part of the design process. Essentially it is about privacy due diligence. DPIAs, on the other hand, are all about identifying data and associated processes and tying that back to the privacy risks associated with that data. This usually entails cybersecurity considerations related to the data.

Key considerations for both DPIA and PIA include defining the types of data and ensuring that sufficient protections are in place to protect that data. It involves knowing who is processing the data and understanding the purpose of doing so. It also involves knowing the governance of that data. Both of these processes are required of data brokers to ensure effective privacy—that and a strong security program.

Privacy, Technology, and Security

If it isn't evident, privacy is very concerned with data breaches—every bit as much as cybersecurity—and for many of the same reasons: loss of business, which leads to loss of customer confidence. The financial penalties combined with people not trusting a source of information can be enough to drive many companies out of business. In fact, 60% of small businesses go out of business 6 months after suffering a cyberattack.[31] Privacy practitioners tend to focus more on the legal requirements than cybersecurity, but there is a strong interdependence between cybersecurity and privacy practitioners. This means that privacy professionals understand the tolerances, the risks, and the requirements for meeting privacy requirements, but they do not necessarily have a strong understanding of the technology, nor the capabilities of the latest tools. As a result, in well-run organizations, the two parts of an organization may be in separate departments, but have a strong relationship.

That said, both privacy and cybersecurity professionals are dependent on technology to accomplish their goals. Privacy professionals tends to be focused a bit more on the governance of data—especially if they are focused on the newer post-GDPR regulations. The background of most privacy professionals is a legal background. They focus on why privacy needs to be in place and what privacy needs to be put in place, but how processes work are a whole other matter. Cybersecurity professionals tend to be focused on compliance, risk, and how to prevent data breaches in the first place. Cybersecurity professionals often have some of the same blind spots as legal professionals in that measuring how to keep track of detailed privacy requirements (especially related to big data) are met. It truly requires strong specialization when dealing with complex data sets. HIPAA provides some common ground for security and privacy practitioners alike as the security rule has specific criteria for defending organizations. Like all laws or compliance frameworks, they need to be updated on a periodic basis—while the old technologies are still relevant, they become dated and less effective, but required nonetheless. This gap can be problematic for organizations that choose to meet the compliance requirements and no more.

Privacy has additional challenges, however, because of how far data science has come. Newer regulations such as CCPA recognize those chal-

---

[31] Robert Johnson III, "60 Percent Of Small Companies Close Within 6 Months Of Being Hacked," 2019, https://cybersecurityventures.com/60-percent-of-small-companies-close-within-6-months-of-being-hacked/#:~:text=In%20fact%2C%2060%20percent%20of,to%20monitor%20suspicious%20network%20activity.

lenges and have done what they can to dampen some of the challenges related to the data. The focus has been on the contractual relationship between organizations, which, in theory, companies are beholden to. The reality is, depending on the country, breaking a United States law may not be taken seriously in the host country. If a data broker were to purchase data from the United States and keep that data in their home country while not doing business in the United States, they may violate CCPA with no one being the wiser. While there are a great number of ethical corporations who will always do the right thing, not all organizations will.

What matters in both cybersecurity and privacy is how technology is utilized. Is the technology patched and up to date from a security perspective? Is it configured properly? What does the architecture of the system look like? Where is it sitting in the environment? What kind of protection does the system have? What requirements need to be put in place to adequately protect the data? How much data is there, and what are the risks related to the data? Privacy will want to know more about the data, who has access, and whether data rights and obligations are followed to ensure legal compliance with the data. It is not that privacy or cybersecurity do not care about the other profession, because the considerations of each profession deeply affect the approach the other profession will take; it is more a matter of emphasis.

Privacy Challenges

One of the challenges that privacy professionals typically have is understanding and working with IT—especially if that professional has a hand in incident response. While there are compliance people who are adept with technology, many of them do not understand technology. Trying to assess the risk related to privacy can be challenging if the subject matter is extremely technical. In these situations, they can lean on IT or security teams to help them better assess the situation. Even then, for some privacy practitioners, this can be a bit much. This is why teamwork is so critical. Everyone has their area of specialization. IT and security people typically do not tend to come from a legal background. They do not understand the intricacies of law and thus do not have the best judgment in those cases.

Working with legal teams to increase the privacy within organizations is a win-win situation for companies. It is an opportunity for team building and for everyone to learn more about their peers and what the overall concerns are from a privacy perspective. It helps to mature everyone on a team by getting everyone to work well together. Meeting regularly to ensure all the parts are working well within an organization only helps to facilitate a better working environment.

Common Technologies

There are some common technologies that privacy and cybersecurity lean heavily on in order to meet the criteria of their professions. The core technologies are encryption, authentication, and databases. This does not mean that these technologies are the only concern or overlap, but that they are the technologies that are most heavily relied upon to achieve privacy and cybersecurity goals.

In today's world, both privacy and security are heavily dependent on encryption, just as the ancient Greeks were dependent on it in battle. Today's battlefield is a little different than what the ancient Greeks faced. It consists of the internet, which means computers, networks, servers, and so on. When you connect into a website, encryption is used there. Browsers, when connected to secure websites, use encryption to make sure that what is transmitted is transmitted securely. Most of the IT protocols for connecting over the internet are also encrypted. Security professionals refer to that encryption as *data in motion*. Since many people are working at home, a VPN also protects data in motion, but at a slightly different level.

Data at rest is also very important. Data at rest comes in two primary forms—structured and unstructured. Structured data generally sits in a database and should be encrypted—especially if it has any kind of sensitive data. The problematic data is the unstructured data. This is data that is anywhere other than a database. This includes email, shared drives, Office documents, flat files, and myriad other locations. This is the data that is the most difficult to secure. The advantage of this kind of data, with exceptions, is that there is less of it than what is located in databases. It doesn't mean that it isn't important. Concentra Health Services, for example, lost a laptop with HIPAA data and ended up having to pay the Office of Civil Rights $1,725,200.[32] In this case, the laptop contained data that was unencrypted.[33] From a privacy and a security perspective, encrypting laptops is a minimal requirement for protecting data.

---

[32] "Stolen Laptops Lead to Important HIPAA Settlements," Health and Human Services Office of Civil Rights, https://www.hhs.gov/hipaa/for-professionals/compliance-enforcement/examples/concentra-health-services/index.html.
[33] Health and Human Services, https://www.hhs.gov/sites/default/files/ocr/privacy/hipaa/enforcement/examples/concentra_agreement.pdf.

Authentication and identity are two sides of the same coin. Part of the reason authentication is so important is attribution—being able to attribute a specific action to a specific individual. If John Doe is making a purchase, that activity should not be linked to Jane Doe. The method whereby we attribute John's action is through authentication. Authentication is far from perfect because of weaknesses in the authentication mechanism. This is why multi-factor authentication (MFA) has been introduced. If one factor is compromised, the password, for example, it does not mean the attacker can gain access to a system because a second factor must also be compromised.

Privacy experts are also interested in attribution, but sometimes for different reasons. Because of laws like CCPA, knowing where someone lives, California for example, affects what laws are applicable to each person. Depending on the size of the company, meeting CCPA regulations can become an administrative burden—one that can be avoided if the person does not live in California.

The Manufacturer's Quandary

Part of the reason we spend so much time looking at the role of privacy is that it really helps to shine a different light on how poor IoMT security affects organizations. It is not just about the hacking, but also the data. That data is not necessarily just related to the PHI. As we learned in Chapter 3, it is also about the anonymized information and how easy it is to connect personal information to that anonymized data in order to re-anonymize that data. As we have explained in this chapter, that data can have an impact on the privacy of that information.

Some manufacturers' IoMT security and privacy are almost appallingly bad. Many of the basic foundations of privacy are completely absent in some IoMT devices. As stated in Chapter 2, it is unfortunate that IoMT grew from the same roots as IoT devices because those security violations also impact the privacy of data and of overall systems. Almost the full list of everything in Chapter 2 under "Historical IoMT Challenges" is not only a vulnerability, but also a privacy violation. Table 6-1 shines a light on these issues.

These vulnerable IoMT devices are antithetical not only to security as described in Chapter 2, but also to privacy. With additional privacy regulations starting to intermingle with traditional security, it only puts additional pressure on hospitals to select IoMT manufacturers with

Table 6-1: Relationship between IoT Violations and Privacy

IOT WEAKNESS	PRIVACY VIOLATION
Weak, Guessable, or Hardcoded Passwords	If you are essentially giving the passcode away, anyone can access the device, which means there is effectively no privacy related to that device.
Insecure Network Services	An insecure network service means anyone on the network can read any of the information from the device. If the network services are insecure, a hacker can easily gain access, which means there is only marginal privacy.
Insecure Ecosystem Interfaces	If the ecosystem interface is insecure, it means that someone with some skill can gain access to the device. It isn't as bad as a weak password, but it is close from a privacy perspective.
Lack of Secure Update Mechanism	If a device cannot be updated securely, it means that it is insecure by default, which makes it easy to compromise a system.
Use of Insecure or Outdated Components	Outdated components mean vulnerabilities, which can be exploited by adversaries.
Insufficient Privacy Protection	By default, this is a privacy violation.
Insecure Data Transfer and Storage	Storing data in a secure way means that anyone with access to the device can take the data.
Lack of Device Management	This is not a privacy violation by itself, but due to the massive effort to update a volume of IoMT devices means that inevitably, it will lead to vulnerabilities, which can lead to a privacy violation.
Insecure Default Settings	This is not the worst violation if the default settings can be changed. But if they cannot, they provide a door for an attacker to go after the data, thus it can be a privacy violation.
Lack of Physical Hardening	The physical hardening is important because access to the device means you can own it. Lack of physical hardening means access to the data on the device, and thus a privacy violation.

stronger security. Until that conscious choice is made to make security as important as the device capabilities, manufacturers will not be appropriately incentivized to create strong security throughout the manufacturing process and post implementation.

Bad Behavior

In this new data economy in a sense, we do not own our own devices and our own information. This is particularly troubling when considering cell phones used in hospitals. Phones only send information back to Google when you say the trigger phrase, "Okay, Google" (or "Hey, Siri" on Apple devices to send to Apple). Any other data is processed on your own phone. That may seem acceptable, but various apps may take a completely different view of that information. For example, if the Facebook app is installed on the system, they may decide to take some of that data and use it internally or sell that data to advertisers. This is why sometimes advertising seems to pop up on Facebook feeds.[34]

But many cellular organizations have a history of flouting regulations, erring on the side of more data being sent. For example, the Federal Communication Commission fined many of the major carriers and collected more than $200 million for violating the Telecommunications Act—providing too much data to advertisers.

It is interesting to note that in *Smith v. Maryland* (1979), the Supreme Court validated that people do not have a reasonable expectation of privacy if we hand that information over to third parties voluntarily.[35] Most apps require that we click an agreement in order to use them. Many of us do not fully understand the information that we are handing over voluntarily.

There are other somewhat sneaky ways that apps can gather information. One such mechanism is the clipboard—where copy and pasted information is on your cell phone. What if it is a password? Many apps today do not clearly state how they are gathering information about what you are doing. GDPR and CCPA, for example, require clear and transparent notifications about how data is collected. Those clear and transparent notifications are not always available on apps as many application developers or even companies may not be aware of the intricacies of those requirements.

---

[34] Sam Nichols, "Your Phone Is Listening and it's Not Paranoia: Here's how I got to bottom of the ads-coinciding-with-conversations mystery," 2018, https://www.vice.com/en/article/wjbzzy/your-phone-is-listening-and-its-not-paranoia.
[35] "Cell Phone Privacy and Warrant Requirements," FindLaw's team of legal writers and editors, 2019, https://criminal.findlaw.com/criminal-rights/cell-phone-privacy-and-warrant-requirements.html.

Imagine some of these challenges in a hospital setting. Even if many major apps do not collect this information, all it takes is one app installed on a mobile device that is used as part of the overall system to create privacy violations that few are aware of. Apple and Google have been removing some malware from their respective app stores, but it begs the question about how many of these kinds of apps are missed.

In the end, privacy and security are very much intertwined with one another—especially where people make assumptions about what is or is not private, which may not reflect the subtle nuances that are made either legally, by contract, or by companies or potentially hackers that could be using an app for their own gain.

In Summary

Privacy is clearly becoming more complicated with each state passing their own laws and interjecting their own perspective onto the scene. Despite the differences of approach, all of those individual laws (and attempts) point to the fact that we need stronger privacy and data governance within the United States. California and Vermont set up the seeds to better understand the roles and complexities of data brokers—and the challenge related to the data they have, the mistakes, the de-anonymization of HIPAA data, and so on. As a country we are just beginning to understand the pros and cons that big data represents. How will medicine 2.0 advance given these privacy challenges? These are part of the challenges we are struggling to find the right balance for.

From a hospital perspective, the new laws create additional challenges because the penalties keep going up along with the vulnerabilities in IoMT devices. As mentioned at the end of the last chapter, there has to be a breaking point. As a society, we are beginning to care more and more about our privacy, which means the laws will probably become stricter and the fines steeper as time goes on.

The Short Arm of the Law

The FBI has built up substantial expertise to address cyber threats, both in the home-land and overseas. Here at home, the FBI serves as the executive agent for the National Cyber Investigative Joint Task Force (NCIJTF), which joins together 19 intelligence, law enforcement, and military agencies to coordinate cyber threat investigations.

—James Comey

Cybercrime, if it were an economy, would be the third largest economy behind the United States and China. Experts believe that the damages will be $6 trillion in 2021 and up to $10.5 trillion by 2025. By contrast, the United States GDP is $21.5 trillion. Cybercrime represents the greatest redistribution of wealth in existence. Experts say that cybercrime is more profitable than the global drug trade. From that perspective alone, it is not surprising that it is so common.[1] It helps to explain why hacking occurs so regularly and why covered entities are often the target of attacks. It also brings to light why IoMT is such a huge problem for covered entities—as we'll see throughout this chapter.

But let us look at how successful the FBI is when considering traditional crimes. Looking at 2018 statistics, the FBI is relatively successful. Ninety

---

[1] Steve Morgan, "Cybercrime to Cost the World $10.5 Trillion Annually By 2025," 2020, https://cybersecurityventures.com/hackerpocalypse-cybercrime-report-2016/.

percent of the defendants plead guilty; only 2% go to trial and 2%. Of those 2%, 83% are convicted, and only 8% of the cases are dismissed.[2]

By contrast, only three in a thousand cybercrime incidents lead to an arrest.[3] That is a very marked gap. More than likely that is a drop in the bucket compared to the actual number of attacks—most not being reported. Most companies are so inundated with attacks that even having the time to report the issues to the proper authorities can become a tremendous challenge.

The purpose of this chapter is to explore the interrelationship between the types of hackers as they relate to the law, what the limits of the law are, and how those limits relate to enforcement mechanisms. This will lead us to better understand the challenges related to law enforcement and why there are so many hacking attempts against organizations today. Ultimately this provides more background information as to why covered entities and the security of IoMT is such an important link in the security chain—especially as it relates to hospital security.

Legal Issues with Hacking

Obviously, unauthorized hacking is illegal in the United States. But what are the laws that help to protect organizations from hackers? How do those laws apply, and why are they important? How do they help law enforcement agencies stop any of the myriad forms of cybercrime? What are the various types of hackers, and how do they relate to the law?

From a legal perspective, there are three types of hackers—white hats, black hats, and gray hats. White-hat hackers are the hackers who have permission to hack sites as part of their job function or through an agreement with other organizations. Without that permission, they are doing something illegal. Gray-hat hackers are a bit different. They do not have permission to hack an organization, but they alert the company to the found vulnerabilities so that it can resolve them before a disreputable individual or organization finds them. The black-hat hackers

[2]John Gramlich, "Only 2% of federal criminal defendants go to trial, and most who do are found guilty," 2019, https://www.pewresearch.org/fact-tank/2019/06/11/only-2-of-federal-criminal-defendants-go-to-trial-and-most-who-do-are-found-guilty/.
[3]Allison Peters and Anisha Hindocha, "US Global Cybercrime Cooperation: A Brief Explainer," 2020, https://www.thirdway.org/memo/us-global-cybercrime-cooperation-a-brief-explainer.

are the truly disreputable hackers that use their knowledge purely for personal gain, such as stealing the data, adding ransomware, or adding malware for the purpose of reselling the access.

How hackers are perceived really relates to not only permission, but also the law. In addition to exploring some basic categorizations of hackers, we will also explore some United States laws to help put things in perspective and what some of those common considerations are.

White-Hat Hackers

For white-hat hackers, usually called penetration testers, paying explicit attention to what is allowed via the contract is absolutely essential. Being very explicit in the contract and educating the employees who are performing that hacking about their role is critical. Even with this kind of careful consideration, white-hat hackers can get into trouble.

On September 11, 2019, two penetration testers working for Coalfire were performing an authorized penetration test of the physical security of Iowa's Judicial Branch. They set off a physical alarm that resulted not only in an arrest, but felony charges—despite having papers stating that they were authorized to perform the action. The two penetration testers were eventually acquitted, but not until they had gone through something of an ordeal.[4] Even though this was an authorized action on the part of the Coalfire employees, they were perceived to be gray-hat or even black-hat hackers from the perspective of the law—at least for a period of time.

It should be noted that this is not the normal situation for white-hat hacking. In fact, white-hat hacking is a typical part of most compliance requirements and every good security program. As mentioned in Chapter 4, on UL 2900 compliance, the manufacturer of an IoMT device ended the test related to UL 2900 with a penetration test to see if the device could be hacked or not.

Gray-Hat Hackers

The story of the gray-hat hacker can get a bit more complex than simply hacking and reporting. What happens if the company does not acknowledge the problem? What if the gray-hat hacker expected to get paid for

---

[4]Kelly Jackson, "Pen Testers Who Got Arrested Doing Their Jobs Tell All," 2020, https://www.darkreading.com/vulnerabilities---threats/ pen-testers-who-got-arrested-doing-their-jobs-tell-all/d/ d-id/1338570.

finding and reporting the vulnerability? Years ago, often the gray-hat hacker was interpreted in the same way as the black-hat hacker and was sometimes arrested.

Today, the landscape has changed somewhat. Some companies offer bug bounties that reward people who find and disclose vulnerabilities responsibly. They have a responsible disclosure program, which includes nondisclosure clauses for the vulnerabilities that are found. Some companies will provide monetary rewards and/or have a recognition program for those who contribute vulnerabilities, and some companies may hire a contributor to help resolve the issues they find. Not all companies have such rewards, however, and not all companies do something about the information they receive.

From an IoMT perspective, manufacturers are hit or miss. Some manufacturers, such as those that follow UL 2900, are more likely to have responsible disclosure policies. Other manufacturers that are not as diligent with their approach are not as likely to be as appreciative of the capabilities of the gray-hat hackers.

Other gray-hat hackers actively attack black-hat hackers by disrupting their malware, patching systems (you read that right), or otherwise causing mayhem to black-hat hackers. A well-known example of this is the Welchia (also known as the Nachi worm). It was designed to delete the blaster worm and patch the vulnerabilities that made blaster possible. While accessing computers is clearly illegal, it is sometimes done for a good cause. Some organizations shut down as a result of being infected with Welchia.[5]

Sometimes gray-hat hackers only wish to make an important point, so they break the law. For example, Samy Kamkar, a felon who likes to hack, is concerned with the connected world. He and a reporter, Laura Sydell, were permitted to break into a colleague's car and take it for a ride. Standing a few feet away, Samy was able to break into the car with relative ease simply by using a wireless Bluetooth device to hack the car—all to make a point about the challenges of the connected world.[6]

In the end, gray-hat hackers have a place in the security ecosystem—it is a matter of how companies want to integrate them into their security strategy. They are plainly breaking the law—specifically the Computer

[5]Wikipedia "Welchia," accessed December 16, 2020, http://virus.wikidot.com/welchia
[6]Laura Sydell, "The 'Gray Hat' Hacker Breaks Into Your Car—To Prove a Point," 2018, https://www.npr.org/sections/alltechconsidered/2018/02/23/583682220/this-gray-hat-hacker-breaks-into-your-car-to-prove-a-point.

Fraud and Abuse Act (CFAA), which we will describe in a following section. Companies can choose to work with gray-hat hackers or prosecute them as part of their strategy.

Black-Hat Hackers

As mentioned, the black-hat hackers are the hackers who violate the law for personal gain. They are not concerned with carefully crossing the line as the gray-hat hackers are. They also are not given the semi-warm welcome that gray-hat hackers can be given. They are the ones responsible for many of the major attacks and incidents that hit the news. They will create malware, use ransomware, and quite often are willing to cross social and/or legal boundaries that others would not cross. The vast majority of attacks related to covered entities and IoMT are carried out by these black-hat hackers.

Computer Fraud and Abuse Act

The Computer Fraud and Abuse Act (CFAA) was created in 1986 in response to the Comprehensive Crime Control Act's (CCCA) failures to deal with the growing challenges of the burgeoning digital age. Clearly crimes were being committed, but the CCCA was not clear enough for these then-modern crimes. In fact, the CFAA was amended numerous times over the years to keep up with the growing and changing face of cybercrime.[7]

Some of the key provisions of the CFAA include the theft of property via a computer, the alteration, damaging, or destroying of data, utilization of malicious code (such as viruses and malware), and DDOS attacks. The CFAA also criminalized the trafficking of passwords and similar items. It also included simply accessing a computer without authorization. This is part of the reason so many cybersecurity frameworks include requirements about having banners on the system. Hackers who gain access cannot claim that they were unaware they were accessing a prohibited system.[8]

---

[7]Published by Office of Legal Education Executive Office for United States Attorneys Prosecuting Computer Crimes, 1979, https://www.justice.gov/sites/default/files/criminal-ccips/legacy/2015/01/14/ccmanual.pdf.
[8]Ibid.

The Electronic Communications Privacy Act

The Stored Wire Electronic Communications Act and the Electronic Communications Privacy Act are sometimes referred to as the Electronic Communications Privacy Act (ECPA) of 1986. The ECPA is partially in response to the Federal Wiretap Act of 1968 being outdated in the electronic age. The key purpose of the ECPA is to protect electronic communications including email, telephone, and stored communications. It even protects the IP address of the communications.[9]

Cybercrime Enforcement

United States laws are a fantastic start to dealing with cybercrime, but they are far from enough. Cybercrime is not just a national problem, but an international one. Traditional crimes do have corollaries to cybercrime. In fact, the Government Accountability Office (GAO) created a comparison of the relationship between traditional crime and cybercrime, as illustrated in Figure 7-1.

The information that the GAO provided for Figure 7-1 is just a starting point, but it does demonstrate that many traditional crimes can be committed internationally because they are committed over the internet. In fact, the GAO report that this was based on, although from June of 2007, in effect, illustrates the challenges of legally handling international crimes.[10] Some countries do not have cybercrime laws as formal as those of the United States. Still others selectively apply the law. If it is against their country and we detect it, they will apply the law, but if it is against another country (the United States in this example), they are not as interested in applying the law. This unequal legal playing field encourages the threat actors to continue their international crimes with relative impunity.

Jason Healey, of the Atlantic Council, discussed at length some of the positions that various governments held related to cybercrime, referred

---

[9]U.S. Justice Information Sharing Electronic Communications Privacy Act of 1986 (ECPA), https://it.ojp.gov/PrivacyLiberty/authorities/statutes/1285.

[10]United States Government Accountability Office CYBERCRIME Public and Private Entities Face Challenges in Addressing Cybercrime Threats, 2007, https://www.gao.gov/new.items/d07705.pdf.

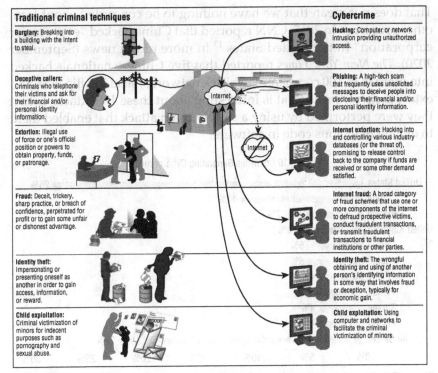

Figure 7-1: Comparison between traditional crime and cybercrime

Source: United States Government Accountability Office CYBERCRIME Public and Private Entities Face Challenges in Addressing Cybercrime Threats, 2007, https://www.gao.gov/new.items/d07705.pdf.

to as "The Spectrum of state responsibility."[11] The spectrum ranges from cybercrime being "state-prohibited" to "state-executed." It also includes countries that ignore, encourage, and sponsor cybercrime.[12] While this is not a complete list, it does serve to illustrate some of the legal challenges of working with various countries.

But how serious of a problem is international cybercrime? Figure 7-2 shows the top 10 countries that are generating cybercrime. The United States, by far, is generating more cybercrime than any other country.

---

[11] Jason Healey, "Beyond Attribution: Seeking National Responsibility for Cyber Attacks," https://www.atlanticcouncil.org/wp-content/uploads/2012/02/022212_ACUS_NatlResponsibilityCyber.PDF.
[12] Ibid.

That does not mean that we have nothing to be concerned about from other countries. In 2015, CNN reported that China hacked "every major corporation" in the United States.[13] In more recent news (September 2020), *The New York Times* reported that five Chinese nationals hacked into more than 100 companies to hijack networks, steal intelligence, and extort their victims. What is interesting about these 100 attacks is that they were performed by using a supply chain attack that enabled them to embed malicious code in software.

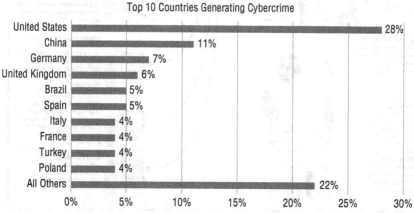

Figure 7-2: Top 10 Countries generating cybercrime

From another perspective, extrapolating data from the Verizon Data Breach Investigation Report, North America is hit with 68% of incidents and 55% of data breaches, which means that North America is being targeted more than its fair share. And the large percentage of these attacks are toward the United States.[14] Clearly there is strong cause for concern as a large number of attacks against North America, and especially the United States, are from international sources.

The effect of these international crimes is absolutely devastating. Only 3 in 1000 cyber incidents reported to the FBI lead to an arrest.[15] The ability of other countries to enforce cybercrime laws in the United

---

[13] Jose Pagliery, "Ex-NSA director: China has hacked 'every major corporation' in U.S.," 2015, https://money.cnn.com/2015/03/13/technology/security/chinese-hack-us/.

[14] Verizon Data extrapolated from the Verizon Data Breach Investigations Report

[15] Allison Peters and Anisha Hindocha, "US Global Cybercrime Cooperation: A Brief Explainer," 2020, https://www.thirdway.org/memo/us-global-cybercrime-cooperation-a-brief-explainer.

States may not be much better. What many criminal organizations do is spread their attacks outside of the countries they are from, which requires the cooperation of law enforcement across multiple countries to seriously disrupt a cybercriminal organization.

In the end, with current levels of cooperation, there is only so far United States laws can go toward dealing with an international problem. Global problems require global cooperation. In many cases, nation-states take an active interest in hacking other countries. If their self-interest lies in hacking other countries, garnering their cooperation can be a challenge. For example, in September 2015, President Obama and President Xi Jinping of China agreed to take steps to address cybercrime.[16] There was a slowdown in hacking for a short period of time from China, but that was over within a few months. A *Wired* article pointed out that what that agreement accomplished was changing the behavior of the hacking attempts, but that China still could accomplish their goals in a diplomatically acceptable manner.[17]

China is only one example out of a whole planet full of different maturities and strategies related to cybercrime. That said, there has been significant progress because of the Council of Europe's Convention of Cybercrime (also known as the Budapest Convention), which 65 countries have signed—including the United States. There are some stark differences in approach, however. Russia and China, for example, prefer a more authoritarian model to the Budapest Convention. Many countries are concerned with human rights violations related to their model. This obviously brings additional challenges that need to be carefully considered.[18]

Results of Legal Shortcomings

If it isn't obvious already, the end results of the global legal shortcomings are absolutely devastating—not just against covered entities, but against almost any government or business that is dependent on computers and

---

[16] BBC News, "US and China agree cybercrime truce," https://www.bbc.com/news/world-asia-china-34360934.

[17] Andy Greenberg, "China Tests the Limits of Its US Hacking Truce As the Trump administration reups an anti-hacking agreement with China, security researchers say China is inching its toes up to that red line," 2017, https://www.wired.com/story/china-tests-limits-of-us-hacking-truce/.

[18] Allison Peters and Anisha Hindocha, "US Global Cybercrime Cooperation: A Brief Explainer," 2020, https://www.jstor.org/stable/resrep25041?seq=4#metadata_info_tab_contents.

the internet. The fact that some covered entities also have IoMT only amplifies the challenges they face—it takes an already bad situation and makes it much worse. The reality is that these legal shortcomings allow hackers to act with relative impunity—doing anything that they may want. With hacking being such a profitable trade, the spoils of which are only amplified by the vast "treasure troves" of data in and around IoMT devices, makes covered entities a prime target for hackers.

Add to that the fact that hospitals are absolutely critical in order to save human life—especially during a pandemic, when they are often willing to pay the ransoms in order to stay in business. Imagine a hacker ransoming an IoMT device that is a respirator keeping someone alive. What would you do as the leader of a hospital? Although paying ransoms is against the best interest of everyone (it encourages hackers to ransom other organizations), it may be in the interest of a particular hospital to pay a ransom rather than letting people die.

In the end, the short arm of the law costs countries billions of dollars. In many situations the relative weakness of law enforcement means that individual corporations need to have higher cybersecurity to compensate for this uneven arrangement between attacker and victim. In short, a strong cybersecurity posture is a must have and not "a nice to have" to protect today's modern businesses.

One of the places that we are beginning to see the effect of the higher costs is in the cybersecurity insurance industry. Rates have been escalating in recent years—partially as a result of the kinds of targeted attacks against organizations. More companies are moving toward cybersecurity insurance, especially as ransom demands become larger and more targeted toward specific industries—including healthcare.

In Summary

From a covered entity and IoMT perspective, this chapter really brings to light the reasons why cybercrime is so common. Until we develop stronger international agreements, it is more important than ever to protect our organizations and IoMT from black-hat hackers—both foreign and domestic. While significant strides have been made in international cooperation, there still remains a substantial cybercrime enforcement gap that allows black-hat hackers to act with relative impunity transnationally.

While stronger cooperation is absolutely critical to any go-forward strategy, it is not just about the cooperation, but the ability of countries to follow up on cybercrime incidents from an international perspective.

Many of the countries that have signed the Budapest Convention have internal struggles of their own, which makes it challenging to bring international cybercriminals to justice. Weighing those concerns against privacy concerns is a challenge we will be working with for ages to come.

In the meantime, it is no secret the ransomware demands have been increasing along with fines for data breaches. The stakes continue to climb higher, making cybersecurity a higher priority, especially within larger covered entities. But before we explore the cybersecurity angle, it is important to understand another influence—the threat actors, their tools, and their methodology.

CHAPTER

8

Threat Actors and Their Arsenal

The fact of the matter is that the United States faces real threats from criminals,
terrorists, spies, and malicious cyber actors.
—James Comey

So far, we have talked a bit about threat actors in general, but only insofar as they relate to the law. It does not provide a strong picture of who the face of the metaphorical enemy is from a cybersecurity perspective. Providing greater insight into these threat actors starts to create a better picture about why cybersecurity is so challenging to many organizations—in fact, it is absolutely critical. Each threat actor has different goals and objectives, which means the tactics they use are sometimes different. Some threat actors are nation-states and have the full backing of the country they live in. The resources for these threat actors is far greater than those of another threat actor, which helps them to provide the resources and opportunities to accomplish their goals.

That leads us to our next point. As a result of the backing a threat actor has, the tools available in their repertoire can be vastly different from actor to actor. Knowing these distinctions can help organizations better prepare for the range of adversaries that covered entities may face.

The Threat Actors

Oftentimes the media portrays hackers as a general stereotype of a teen or early-twenties male sitting in their mom's basement, hacking organizations for the fun of it. While undoubtedly a small number of hackers do fit this profile, the vast number of hackers that most organizations need to be aware of are not these kinds of unorganized amateur players.

Amateur Hackers

There are several names used to describe hackers that are relatively new to hacking and may not be well versed in the hacking arts. These include script kiddies, green-hat hackers, and so on. Generally they do not have the risk profile that most CISOs are concerned about due to their lack of skill. That said, many of them have access to tools and capabilities they can pull from the deep web or the dark web (which we will explain in a few pages), which can quickly make them a bigger risk than they would have been previously.

Insiders

Insiders are actors who work for the organization whose actions, either intentionally or inadvertently, lead to a breach. Unfortunately, healthcare organizations have the largest number of insider risks, with 48% of the breaches caused by insiders sending emails or postal correspondence containing PHI to the wrong address. Another high risk for healthcare organizations are lost and stolen assets. Lost assets are exactly what you might think. An employee or contractor lost a laptop that contained PHI. Stolen assets are similar, but it is a confirmed case where someone stole a device that contained PHI. As a result, putting the appropriate security on assets is absolutely critical.[1]

These are the not only types of insider threats. In fact, IT staff can misconfigure systems leaving them exposed. In the first chapter we spoke about the S3 buckets from Amazon. This is but one example of misconfiguration issues. Firewalls, operating systems, any type of security gear can be misconfigured and lead to a data breach. These are quite often innocent employees with good intentions who make a mistake that anyone can make.

---

[1] Verizon 2020 Data Breach Investigation Report

Unfortunately, these are not the only kinds of insider threats to consider. As healthcare organizations begin to set up more portals for patients to access their data, there are larger risks around the development of the software, which, if not done securely, can inadvertently leave a wide-open door to hackers. There are a number of these kinds of vulnerabilities that can affect an organization—and not just in software.

In some cases, which are less common in healthcare, there can also be the malicious insider who wants to steal PHI, PII, or credit card data from the organization. They actively take advantage of an organization's vulnerabilities to steal data for nefarious purposes. These kinds of attackers quite often have access to privileged information and thus are often more difficult to detect.

The insider risks, whether malicious or not, represent a tremendous risk for healthcare organizations. Protecting them against these kinds of attackers often takes additional controls beyond the compliance requirements of HIPAA.

Hacktivists

Hacktivists (hacking and activism) are hackers who hack other organizations to make a moral point. They often are viewed as a shade of vigilantism because their motivations are not usually for profit but for social causes. The goals vary depending on the group, but they are known to support such causes as protecting free speech, protesting capitalistic ventures, protesting governmental acts of war, and so on. There is disagreement among various hacktivist groups about which causes can be supported and which methods are considered acceptable and which are not in which circumstances.[2] Nevertheless, they represent another type of hacker that luckily most hospitals do not need to be overly concerned with compared to other industries.

Hacktivists can utilize reasonably sophisticated mechanisms to do their work, but in other cases, they utilize social media to encourage others to aid them with their causes. In some cases, they will encourage people to download a simple tool to perform a distributed denial-of-service (DDoS) attack against larger organizations. In this case, an individual hacktivist poses very little risk to organizations, but in large numbers, a DDoS attack can be quite devastating against some organizations.

---

[2]Jake Frankenfield, "Hacktivism," 2019, https://www.investopedia.com/terms/h/hacktivism.asp.

Advanced Persistent Threats

Both organized crime and nation-state attacks are the most sophisticated of the attacks on the internet. Both are referred to as advanced persistent threats (APTs). APT threat actors are well funded to accomplish their goals. They represent the most sophisticated attacks because they have the resources to invest in properly targeting their organization to achieve their goals. There is an age-old statement that organizations need to be right about protecting their organizations 100% of the time while the criminal only needs to be right once. APT actors are the reason why. They have the time and resources for picking their targets.

Organized Crime

There is no universally accepted definition of organized crime, but generally speaking, it is well funded by people willing to pay for illicit activities such as hacked passwords, DDOS attacks, an already compromised server's credentials, and so on. In some cases, organized crime is self-sustained by corrupting of public officials and the use of threats and intimidation to maintain their base of power. Organized crime syndicates have different focuses depending on the organization. Sometimes they engage specifically in cybercrime, while other organizations perform a mix of traditional crime and cybercrime. Some organized crime groups are transnational, which means that the cooperation of law enforcement agencies from multiple countries may be required to take them down. No matter the organization, there is usually a kingpin at the center directing the different aspects of the organization.[3] The kingpins call the shots, set up the websites, and direct other threat actors and dictate the services that a particular organization will have.

Many organized crime syndicates see themselves as entrepreneurs rather than criminals, in that they have a product or service that they need to market. Sure, they may be doing something illicit, but they pride themselves on the quality of their product and/or service. In this way, experience and/or reputation is just as important in the criminal underworld as it is the normal commercial world. In fact, in some cases having a smooth-looking website is absolutely critical to making a sale—just as that is important for modern commercial entities.

---

[3] Steve Ranger, Cybercrime kingpins are winning the online security arms race, https://www.zdnet.com/article/cybercrime-kingpins-are-winning-the-online-security-arms-race/.

A good example of this in Brian Kreb's book *Spam Nation*. In it, he talks about the Russian mafia that buys drugs from India and then resells the drugs through supposedly Canadian pharmacies online. In this case, Americans tend to trust Canadians and believe that the drugs are safe so in combination with a slick-looking website, Americans purchase pharmaceuticals from these "Canadian" pharmacies for far cheaper than what could be obtained from legitimate sources in the United States.[4] Sometimes those drugs are cheap knockoffs and can be very dangerous.

Whatever their business model, these organizations have moved toward the internet and focus more on cyber rather than traditional crimes, because they are more likely to get away with them. Traditional crimes leave a bigger footprint that makes them easier for investigators to track. Further, being outside the reach of the law has certain allure for those committing cybercrime.

While there is the occasional nation-state attack against healthcare organizations, organized crime is one of the most prevalent threat actors to healthcare companies second only to insider threats. Given their laser-like focus on profit and the value of healthcare records on the black market, this should not be a surprise.

Nation-States

Nation-state actors are some of the most feared hackers around the world. The men and women who engage in this kind of hacking are given a license to hack companies or governments around the world—whether or not it is illegal in that part of the world. Some do it for fun, while others do it out of a sense of nationalistic pride. Often, they have access to some of the best tools available, which means they can be the most challenging threats to thwart for cybersecurity professionals.

The goals of nation-state actors tend to be very specific. Sometimes the goal is espionage. A nation-state could steal a billion dollars of research that could take 10 years to create by utilizing a $10,000 hacker. While dishonest, it is an extremely efficient way of getting the same information without spending a billion dollars.

In some cases that means corporate espionage so their companies win out in business negotiations, and other times this means gathering national secrets. In these cases, the nation-state attackers may attack government agencies with the intent of gaining information—if a country understood

---

[4] Brian Krebs, *Spam Nation*, page 59, *Sourcebooks*, 2014.

the strategy of a potential aggressor prior to the start of a war, they could adjust their strategy to compensate for what the enemy is doing.

In the 2016 United States election we saw another angle where Russia was focusing on information warfare in the attempt to change the outcome of the election. This is a different use of cyber-power and focuses on understanding the social forces at play with an attempt to accentuate and tweak the belief systems sufficiently in order influence people's behavior.

With the massive resources that nation-state attackers have they also can invest in understanding how to hack organizations—even if they are using the latest technologies to defend themselves. They can test the tolerances of the artificial intelligence and machine learning techniques in order to develop malware that will not be detected. This makes nation-states among the most dangerous of adversaries. No government will want to turn in their own hackers on principle. More than likely those hackers will be closely guarded secrets of the state.

While nation-state attackers are often not the first concern of most healthcare organizations, occasional intrusions are enough to scare almost anyone in healthcare because of their ability to cut through many of their defenses. The deficient cybersecurity in IoMT devices is a veritable playground in that a nation-state could get in and do whatever it wanted without anyone being aware of their presence. Defending against nation-states should be the bar that companies set to defend against in case they do attack.

To further this point, nation-states and organized crime are both easily able to create their own malware from scratch that can modify itself with every iteration, making it invisible to traditional antivirus defenses. If covered entities can defend themselves against state attackers, they can defend themselves from almost anyone.

Nation-States' Legal Posture

More really needs to be said about nation-states, however. It is not just about the raw ability of the nation-states to hack other countries, it is also about the laws and enforcement of those laws within nation-states. In some cases nation-states will not perform unauthorized hacking against other nations, but will farm out that responsibility to threat actors in their country (or sometimes to international organized crime) to accomplish their goals. In these cases, nation-states are active sponsors of cybercrime—often against the United States and other countries.

Still in other cases, a country will use law enforcement against their own people if and only if the perpetrators are attacking their own country. Usually, the criminal elements are highly aware of this so they can act with impunity against other countries so long as they do not harm their own. Obviously, this creates a number of enforcement challenges, but it explains, at least in part, why hacking is so much on the rise in recent years—there is a tremendous amount of money and no downside to hacking other countries.

The Deep, Dark Internet

Many of us think of the internet as a way to conduct commerce. Indeed, that is true for most of us, but there are actually a few different layers to it that are important for our story. The part most of us are familiar with we'll refer to as the "surface web" or just "the internet." In reality, there is much more to the internet than just websites. Many businesses have layers of interconnections with another where they share information through a variety of technical means. These are all part of normal business operations. Sometimes these connections are accessible from the internet, but not identified by search engines. This is part of something called the deep web.

While the deep web has many legitimate business purposes, many of the sites are created by cybercriminals in order to lure unsuspecting victims to websites for criminal intent. Often phishing or other techniques provide links to these malicious sites, but other times cybercriminals use a technique called typosquatting to have a website with a name almost the same as a legitimate website, but are easily mistyped by an unsuspecting victim. These sites often have malware designed to infect the computer of an unsuspecting victim. Some of these sites are accessible via search engines that capture malicious sites as legitimate sites.

A step further into the internet is the dark web. While there are actually many different dark webs, the most common definition of the dark web being an overlay of network anonymizers that hide any system and people from the open internet. The most common of these anonymizers is Tor—also known as the Onion Router. Tor's mission is to advance human rights and freedoms by providing a place where people can speak freely without monitoring.[5] In fact, in times when governments have cracked

---

[5] Tor Project, https://www.torproject.org/download/.

down on users, Tor's popularity rose. For example, in Iran, the number of users went from 7,000 in 2010 to 40,000 two years later to avoid the state eavesdropping on their communications.[6]

Unfortunately, Tor has been used for a number of illicit services that are often for sale by organized crime. This includes services like hacking, pornography, drugs, and so on. Stolen credit cards, healthcare data, and a wide number of other services can be bought and sold as well. One of the other things that can be bought here are systems that have been hacked. The typical cycle of hackers is that they hack into organization, get what they want from the site over a period of months, and then sell that connection to someone else to use. This way, they make money twice on their access, and they gain the benefit having it appear as though other adversaries were responsible for the attack if that open connection is ever used.

Tor has other benefits for cybercriminals, too, because they can hack websites through Tor, which reroutes the traffic flow of the computers they are on. In this way many websites do not know where the connection is actually coming from. A cybercriminal could be sitting in a small United States city, but the traffic seems to come out of Germany (as an example), which helps to create additional anonymity about their illegal activities.

One of the unfortunate consequences of such an open market on the dark web is that like the real world, there is an abundance of sharing—some through purchase of tools or services, some through the various forums. This means that an amateur hacker could easily purchase powerful tools used by APT hackers on the dark web. This includes everything from malware to various services. Indeed, that is exactly what we see happening. MimiKatz, a popular credential stealer, is used by hacking organizations around the world. For example, it is used by North Korea, Russia, China, Iran, and Vietnam.[7] Even if one version of MimiKatz can be detected by antivirus tools, a few small tweaks can make it virtually invisible from old-school signatures.

Because of all the illicit activity on the dark web, many security companies have taken to monitoring it and getting to know some of the key

---

[6]National Public Radio, "Going Dark: The Internet Behind the Internet," 2014, https://www.npr.org/sections/alltechconsidered/2014/05/25/315821415/going-dark-the-internet-behind-the-internet.
[7]SBS CyberSecurity, "TOP 25 THREAT ACTORS - 2019 EDITION," https://sbscyber.com/resources/top-25-threat-actors-2019-edition.

threat actors in order to create services to help warn organizations of pending attacks. Governments, too, are investing their time on the dark web for some of the same reasons. While the initial intentions of Tor were lofty, it has obviously attracted the attention of hackers for other reasons.

Tools of the Trade

We have already started to explore how tools are shared through the dark web and how some of the attacks against organizations are hidden, but there are a whole range of tools in the arsenal of the various adversaries. They did not evolve overnight. They had to be constructed over a period of time as people thought of them. It is interesting to note that the basic concept did not begin with completely harmful intent. As with the Tor network, many of the activities took on a life of their own.

Before we begin, it is helpful to provide historical context. Viruses have partially become the generic name for malware—but viruses are only one type of malware. The other common types of malware include worms, Trojan horses, rootkits, spyware, adware, and ransomware. They each have their own peculiarities, but suffice it to say the antivirus is considered the blanket program to protect against all the types of malware—with a few exceptions over the years.

What is important for our story is that there has been a tremendous amount of evolution related to malware over the years. If we go back to January 1986, the first PC virus was written by Baset and Amjad Farooq Alvi (17 and 24 years old at the time) who became aware that their software was being illegally pirated. Pirating, in this case, refers to software that is copied, distributed, or used in an unauthorized manner. If someone installed the pirated software, the brothers developed a mechanism to detect if the software was pirated or not and if it was pirated, the software would copy the virus onto the computer and alert the owner that their computer was infected. Their goal was simply to protect their software from being pirated.[8] So viruses back in the '80s were obvious—often doing things to catch people's attention. Because

---

[8] Norton Lifelock Employee, "When Were Computer Viruses First Written, and What Were Their Original Purposes?" https://us.norton.com/internetsecurity-malware-when-were-computer-viruses-first-written-and-what-were-their-original-purposes.html#:~:text=In%20January%20of%201986%2C%20the,years%20old%20at%20the%20time.

malware was so obvious for the next few years, often all one needed to protect their computer was a firewall and antivirus. As we will explore throughout the rest of this chapter, that is no longer true today.

Since 1986, malware has changed significantly. The aims and goals of modern malware developers are nowhere near as benign as two brothers trying to prevent others from pirating software. Now the malware, with the exception of ransomware, is far stealthier than it ever was in the past. Some of the goals are getting back into systems, stealing intellectual property, stealing data, and espionage. Let us take a closer look at the types of malware, though, because they each can affect IoMT, and the covered entities, in different ways.

Types of Malware

Understanding the types of malware and how malware relates to covered entities and IoMT in particular helps to give a fuller perspective about the challenges of protecting environments because of the weaknesses within IoMT. While really bad for any environment, the weaknesses of IoMT amplify the problems that malware poses. As we go through and analyze each type of malware, we'll tie in how different kinds IoMT devices are affected by the malware landscape.

Despite being the oldest type of malware, viruses are still quite common and have certainly evolved to fit the times. Today's viruses are almost uniquely suited to handle the complex infrastructure of today's IoMT. First, they are able to adapt to environments very quickly. If one capability is not available on a system, they can try a list of many other ways of gaining access to a system or finding information about a system they are already on. This means that depending on the peculiarities of an environment, a virus may behave differently. When cybersecurity experts say that the hacker only needs to be right once and the cybersecurity expert needs to be right 100% of the time, this is a tiny part of what they mean.

Viruses are also polymorphic. This means that not only can they adapt on a specific system or a specific type of system, they can also be effective on different kinds of systems. For example, they can move from a cell phone to a personal computer. How many people charge their cell phones while connected to a personal computer? While very convenient, it is also an attack vector. If someone innocently gets their mobile device infected by a virus due to malvertising, they then could inadvertently infect their computer. So not only can applications be infected through the cell phone, they also then infect IoMT devices that are computers or are perhaps just a few jumps away from infecting a system on a corporate network.

Worms are self-replicating standalone programs that replicate over a network by jumping from machine to machine. One of the first worms to gain the attention of the media was the Morris worm. Its intent was to point out flaws in systems—especially related to weak passwords—but it had some coding flaws and ended up spreading much faster than anticipated and reinfecting machines, rendering them useless.[9]

Trojan horses, much like their physical namesake, are programs that are designed to look appealing, but have a payload that can be used to accomplish nefarious aims. Any of the applications for cell phones in the Google or Apple stores that contain malicious code are considered Trojan horses. Both stores have made considerable efforts to remove Trojans, but sometimes it is difficult to tell if a particular app has malware or not.

Rootkits, also referred to as command and control (C2, C&C, etc.), are software used to stealthily provide unauthorized access to a system. They allow an attacker to gain access again and again without needing to hack into the system. It is as though someone added a hidden door to your house that you have no idea about that would allow them to remain nearly invisible whenever they entered. Often, rootkits are embedded within other applications, which makes them very difficult to remove. For the IoMT Windows systems that do not permit protective software, rootkits are the mechanism of choice for many cybercriminals.

Keyloggers are concerning on many levels. They are what makes it possible to steal usernames and passwords. Typically, they sit on a machine and record what keys you type. If you type a website name, then an email address followed by a random word, phrase, or character set, the owners of the keyloggers have captured your username and password. If you are on a network, they can then use that username and password to log in to not only your machine, but also other machines if that username and password combination is reused. That is a tiny bit like identity theft, as that account can be used to log in to multiple machines in many environments. In a hospital setting, cybercriminals can then infect other machines—including IoMT. If an administrator ever logs in to an EHR, the owner of the keylogger will have just handed over the keys to all of a covered entity's data.

Spyware is part of a large family of malware that includes everything from adware to stalkerware, stealware, system monitors, and so on. What all of the various types of spyware accomplish is spying on devices and the users—and some are more nefarious than others. Adware, for example, is geared toward seeing what sites you visit in

---

[9] Wikipedia, https://en.wikipedia.org/wiki/Morris_worm, accessed December 4, 2020.

order to target advertisements. Stalkerware is a bit more insidious as it allows the attacker to see all the text messages and phone calls on someone else's phone. Stealware takes credit for websites you visit in order to earn advertising dollars. Some spyware includes keystroke loggers, but more aggressive versions, called system monitors, record everything happening on a device. Whatever the form, cybercriminals love spyware. It allows them to gain everything they want so they can accomplish their objectives.

We have already spoken about ransomware throughout this book. Some of it blocks access to a specific computer, while other ransomware encrypts systems so that the system does not function. Because companies are willing to pay the ransoms, attackers keep using ransomware as a tool to obtain their objectives.

Malware Evolution

The efficacy of the various forms of malware have improved over the years. One of the ways malware has jumped around traditional antivirus tools is by being metamorphic. This allows the virus to slightly rewrite itself to alter the signature with each computer. Another capability of malware is polymorphism, which allows it to change its behavior based on the environment. This means it can function on a phone or a computer. Webroot found that 97% of malware today is polymorphic.[10] Another common capability is for malware to be fileless—most of their nefarious actions occur in memory and not on the computer. In this way, the activity is largely hidden. While they usually have a small presence on the system, many traditional antivirus systems will not pick up on these kinds of behaviors.

Some malware can protect itself either on an existing system or by downloading parts of itself from various locations repeatedly. Deleting one part of the malware means that it compensates by reinstating the malware in other parts. Some utilize other kinds of evasion techniques so they are not detected—even against some of the advanced capabilities of machine learning in next-generation antivirus tools.

This is far from the end of things. We have been defining the capabilities of malware as if there is a clean division between the various definitions. Most of the time, malware may have two or more capabilities and

[10] Nate Lord, "What is Polymorphic Malware? A Definition and Best Practices for Defending Against Polymorphic Malware," 2020, https://digitalguardian.com/blog/what-polymorphic-malware-definition-and-best-practices-defending-against-polymorphic-malware.

accomplish multiple objectives at the same time. It truly has become an advanced game of cat and mouse between attacker and defender—and the attackers seem to be winning.

In 2014, Symantec (now part of Broadcom) famously declared that antivirus is dead because it only caught 45% of malware attacks.[11] Outside of the technical industry that might seem absurd. Traditional antivirus is signature-based. Think of a signature as a digital fingerprint, and each piece of malware has a different signature (fingerprint). Antivirus blocks that malware if the signature matches a known bad signature, but if that signature is not recognized, the malware actions are permitted. The hackers began to figure this out, so they started to create customized malware that would evade the detection of antivirus.

Too Many Strains

It would be a fallacy to think that these are isolated problems because not many people know how to create malware. Unfortunately, nothing could be further from the truth. Figure 8-1 shows you the statistics from

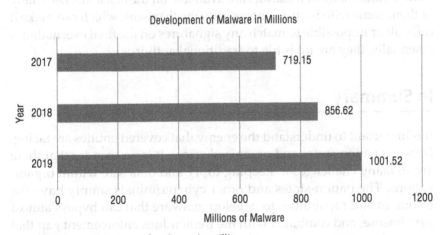

Figure 8-1: Development of malware in millions

Source: AVTest Malware www.av-test.org/en/statistics/malware

---

[11] Samuel Gibbs, "Antivirus software is dead, says security expert at Symantec," Information chief at Norton developer says software in general misses 55% of attacks and its future lies in responding to hacks, 2014, https://www.theguardian.com/technology/2014/may/06/antivirus-software-fails-catch-attacks-security-expert-symantec#:~:text=Antivirus%20software%20only%20catches%2045,a%20senior%20manager%20at%20Symantec.&text=Malware%20has%20become%20increasingly%20complex%20in%20a%20post-Stuxnet%20world.

the last three years as reported by the AV-Test Institute—over a billion pieces of malware were created in 2019 that we know of.

Stop and think about that from a practical perspective. How many people does it take to create millions of signatures every year? How do companies know about all of those strains in time to stop them? How big will the antivirus software become if they are adding these many signatures each year? How much will the system slow down as a result? At a certain point, it becomes not just impractical, but almost pointless. The 2014 Symantec proclamation that traditional antivirus is 45% effective is much lower today than it was yesterday from a number's perspective alone. If you consider the time lag it takes to write a signature and then stop the malware, there are clearly challenges. Obviously, a new strategy is required to keep up with the onslaught of malware.

Malware Construction Kits

We do not need to make the case that malware is a major problem. Today, malware construction kits make creating malware as easy as clicking a few buttons, and many of these kits are available on the black market. Many of them come with built-in obfuscation mechanisms, which can make it difficult or impossible to match any signatures on the final executable—essentially, they are invisible to traditional antivirus.

In Summary

It is important to understand the enemy that covered entities are facing. Between nation-states and organized crime, it is no wonder that there are so many challenges to keeping IoMT and data safe within organizations. The nation-states and other cybercriminals simply have the resources and capabilities to develop malware that can bypass almost any defense, and combined with the tremendous enforcement gap that exists when it comes to apprehending international attackers, it only adds to the overall challenges.

For those outside of the cybersecurity profession, much of this information is new and probably an eye-opener. It really starts to paint a picture as to why protecting IoMT and our data is so difficult. Cybersecurity professionals can do everything right and make no mistakes, and then someone inadvertently clicks a link and it is game over for the organization and everyone's personal data.

But these are not the only options for cybersecurity professionals. There is a whole host of things cybersecurity professionals can do to defend IoMT and data within organizations. What is cybersecurity, though? We have thrown the word out there, but we have not attempted to define what it means. This is what we will explore in our next chapter.

Part

II

Contextual Challenges and Solutions

We have taken the time to thoroughly explore the context that covered entities, data, and IoMT are in and how those risks ultimately affect us. Having that background paints a fairly realistic picture of the context, but not the specific day-to-day contexts of IT environments nor the associated solutions.

The reality is that while some IoMT devices are relatively secure, many are downright insecure with the manufacturer actively blocking covered entities from performing updates, installing protective software, and/ or configuring the devices to best protect the organizations. As a result, a holistic approach needs to be taken to protect these IoMT devices.

Of course, this is not the only consideration. The fact that many IoMT devices are kept for years—far past the warrantee or the manufacturer's ability to patch the devices. While smaller devices for people are often upgraded more quickly, larger, more expensive devices can be the pro-verbial bane of cybersecurity professionals due to the vast number of vulnerabilities and devices that are simply not fixable. This means a longer-term strategy must be utilized to protect IoMT devices, our data, and our hospitals.

As you read through this section, keep in mind that it is presented in logical nuggets. The same types of considerations, often the same tools, can be used in multiple contexts to explore different aspects of cybersecurity. This part of the book is a bit more technical, but efforts were made to keep things as easy to read and understand as possible.

Enter Cybersecurity

As we've come to realize, the idea that security starts and ends with the purchase of a prepackaged firewall is simply misguided.
—Art Whittmann

We have been talking at length about the challenges of IoMT devices and how they affect the security of our covered entities, our data, and sometimes our lives. Obviously, many traditional methods of protecting systems are not possible when considering IoMT and how covered entities have very thin budgets, and traditional cybersecurity protections are not a possibility given the circumstances. As a result, other methods must be used to protect our institutions because with each passing day the situation related to hospitals seems to get more dire—in part due to IoMT devices themselves, but also due to the evolution of technology and the various threat actors that profit off the vulnerabilities a system might have.

But that evolutionary perspective related to technology has an amplifying effect on the challenges of IoMT over the long haul. Problems that started small sometimes grow much larger over time. Those minor mistakes of yesteryear become major cybersecurity challenges today. It is critical to understand those challenges and how they create problems to help us see more clearly the possible paths ahead.

Those paths forward are the ones cybersecurity professionals follow for protecting organizations. Understanding what cybersecurity is, the various disciplines that comprise cybersecurity, and how security professionals think about protecting IoMT, data, and organizations, starts to paint a picture about how and why the mistakes of yesteryear can be corrected, thought about, and ultimately executed on.

That said, cybersecurity, like any profession, is a deep and vast field of expertise. Any of the topics we touch on could be the focus for a lifetime—just as there are different kinds of engineers or doctors. We cannot hope to adequately cover all the aspects of cybersecurity in one chapter (let alone one book), so we are going to skim the surface of some of the major aspects of information security to give readers an idea of some parts of the profession and how they apply to protecting IoMT and covered entities.

What Is Cybersecurity?

If you ask a hundred cybersecurity professionals what cybersecurity is, you will get a hundred different answers. Everyone has their own nuance and approaches when it comes to cybersecurity. Every one of those professionals will take a different approach in a different context. Also, cybersecurity has evolved considerably over the last 30 years—including the various names of the activities that cybersecurity professionals engage in. Keep in mind that many organizations take widely different strategies for protecting their business Cybersecurity is not a profession with a great deal of conformity—especially in the United States. The goal here is not to provide a definitive definition or approach to cybersecurity, but to create a general understanding of the various aspects of the profession with the understanding that it has evolved over a period of time. Sometimes that evolution is on divergent paths. While sometimes that divergence can be an indicator of problems, often a unique approach to cybersecurity needs to be taken to meet the organizational needs. Protecting IoMT devices, due to their particular characteristics, certainly requires a unique approach, which we will learn about over the next several chapters.

Cybersecurity Basics

There are many different definitions of cybersecurity, but there is some basic agreement about what it strives to accomplish. In the simplest of terms, cybersecurity protects confidentiality, integrity, and availability.

Together these are referred to as the CIA triad. Confidentiality pertains to ensuring that the appropriate people have the appropriate access to data. The changes in privacy regulation over the last few years are also extremely concerned with confidentiality, and many processes have been put into place to protect it. Integrity is about ensuring the data has not been altered in any way. From a HIPAA perspective, this is critical. For example, if someone is deathly allergic to a particular medicine and that piece of data is altered or removed from the person's medical record, it could be fatal. Finally, availability is about the data being available when needed. HIPAA is so concerned about the CIA triad that they require risk assessments to also include an assessment of CIA.

There is one definition of cybersecurity (using the old information security moniker) that provides a description that may be a bit easier for people to understand:

Information security is the practice of defending information from unauthorized access, use, disclosure, disruption, modification, perusal, inspection, recording, or destruction, regardless of what form that information may take."[1]

Compare that definition with the definition that the Cybersecurity and Infrastructure Security Agency (CISA) utilizes:

Cybersecurity is the art of protecting networks, devices, and data from unauthorized access or criminal use and the practice of ensuring confidentiality, integrity, and availability of information. It seems that everything relies on computers and the internet now—communication (e.g., email, smartphones, tablets), entertainment (e.g., interactive video games, social media, apps), transportation (e.g., navigation systems), shopping (e.g., online shopping, credit cards), medicine (e.g., medical equipment, medical records), and the list goes on. How much of your daily life relies on technology? How much of your personal information is stored either on your own computer, smartphone, tablet or on someone else's system?"[2]

What is starkly different about the two is that information security is about protecting data in all of its forms, including printed information. Any document with sensitive information should be either shredded or put in a bin for shredding. Cybersecurity focuses more on the risks of electronic information; hence, the term cybersecurity is now in vogue.

---

[1]I cannot find the original quote for this, but years ago it used to be everywhere.
[2]Cybersecurity & Infrastructure Security Agency Security, "Tip (ST04-001) What is Cybersecurity?" 2009, https://us-cert.cisa.gov/ncas/tips/ST04-001.

As far as these definitions go, they still do not fully describe what cybersecurity is. The reality is that cybersecurity is an ever-expanding interdisciplinary set of practices designed to protect data, especially electronic. Saying what cybersecurity does is far from enough. Understanding the how is just as critical, as that will help to shape the entire section of this book. Part of the overarching goal of this book is to discuss how to protect IoMT devices—especially given the fact they have some unique characteristics that make them more difficult to protect.

But this is also tied into the evolutionary nature of covered entities—especially over the last five years—as IoMT has grown substantially in numbers, so too have the risks, partially in relation to the challenges of the past. Understanding the key disciplines of cybersecurity will help us elucidate the means by which we can protect both IoMT and our healthcare from our adversaries.

Cybersecurity Evolution

Cybersecurity, as it started to differentiate from IT, was originally called IT security. People who would do IT security were generally involved in the parts of IT related to protecting the organization—the firewalls, antivirus, incident response, security training, and so on. Of course, every company was different, but the purpose of the process was "just get it done," which sometimes means cutting corners. Things work, but they may not be secure. This is seen all the time in organizations—especially if an executive is complaining something isn't working. Taking the time to figure things out the right way is not really an option due to time constraints. When resources are thin and there is a time crunch, it is a perfect recipe for creating problems that, quite often, do not get resolved. Even today, IT is fantastic at getting things to work, but not always so great at preventing security issues—even big companies struggle with some of the basics of IT security.

Obviously, IT security by itself is not enough. Compliance was the new answer. It slowed down IT and put some guardrails on the processes to ensure things would be done with more due diligence—not perfect, but it was a step in the right direction. Among some of the requirements was change management, which essentially involved creating a ticket that states exactly what the change is that is being made, getting approval in the ticket, and allowing the change to take place per the rules of the organization. While this description is woefully inadequate for many organizations, it does show that a measure of due diligence is required. Changes are not made on the fly without managers knowing they are taking place.

But this is not the only change that compliance models brought to the table. Many of them required periodic validation of certain IT systems. An excellent example of this is the review of firewall rules. It is more complicated than this, but essentially firewall rules define what communication is permitted within an organization. What often happens in those crunch situations mentioned previously is that too much communication is permitted. Reviewing the communication pathways allows organizations to periodically see where mistakes are made and what needs to be done to resolve them. There are several other examples of periodic validation within organizations, but you begin to see the value of that validation after catching mistakes.

Having the person who is responsible for changes to the firewall communication reviewing their own work is problematic, as everyone has blind spots about their own work—including myself. Also, some people may be incentivized not to report their own problems and may just sweep them under the metaphorical rug, with or without the intent to deal with the changes later. Even today, these kinds of problems pop up regularly within organizations. The solution is to have separation between the person doing the work and the person doing the review. This separation is also important for other reasons such as insider risk. One person can act by themselves and sweep things under the rug, but it is less likely that two people will act together for the same goal. In addition, knowing that someone is reviewing your work means that you will probably strive to do a better job and not just "get it done."

But these seemingly small changes required a different set of skills—reviewing skills. The review process creates the need to differentiate IT from security. IT security is getting work done across an organization to protect that organization. These new sets of skills needed new roles and new designations. Eventually organizations settled on the phrase "information security." These information security professionals cared a great deal about compliance—indeed so do many businesses—because it was the way to protect organizations.

Probably unsurprisingly at this point, companies continued to be hacked, costing them a tremendous amount of money despite environments being certified for compliance. Eventually the phrase "Compliance does not equal security" was echoed by security professionals everywhere—almost as a mantra that things needed to change. Indeed, that is true because obviously crime still pays, which is why so many criminal organizations continue to hack every organization—not just covered entities. The old compliance models were important foundations for cybersecurity, but as they became stale with age, they certainly did not keep up with the new technologies that were beginning to blossom throughout the industries.

It is interesting to note that the term *information security* is still often used. For example, the head of a cybersecurity department is usually called a chief information security officer (CISO). While there are certainly variations, that is the title that many cybersecurity professionals seek and where we are today.

Key Disciplines in Cybersecurity

In theory, there should be only three reasons that cybersecurity professionals engage in any activity—compliance, risk, or business. The importance of each of these is dependent on the business context. Cybersecurity is, and should be, a business enabler. Protecting devices helps to protect businesses not only from things like data breaches or ransomware, but also from lawsuits, losing the ability to take credit cards, and a host of other considerations. Part of the way cybersecurity protects organizations is by being compliant—either from a legal standpoint (such as HIPAA) or from any of the security compliance models that the business may choose to follow for other reasons. As mentioned earlier this chapter, compliance is not enough to protect organizations, so most intelligent businesses also look at cybersecurity from a risk standpoint. Assessing risk is really more of an art than a science, but the more holistic your perspective, the better the assessments will be. If the assessor is very knowledgeable about all the disciplines of cybersecurity, they will have a deeper, more meaningful assessment. Business requirements are a bit more open ended, but can be a whole range of possibilities depending on the agreed upon relationship. Sometimes they bleed over into other disciplines in cybersecurity depending on the context. Sometimes, there are really strong cybersecurity requirements built into the contract.

Compliance

Let us start out by exploring compliance a bit more. Why is compliance important at all? Shouldn't all businesses just do the right thing and protect data? Indeed, that is true in many organizations that have competent security people who take a risk-based approach to cybersecurity. Unfortunately, not all companies take this approach. As a result, federal, state, and local laws are passed to better protect information—each in their own way. They help to provide requirements for protecting information. They become a legal standard to judge organizations in the case of a breach. Smart compliance frameworks, such as HIPAA, include risk assessments as part of the overarching process. We'll talk about risk soon, but risk gives businesses a way of saying that more needs to be done above and beyond the requirements of compliance. For companies that are not compliant, but striving to become compliant, these laws can also act as guidance to determine which projects to start on first.

That said, many cybersecurity experts dislike compliance because not only are all requirements not equal, but newer technologies are sometimes a better investment than older methodologies that compliance or laws may provide. This can create some tension as cybersecurity experts and businesses as a whole must sometimes make decisions that may be legally expedient without investing in the new technologies. These are some of the challenges that covered entities must face that ultimately impact the security of both IoMT and covered entities—some of this may relate to the size of the organization and the amount of data.

Typically, when it comes to compliance, the larger the covered entity, the more complex the compliance requirements are. HIPAA applies to all covered entities, but the reality is that a small office may not or cannot fully meet HIPAA requirements. What most small offices do is meet the privacy requirements and employ a few things like a firewall and antivirus. Large hospitals usually have a compliance team and a cybersecurity team to help protect the environment. Indeed, that is what is required to protect both IoMT and hospitals.

Many hospitals also accept credit card payments. In these cases, they need to meet the Payment Card Industry Data Security Standard (PCI DSS)—often referred to as PCI for short. While there are some parallels between HIPAA and PCI, PCI's main goal is to protect credit card transactions. For small organizations they will utilize devices that encrypt the transaction automatically and provide a receipt so the risk is reduced. Larger organizations will do the same, but they often want to keep the credit card number on file so customers do not need to input their credit card every single time. In these cases, more rigorous PCI requirements come into play. The larger the number of credit card transactions taking place and the larger the amount of data, the more stringent the requirements. These requirements can also be a big boon for both hospital and IoMT requirements. For example, PCI has very strict firewall requirements (stronger than HIPAA) that can help protect both. In this way, adding additional compliance requirements onto an organization can help protect covered entities.

We have already spoken a bit about HITRUST as a compliance model in that meeting the requirements is considered equivalent of meeting HIPAA in the eyes of the law. It is also helpful for meeting other frameworks as they can be built into the HITRUST model. This makes the compliance process simultaneously a bit easier and a bit more difficult. HITRUST is very strict on its scoring mechanism, which means that requirements baked into HITRUST from other compliance models can add to the number of requirements that must also follow the HITRUST scoring model. HITRUST is a risk-based model like PCI, and the more data and records received, the more requirements are in place. While not all requirements within compliance are made equal for protecting IoMT and hospitals, there are advantages to following compliance models in general.

From here, there are number of other compliance models that may be applicable depending on the requirements of the organization. In many cases, the compliance models may not be immediately intuitable—even for those that are experienced in cybersecurity. Without going into too many details, each type of compliance does indicate a reduction in risk, which provides a level of assurance for organizations. Sometimes HIPAA or HITRUST are not the measure that organizations use when looking for assurance that their data will be reasonably safe. Some of the disciplines identified in the following sections are also in many different compliance frameworks—including HIPAA.

Patching

Patching refers to updating systems and is a critical method for protecting them—including IoMT systems (where applicable). It is essentially applying updates to systems much as updates are applied to a home PC. Some patches provide features and functionality while others remediate weaknesses in the system. Patches can be applied to just about every system. Not only can home systems be patched, but also servers, network devices, applications, databases, and some IoMT devices.

Technically, patching is part of IT and not cybersecurity, but the security teams care about patching because it helps to reduce risk within organizations. Patching is very much a part of compliance for precisely these reasons, and it is probably one of the biggest indicators of problems within organizations.

Patching may seem like an easy task on a home computer, but when you consider the numbers and types of systems that exist and the fact that quite often some patches can be centralized and others not, it creates challenges due to timing and resources—especially if the business has a high expectation for the systems to be working all the time. In fact, many hospitals strive for close to 100% uptime for most systems as they are mission critical. Working around that can become challenging. Alternatives are to have alternate infrastructure on standby, which is not always possible.

Antivirus

For decades we have realized the importance of antivirus. It became an old standby that not only prevented viruses, but also removed viruses that it found on the system. It was so obvious of a way to protect systems that every cybersecurity framework required that antivirus be installed. It became a staple of every IT program. The effectiveness of antivirus programs began to fade because the viruses and malware grew so plentiful (it is relatively easy to modify a signature) that the old signature-based approaches were no longer as effective. As a result, a new breed of next-generation technologies began to appear. They made some marginal inroads toward blocking malware and viruses, but the cybercriminals creating malware and viruses were too sophisticated and were working around these next-generation antivirus technologies.

To meet that need of protecting organizations, there was a fundamental shift away from the protective antivirus technologies of yesteryear to a new breed of tools that were much more adept at detecting malware because they used machine learning to detect problems on existing systems. What is lost with these new technologies is the ability to block the problems as effectively as before. This created a great deal more work for organizations because they then needed to manually go in and remediate the problems. While some organizations could respond in a timely fashion to these kinds of intrusions, many organizations could not keep up—thus services were born to help manually remove any detected problems 24x7x365. This is a huge boon to organizations that are based only in the United States because the around-the-clock support means that people can sleep while trained professionals remediate problems automatically.

Network Architecture

Just as there are multiple architectural styles and requirements for buildings, the same holds true for networks. Compliance, with exceptions, tends to focus on having something called a De-Militarized Zone (DMZ). From a network perspective it means that there is at least (depending on the framework) a logical separation between the web servers and all other servers such as database servers (where data is stored). While these are great requirements, they only marginally help organizations address the challenges that IoMT brings to the table. They can help to slow attacks from IoMT to internal websites, but that is the extent of the value from an IoMT perspective. If the IoMT device is compromised, the data on the website will be compromised through the device.

Application Architecture

The architecture of applications goes hand in hand with network architecture—especially with web servers. The purpose of the DMZ is to act like a barrier between the communication zone and internal zones. Data should only pass through this zone on its way to another zone in order to protect it from hackers as the sites are exposed to the open internet. It is the most likely place to be compromised from outside attacks.

Threat and Vulnerability

So far in our journey we have spoken a great deal about the vulnerabilities that IoMT devices have. That is a very important consideration when looking at how organizations are attacked. As mentioned in Chapter 5, the cumulative vulnerabilities of IoMT create greater and greater risks for organizations. Vulnerability management, for IoMT devices that allow agents to be installed and can be upgraded, these standard vulnerability management practices are fantastic. A vulnerability management scanner scans the system and then reports back a list of vulnerabilities with recommended remediation. It is an integral part of the remediation strategy of many cybersecurity programs—in fact, a critical one.

Almost expectedly at this point, for IoMT devices, the standard technologies for vulnerability management are not always applicable. For example, many of today's vulnerability management tools require an agent to be installed on the system. There are agentless vulnerability scanners, but they produce false positives—a vulnerability will appear to be there, but in reality, it is not. This was the problem with vulnerability scanners from 20 years ago that were not agent based. Agents, while not perfect, significantly reduce the false positives. Those false positives can create busywork, which can build some resentment because "real work" needs to be done. False positives can create work for both IT and security teams, which does not have material value except to rule out the false positives.

There are alternative strategies to search for vulnerabilities, such as monitoring the network packets of some of the existing systems. Each vendor uses a slightly different approach to handle some of these problems. Some are specifically geared toward monitoring IoMT devices on the network and will report on systems that have old operating systems (which usually means vulnerabilities, just as a home system often usually does) and possibly recommend solutions. Still other packet solutions are geared toward monitoring for anomalous behavior and blocking if there are issues. Each covered entity, specifically hospitals, will need to determine the best strategy for monitoring IoMT given the specific mix of IoMT challenges for their organization.

Another challenge that organizations relates to the fact that many IoMT devices cannot be upgraded, which means that being aware of the problem does not mean the vulnerabilities can be remediated with a standard patching process. It is more of an indicator of risks that organizations face, so alternate approaches can be taken to defend the IoMT and hospitals.

Traditional vulnerability management, while valuable, may yield different results depending on the mix of IoMT within a hospital. As a result, sometimes different strategies may need to be employed. Clearly, a one-size-fits-all approach to IoMT is insufficient to meet the requirements of today's systems, especially when considering vulnerability management.

Identity and Access Management

For most compliance frameworks and also in the minds of most cybersecurity professionals, Identity and Access Management (I&AM) is a critical aspect of securing an organization. Part of the purpose of I&AM is to tie a person's identity to authorized resources. When someone uses a username and a password, there is reasonable assurance that the access related to that username and password came from that account. In this way, so long as the account is set up properly, confidentiality is reasonably assured. It is a way of attributing electronic behavior to a specific person. The stronger the authentication mechanism, the more trust in the identity, the more confidentiality is affirmed. In many cases this also means integrity is affirmed as well.

Many readers may use multi-factor authentication (MFA) when logging on to specific accounts. What that second factor is depends on the organization, but it can be anything from a token connected to the computer, scanning a QR code, or an extra set of numbers that randomly change when typing in a password. No matter what is used, they add another level of assurance that the authentication is safer with multi-factor authentication than without.

But this is not the only part of identity and access management—it also boils down to enabling, disabling, and deleting accounts at the right time with the right level of access. For those outside the IT world or for people only experienced with smaller environments, this may seem like a very easy task that should not take a great deal of time—just disable the account. The reality is that for larger organizations, there may be multiple environments or one-off systems that are connected to a centralized identity authority. Sometimes there is that connectivity, but the individual systems require altering access at the system level, which relates to specific system configurations and not something that is individually configurable. As a result of these kinds of issues (and many others), getting the right identities at the right level at the right time can begin to create a number of challenges within organizations.

If you then consider emergency situations or a host of other challenges, it is easy for organizational identities to get disorganized over a period of years. IoMT can also create additional challenges as some of the systems will not connect to traditional identity directories. Add in consultants and contractors with temporary access, and the challenges can multiply rather quickly. There are a couple of different answers to these kinds of challenges, such as tools to govern the addition and removal of accounts across a range of systems, but also to review accounts on a periodic basis—some of which can be accomplished by accompanying products and or processes. This governance process is typically validated by the information security teams.

Monitoring

Monitoring is a way of detecting what is going on in an environment. There are a whole host of different tools that can be used for monitoring, which will be discussed in future chapters, but from a compliance point of view, the monitoring typically means two different types of monitoring— monitoring of logs from various devices and monitoring of devices such as Network Intrusion Detection System (NIDS).

Logs are records of what happens on a system. Typically, the key systems that are supposed to be monitored are firewalls and servers. Depending on the framework, this can (and should) include any system that holds sensitive data. This means that databases and applications that process data need to be included in this overall process. They are used by various systems and services for two primary purposes—to detect problems that are happening on a system in near real time and for forensic purposes to determine what has already happened on a given system.

In larger enterprises such as hospitals, logs are centralized and monitored either by an internal system referred to as a Security Information Event Management (SIEM) system or by utilizing one of the various services that extend the capabilities of an existing SIEM or replacing the SIEM with one of the various options that are on the market. We will touch on the various details related to log monitoring and options in Chapter 16. What is important here is to keep in mind centralized logging and the ability to detect hacking or potential breaches through the use of log monitoring. It is a discipline unto itself and cybersecurity professionals strive to seek the right balance of monitoring given the array of options.

Incident Response

Related to monitoring is the discipline of incident response. The first phase of many events is to look at the log (or often sets of logs that the SIEM turns into an alert) to determine the veracity of the alert—to determine if the event is a false positive or a true positive. A false positive is an event where an alert was sent, but it was not indicative of the event that took place. A true positive is a case where the event actually took place and has been validated. In some cases the information is very clear, but in others, the information is not very clear, and the case must be investigated. In other cases, an event was a true positive, but it was expected (and often authorized)

Depending on the type of event, the severity might be high enough to make it a business concern. In these cases, there should be a plan to determine what situations are serious enough to alert the business about. This plan, unsurprisingly, is typically referred to as an *incident response plan*. Most compliance frameworks require that the incident response plan is tested on a yearly basis. This ensures that everyone remembers the process for testing and what the formal approach would be to resolve incidents.

Hopefully, for most incidents in an organization, the formal incident response plans do not need to be followed. Instead, what are followed are highly technical plans to handle very specific types of incidents. These are referred to as *playbooks*. Mature organizations will automate these responses with tools as much as possible, while less mature organizations may informally define responses to specific incidents.

Digital Forensics

Often tied into the incident response process is digital forensics. Digital forensics, like its medical counterpart, is the process of collecting data to determine what happened related to an incident and/or prepare it for going to court if required. Most mature organizations develop incident handling techniques, designate evidence custodians, and have other practices to store data for organizations. Digital forensic tools go hand in hand with e-discovery tools, which can be used to store and/or collect evidence within organizations.

The output of these investigations can help organizations determine what happened, if a particular event was contained, and so on. It can also help determine if an incident response plan needs to be triggered or if the report should go to a law enforcement agency.

Configuration Management

Configuration management is the cornerstone of any good IT program, but from a cybersecurity perspective, there are a few key things that are critical. Like IT, cybersecurity is concerned about how those changes are made—that they are made through a change management process that is consistent, that they are verifiable, that they take into account emergency contexts, and that they have the right levels of approvals from both IT and cybersecurity. Every cybersecurity framework has at least a few change management requirements.

While the how is critical, so is the what. Starting from a security baseline is essential while building a configuration management program. A security baseline is essentially a set of security configurations to ensure that the system is as protected as it can be given the context. Most people who work in corporate settings are familiar with password rules: at least one uppercase letter, one lowercase letter, one special character, and one number. These types of configurations (and many more) are all configurable in many systems. For commercial entities such as hospitals, the Center for Internet Security (CIS) has configuration baselines that have these configuration settings built in. Essentially, they are guides on how to build systems securely. As an individual or a company, you don't have to re-create the wheel by trying to figure out what is and is not secure across an array of platforms. The CIS baselines provide that starting point from which a configuration management program can be built. It should not be the end state, as both systems and standards change over time.

These guides can also be applied against a large array of systems—including cloud systems. Servers, workstations, databases, internet servers (IIS and Apache for the more technically inclined readers), AWS, Google, cell phones, and so on guide IT and security staff on how to set up these kinds of systems. Remember in the second chapter where we talked about AWS vulnerabilities? Using baselines is an excellent way to mitigate some of those risks.

These kinds of baselines should be a starting point of a cybersecurity configuration management program. For example, knowing what to install is also important. If a system will not be used as a web server, web servers should not be installed. This is in line with a minimal build for a specific system. Minimal builds help to ensure that only the minimal requirements are installed for the systems. Readers who are experienced with Linux may be laughing at such a notion because of cascading installation requirements. Sometimes, in order to get systems to function properly, vulnerable or weak systems must be installed. That is a true statement, but then for those weak systems, what can be done to mitigate those risks? Can the weak components be disabled? Can you block the ports (either locally or on the network) to prevent their general use? In short, it is not a perfect world, but doing what can be done to see that the IT needs are met while securing the system as much as possible given the context is a worthwhile goal.

There are many other programs that can feed into configuration management. Threat and vulnerability are good examples. Oftentimes vulnerability tools include basic CIS configurations. More importantly, the vulnerabilities themselves can sometimes be remediated by simple configuration changes. Adding those changes to the baseline to help prevent future problems is not only logical, but makes good business sense. Penetration testing, quality assurance testing, and a host of other programs can and should help feed into a mature configuration management program.

From an IoMT perspective, sometimes there are no specific configuration requirements. In these cases, it may be a good idea to build the standards internally in a way that makes the most sense for the organization. Admittedly, sometimes manufacturers will not permit any alteration of systems, which makes managing the configurations impossible (or face not having any support for the system). If you do have systems that can support strong configuration management, this is a good place to start.

These kinds of challenges come up all of the time in organizations with all kinds of systems. What is important is knowing how to respond to these kinds of issues within organizations. Do you meet to discuss these issues in an operational board, or do you note the issue and plow ahead—consequences be damned? The heart of cybersecurity is due diligence, which entails having a strong understanding of the facts in order to create a better, more secure environment. Configuration management is only a small part of those challenges that organizations should be facing.

Training

Working with and educating people relates to the human element in cybersecurity—and the fact that everyone has some part to play related to cybersecurity within the organization. It is not just something that a few people in the back office are responsible for. Training is one of the ways that cybersecurity helps with the human defense aspect of the equation. A good deal of that training relates to educating others about the dangers of social engineering and how to handle those kinds of risks. Take email, for example. Emails may have a technical component to them, but fooling others to click on those emails requires a bit of finesse. While the Nigerian prince scam was sufficient 30 years ago, it is often only the butt of jokes today. Today's phishing exercises are much more subtle. They utilize spell checking, use pharming techniques (websites designed to look like a real website, but that actually steal usernames, passwords, credits cards, etc.), send emails that look identical to real emails from the sites, and so on. In some cases, they even impersonate a senior executive by email.

Clearly these are not the only kinds of social engineering techniques. Others include phone calls or in-person communication or disguises. One of the groups of people that often have full access to an environment are the various mail carriers. In fact, one of the most commonly sold imitation uniforms at Black Hat (a famous hacking conference) is the UPS uniform. Think back to what we said in the second chapter—if you have physical access to a box, you own it. Getting access to an environment by using a uniform is very common. In fact, fake uniforms are very popular at hacking conferences.

Risk Management

Of all the disciplines in cybersecurity, risk management is probably one of the most important. Compliance is continually playing catchup with where the information security world is at. The tools and capabilities can be years behind where the technology world is. The way to get beyond that compliance-only mindset is through influencing others to understand the risks within an organization. The reality is that new and innovative technologies are coming out very quickly. There is a huge market demand for this because APT actors such as nation-states and organized crime are winning the cybersecurity battles. The new spate of ransomware attacks demonstrates all too clearly the problems with current tools, techniques, and practices.

Robust risk management can also help to provide clarity to organizations. A CISO can mention a hundred problems, but most organizations cannot focus on a hundred problems. They can focus on a few at a time. If you distill down the major problems within the organization to five, senior management is more likely to agree to start working on those five major initiatives.

In Summary

While this chapter was far from complete and excludes several positions within cybersecurity, it does start to offer the flavor of some aspects of information security and what it entails—especially considering IoMT. Astute or experienced observers will have noted that there is an undercurrent of due diligence that is pervasive throughout all of these disciplines. If there is one thing that separates IT from cybersecurity, it is due diligence—slow down and think about the decisions that are being made.

It is important to note here that no one has all the answers and everyone's opinion is important. Thinking about those processes can be a huge advantage. One of the typical flaws of IT is that it does fully take into account the security needs. Conversely, security often is short-sighted about IT considerations. Both teams need to work together, along with the business, to ensure that an optimal strategy is utilized to produce the best business outcomes. As long as all sides are working together toward a common goal, progress will be made. Challenges that IoMT have often can be met with conventional wisdom, but sometimes alternate strategies are the best way to handle a tough situation.

CHAPTER

CHAPTER

10

Network Infrastructure and IoMT

Information technology and business are becoming inextricably interwoven. I don't think anybody can talk meaningfully about one without the talking about the other.

—**Bill Gates**

We have taken a great deal of time to discuss how IoMT devices are vulnerable, how they do not meet HIPAA or other privacy regulations, how those systems can be used to compromise other systems, the challenges related to anonymized data, and more. While these are fairly recent issues, the problems center more around the sheer volume of IoMT devices, which has blown the problems further out of proportion from where things were five years ago. We had strategies for handling these problems more than a decade ago, but more often than not, these strategies are not implemented. In Chapter 5, we clearly saw the results of what were small missteps yesterday and how they became greater problems today. As a result, in these next six chapters we'll be looking at the mistakes that many covered entities are guilty of that have helped to exacerbate the existing problems.

The first topic on this leg of our journey is network infrastructure. Network infrastructure is particularly important as many IoMT devices are not capable of using traditional defenses to protect themselves. As a result, network defenses are even more critical for protecting these kinds of devices.

Just because we are starting to focus on the IT infrastructure does not mean the business isn't important. On the contrary, the business is absolutely critical. It is just that, as Bill Gates points out, IT and business are "inexorably interwoven," and this part of the story is important to understanding IoMT risks. With Medicine 2.0, that is becoming more and more true with each passing day. If you don't understand the business, you have no way of knowing if the existing infrastructure is adequate, where it needs to be improved, and how it needs to change.

Of course, as we are talking about IoMT devices that are not always that secure, we'll be advocating that the business needs to modify its IT and/or security strategy as a result of the vulnerabilities in IoMT. To that end, over the next several chapters, we'll explore the mistakes of yesteryear in order to clearly elucidate why they are challenges in order to present solutions. In this way, the solutions may start to make more sense with a broader context.

In the Beginning

Some of the problems covered entities are having with IoMT are partially related to the relatively slow evolution of things. In Chapter 1, we spoke about how long it takes companies to change. Organizations tend to change slowly over time, and because of the ACA, IoMT has drastically changed within a relatively short period of time. It takes both manufacturers and covered entities time to fully understand the impacts of those changes and then even more time to change the general culture—in this specific case to a more cybersecurity-minded culture. But let us explore what that means with how technology evolved and how that has influenced the IT/cybersecurity culture today.

If we step back in time 50 years, the world was a much simpler place from an IT perspective. The technologies were comparatively simple and the data tended to be inconsequential compared to today. Our goals were to get things to work, not to think about the intricacies of nation-state actors attacking us. If you had a firewall and antivirus, you were adequately protecting your systems from attacks. In the early 1980s, the first books of the *Rainbow* series were released—they were essentially early cybersecurity guides the Department of Defense used to protect systems. But for many companies, the need for such sophisticated guidance was not heard of, nor was it as needed as it is today. Many organizations did not even see the value of antivirus when antivirus programs were first released. They had to learn about its importance when their systems started going down. Those were in the early days when mayhem was often the goal of the attackers and not the subtle machinations of modern organized crime or nation-state actors.

Still, this beginning is important to realize because the after-effects of this kind of thinking is still with us today—partially as a result of the lack of cybersecurity education in schools, as mentioned in Chapter 1. The cybersecurity of many organizations today is no different than the security from yesteryear. Today, as the result of almost constant news about organizations, people have become numb to the news—some companies are not overly aware of the need for cybersecurity other than basics such as a firewall and antivirus. The same is true for some covered entities.

Networking Basics: The OSI Model

Before diving too much deeper into networks and what the challenges are, it is important to better define some of the basics of what a network is. Most of us are familiar with home networking capabilities. A service provider gives us a link to the internet, through either a physical connection, a category 5 (CAT 5) cable, or a wireless connection. It may seem fairly simple for the home user, but a lot is going on underneath that connection. The International Standards Organization created the Open Systems Interconnection (OSI) model to explain how network communications take place. Because this is not intended to be a deep-dive book on networking, we'll provide a simplistic version for ease of digestion. Traffic traverses a network via a packet, which is a little like a container of information. Each container can only hold so much information, so it must be broken up into packets:

- **Layer 1: Physical**—The physical layer is all about the physical connection—the physical stuff as it connects the system to the internet. All home networking has a physical layer. All cloud resources, all websites, all cell phones, Wi-Fi connections, and so on have to traverse a physical layer at some point—even if the initial communication is not over a physical device.

- **Layer 2: Datalink**—The datalink layer is all about mass connectivity. Wireless communication occurs over this layer. There is also something called a switch. It allows devices to communicate with one another if they are part of the same physical or logical network without going to another layer. This is referred to a Local Area Network (LAN). If logical segmentation is used to create different virtual networks, this is called a Virtual LAN or VLAN. Some firewalls can be configured to be at this level, but typically are not used in this capacity.

- **Layer 3: Network**—The network layer provides the groundwork for systems to communicate with one another from one LAN to another. If you have heard of Internet Protocol (IP) addresses, the IP address is kind of like a phone number. It allows connectivity that traverses more than a VLAN. Most communication here is via something called a router, which routes traffic from one IP address to another. Firewalls and many other network devices are typically found at this level.

- **Layer 4: Transport**—Network traffic must utilize a transport mechanism. The two primary mechanisms are via Transmission Control Protocol (TCP) or User Datagram Protocol (UDP). TCP is generally referred to as connection-oriented. If a packet is lost, the system will resend it. This way, everything that is sent is received (with some exceptions). UDP is a set and forget protocol. It sends the packet out, but once it is sent, it does not validate the packet has been received. The original intended purpose of UDP was for voice communications. You can't resend part of a voice transmission at a later point in time because it will garble the message.

- **Layer 5: Session**—Generally speaking, a session is what is set up between two computers. Authentication of usernames, passwords, and so on take place at this layer, and multi-factor authentication is used on occasion.

- **Layer 6: Presentation**—The presentation layer presents information to the application layer. This is where decryption often takes place.

- **Layer 7: Application**—The application layer represents the applications that are doing the communication. It allows the applications to speak to one another. For example, if you use a browser, the communication will take place via the application layer.

Communication begins at layer 7 and then works its way down to layer 1; then when it reaches another computer, the communication goes up the stack from layer 1 to layer 7. Figure 10-1 shows how communication goes from one computer (or to a server) to another.

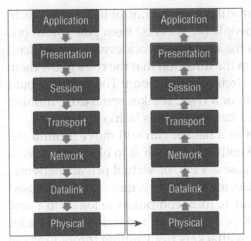

Figure 10-1: Network communication via the OSI model

Mistake: The Flat Network

We have already touched on the flat network from a general perspective, but it is so important when protecting insecure IoMT devices that it is worth doing a deeper dive. Imagine for a moment someone running a marathon on a flat road in sunny, beautiful 70° weather. A trained athlete can get to the destination having perfected only their running skills. Now imagine a marathon whose route includes snowcapped mountains, deep tropical valleys, rivers, the ocean, and often no path. The skills and equipment for the latter case are much more diverse than the former. Which do you think is more difficult to reach the destination? This is why a network that is not flat is so critical.

But what does that mean? What is the logical equivalent of a mountain or a river on a network? Let us start at a very basic level. A flat network, assuming basic configuration, is a Local Area Network (LAN). If the LAN has not been virtualized to produce many LANs without one large open area (a single VLAN across the enterprise), that is a flat network. If there are virtual LANs, this means that instead of one big domain, lots of domains are created. That VLAN can slow down an attacker because they will have to jump from one LAN to another. If they do not know the network, that may take them some additional time to work out the virtual landscape.

That is only the first step, and VLANs are not the mountains in this metaphor. A VLAN would be the hills that the runner would have to go up and down in order to reach their destination. Sometimes a firewall will be used. A firewall can put rules (access control lists for the technophiles) in place to prevent people (or hackers) from going from one VLAN to another. This makes the attackers' work even more difficult because now they can only go in the direction that the rules allow them to go, which slows them down a tremendous amount The firewall would be the equivalent of a mountain or a river. It takes some extra training and equipment to get through a network in this fashion.

Still, this is far from perfect as a hacker can still move around the network, albeit more slowly. Another approach is to block off areas of sensitive data entirely. In this case a VPN, or virtual private network, would be used to gain access. During COVID-19, more people are used to using VPNs because it is a way to force computers to log on to a new network. VPNs, if configured properly, patched, and include multi-factor authentication, can prevent most attackers from getting through. Many companies use VPNs to allow access to sensitive systems—often to servers that contain sensitive data. Extending the metaphor one more step, the VPN would be the equivalent of the ocean the attacker would have to cross. They will need other techniques and tools to get past a VPN.

There are numerous contexts that the flat network can apply to. If a flat network is used between an ordinary workstation and IoMT devices, the workstation becomes a single hop over to the IoMT device and the device can easily be owned. If the IoMT devices are all on the same VLAN, it then becomes easy for an attacker to hop from one IoMT device to another. In the context of the flat network being a web server to the rest of the environment, that too is a big problem because a web server is exposed to the open internet, and depending on several factors, it can be compromised. Then the data can be compromised directly from a database server (lots of data can remain here).

A great deal more can be said here as the technology has come a long way from its humble beginnings, but the point is that a flat network is easy to implement, but also easy to compromise. A single system can become the downfall of a whole environment if the systems are not properly protected. The weaknesses in IoMT only amplify the risks in a flat network by several factors. The more "mountainous" the network, the more the IoMT devices and hospitals will be better protected. It is truly a symbiotic relationship.

As the amount of IoMT devices continue to increase, the more important it will be to have a network that is not flat. One IoMT device in an environment (especially if not connected to an EHR) poses a risk, but the more the number of devices increases in an environment, the greater the risk. The hospitals that have the flat networks will take the least amount of time to compromise as a general rule. Because of this, despite no hard external requirements to have a network with VLANs, the flat network deserves special mention for healthcare mistakes.

Resolving the Flat Network Mistake

It is easy to say but hard to implement that mountainous network. Creating the right number of mountains, rivers, and oceans to fit the challenges that IoMT networks bring to the table is a bit of a balancing act. If separating the IoMT environments increases security, wouldn't creating a separate VLAN for each medical device be the best way to approach a problem? Technically, yes. The more the better, but there is a cost-benefit analysis that has to take place. Setting up each device on its own VLAN is a tremendous amount of work. For example, if a hospital has 100 beds with 15 IoMT devices per bed, that would be 1500 VLANs. It would also mean 1500 different firewall ACLs that would be put in place. That is not reasonable for any organization. What typically happens in situations like that is that the people administering the network create workaround to the problem—even putting in ACLs to completely bypass the problems they have with the solution.

What is typically done in situations like this is that organizations find a reasonable balance between security and IT operational costs. Maybe it would be reasonable to have a VLAN around each ward—each group of rooms with similar functions in order to minimize the damage that attackers can do. If there are 10 beds to each ward, that would mean 10 VLANs. Ten VLANs is far more reasonable than 1500 VLANs and is a reasonable compromise. With a situation like that, the IT staff is less likely to create workarounds. It is also easier to perform due diligence on 10 VLANs than 1500, which means the work has a much greater chance of getting done with far fewer mistakes.

While an infinite number of variations could be created around how to set up VLAN ACLs and the equipment, it is important to think about the environment, what the various challenges are, and how each environment is best protected. The point here is to have a reasonable approach to security where you can and then utilize other tools to compensate for everything else. Organizations have budgetary considerations that need to be taken into account and balanced across the various cybersecurity disciplines. Networking is only one discipline—one that requires work from both the IT and security teams.

Another consideration is to think about both inbound and outbound ACLs. Both are valuable in an organization. Focusing on inbound traffic for a specific IoMT VLAN is good because it helps to shield the individual devices from being compromised. On the other hand, if an IoMT device is being used to surf the web, an inbound ACL will not provide much protection. Obviously, the best strategy is to use both, but if that's not possible, taking into account the capabilities of the IoMT may provide a reasonable compromise.

Alternate Network Defensive Strategies

As there are limitations for protecting IoMT devices from a VLAN ACL perspective, it doesn't mean that organizations are done protecting their business. Many of the following strategies are used by organizations all over the world. They are part of the overall strategy for protecting IoMT and organizations.

Network Address Translation

Network Address Translation (NAT) is usually thought of as an IT need because it was invented as a means of handling the quickly dwindling number of IP addresses available on the internet—specifically related to IP version 4.[1] What it allowed companies to do is distinguish between public and private IP addresses. The public IP addresses that are used to communicate over the internet are the standard for most organizations. Seeing that the public IP addresses were running out, the governing bodies designated some of those IP addresses as private IP addresses, which are used all over world for internal traffic within organizations.

While everyone is using the same private IP addresses, it doesn't mean that everyone will be using the same IP addresses within the same range. There are more than 17 million different addresses available within the private IP address range and there are many different ways to set those IP addresses up, which can make them a little more secure. For the junior hackers, private IP addresses are typically more difficult to hack just due to raw numbers. From an IoMT perspective, this kind of security control is a generic control that protects all systems, not just IoMT.

---

[1] Network engineers are probably aware that NAT is a bit more complicated than this because there is port address translation as well that is usually associated with NAT.

Virtual Private Networks

Many of us are familiar with virtual private networks (VPNs) from using work computers at home to connect to an office environment. That same type of technology is also used for inter-organization connectivity as semi-permanent connections. VPNs provide an encrypted tunnel between the VPN devices (often a firewall). A VPN is one of the best ways of protecting organizations from a man-in-the-middle attack. If IoMT has insecure communication, that IoMT communication should traverse a VPN as much as possible to protect that protocol. At no point should that communication traverse the open internet unencrypted—especially if that communication has sensitive data. Any organization that doesn't may find their data or devices compromised by cybercriminals or nation-states.

Network Intrusion Detection Protection Tools

Network Intrusion Detection Protection Systems (NIDPSs) have been around for a very long time and are a good way of providing extra protection on a network. The basic consideration for them is that they can be set up in detection mode or protection mode. Detection mode simply alerts on network intrusions, while protection mode actively blocks network intrusions. What is great about NIDPS tools is that they look at the packets, not logs. Packets are how all traffic is transmitted over the internet. They contain a great deal more information than logs typically carry, so they tend to be more powerful in some respects than firewalls.

Today's NIDPS tools have a vast array of capabilities. They can detect/block known malware, nations, and the Tor network; import information about threats; deny certain types of traffic; and so on. They are an excellent way of adding an extra layer of protection onto the network. While not specifically geared toward protecting IoMT, they end up protecting IoMT because they protect everything on the network they are on.

Deep Packet Inspection

Deep Packet Inspection (DPI) tools are almost a technological cousin of the NIDPS. Like the NIDPS tools, they fully examine packets and oftentimes can be set up to store packets. The key differentiator between DPI and NIDPS is that DPI uses machine learning algorithms to find problems, whereas NIDPS tends to use a more signature-oriented approach. Both technologies have advantages over the other, and more than likely there will be a stronger merging of these technologies over time.

Web Filters

Web filtering comes in several different forms, but its defining characteristic is the ability to filter websites and web traffic. What this means can vary greatly based on the vender and the product. For example, many firewalls have an add on option to filter websites requests from servers. How they block web requests depends on the firewall, but often the firewall acts as a web proxy—essentially the proxy serves as a technical intermediary between the requester of a web site and the web site itself. Whatever the mechanism, they can categorize websites into types of sites and block according to that type. They can even block known APT sites or brand-new sites (many of which are harmful the first few days they exist). This is another extremely useful capability to limit the outbound communication of systems. While threat actors have the ability to set up web sites on the fly that are unknown to the firewalls, it is an excellent way to limit the damage done by specific systems.

There are more powerful web filters known as Secure Web Gateways (SWGs)—a SWG being a type of web proxy. SWGs can provide granular capabilities for protecting organizations, but they typically take more effort to set up and manage. Almost all have all the capabilities of standard web filters in firewalls. Some have very powerful capabilities such as scanning files that traverse browsers for malware. Others have a sandboxing function that not only scans for malware, but can let threats detonate in a safe environment as a means of detecting attacks. Another modern capability is machine learning to help catch web-based threats that are problematic.

Adding an SWG is critical for most servers and workstations and may be a reasonable practice for some IoMT, but in other cases, an SWG is not possible. In those cases a web filter may be the best practice because it does not require any modification of individual systems. When it comes to securing IoMT, sometimes it is about the best approach for the context and not the best of all possible worlds.

Threat Intelligence Gateways

For most organizations, Threat Intelligence Gateways (TIGs) are not the most common defense, but still part of the network arsenal defending many organizations. TIGs are typically placed external to a network between a firewall and the internet. They are designed to push away the most common attack vectors against organizations so that by the time the traffic hits firewalls, there are far fewer threats for the firewall to contend with. NIDPS used to sometimes be used in this location, but they can require a tuning to be effective. TIGs offer that middle-of-the-road alternative to protecting organizations from threats. From an IoMT perspective, they are a few layers away from most IoMT devices so the benefit is about fewer attackers hitting organizations.

Operating System Firewalls

Operating system firewalls are the firewalls for local operating systems such as servers and workstations systems, and not for the network. Technically this is not a network security control, but it is often used as a compensating control for lack of network protection. Utilization of these operating system firewalls is often referred to as micro-segmentation. It stands in contrast to network segmentation, which is not on the individual server level. What is great about micro-segmentation is that it can be used to defend IoMT systems that vendors will not permit agents to be installed.

Wireless Woes

In a hospital environment, connectivity is everything. Cellular service, depending on the location, can be less than perfect. Also, some rooms may be designed to block wireless service for safety reasons. Sometimes the logistics of a basement floor create the same issue. Whatever the reason, the natural alternative to cellular is Wi-Fi because a Wi-Fi signal can be placed in rooms where other wireless service is blocked. But connectivity is important to patients as well as the hospital. Being able to communicate with connected family members and loved ones while someone is in a hospital is a critical component of customer service. Wi-Fi is part of critical connectivity.

Wi-Fi, like everything in IT, can be challenging to set up properly—especially considering how it interconnects to the environment. Do you set up Wi-Fi to have encryption? What level of encryption? Some IoMT devices, especially the older they get, cannot handle the latest and greatest encryption, so some options for poorer Wi-Fi signals must be provided. With devices taking different levels of encryption it would be tempting to set up different SSIDs with different levels of encryption. There are obvious trade-offs because maybe the devices need to be connected to the same backend network, which can bring additional network configuration challenges. If the network is flat network behind the wireless device, that can be an opening for cybercriminals to expand into the rest of the environment.

In Wi-Fi, the level of encryption matters because many types of Wi-Fi encryption can be hacked almost instantaneously, which means, depending on the transport mechanism (HTTP versus HTTPS, for example),[2] the traffic may be hacked by someone monitoring the Wi-Fi. To that point, anyone within range of the Wi-Fi signal can pick up Wi-Fi traffic, which makes it less secure overall. Using a VPN is the best way to protect traffic over Wi-Fi, but this is not always possible with IoMT devices. Without a VPN, anyone within range of the Wi-Fi can record the traffic potentially putting usernames, passwords, corresponding systems, and associated data at risk.

Whether from a laptop or a cell phone, some of the Wi-Fi issues stem from automatic logins. The reason that is concerning is because hackers can easily fake a Wi-Fi access point, which means the Wi-Fi data may traverse an unauthorized system. If the traffic is unencrypted, usernames, passwords, or worse, data may traverse a hacker's laptop—meaning data may be silently copied without anyone being the wiser. If the IoMT device is connected to an EHR system over the internet, it can provide an attacker with a username and password to gain access to all of the data in the EHR.

In the end, Wi-Fi, like any technology, is far from simple and even very intelligent people can make mistakes setting up a Wi-Fi device. The people part of the equation needs to be considered as part of the Wi-Fi setup. For example, if there are several Wi-Fi SSIDs available, it can be easy to confuse which network a Wi-Fi device should connect to. Some equipment is critical to human life. Do you want to take the time to assess what devices should go on what SSID when a human life is at stake? Sometimes simpler is better as hospitals need to weigh decisions between security of data versus a human life. Wi-Fi design and setup can be one of those occasions.

In Summary

It is important to remember that the large risks that a flat network has. Yesteryear it was problematic, but today, the risks related to a flat network are far higher. The poor security of many IoMT devices has amplified

---

[2] For those who are not familiar with HTTP or HTTPS, HTTPS is the secure encrypted form of HTTP. Like Wi-Fi, HTTP has its own encryption that can be utilized, which means that it can potentially be hacked. Without going into too much detail, security is hard, and there are layers and layers of careful consideration that need to go into securing environments.

the risk—partially due to volume. Trying to remediate the flat network after the fact can be very challenging because once new networks are made, the IoMT (and other) devices need to be moved over after the fact. Being as thoughtful as possible when setting up the network is very critical. It involves multiple teams working together to ensure a reasonable network strategy is in place.

That said, while having an unflat network is important, so are many of the other recommendations that are so common in many environments. Ultimately, the right thing to do depends on a tremendous number of factors. What kind of data is flowing over the network, the interconnectivity of the various types of systems, how much data, what additional compliance is in scope, and what other controls are in place are all relevant considerations when determining the strategy for protecting IoMT.

CHAPTER

11

Internet Services Challenges

Navigating a complex system of cloud computing with an enterprise cybersecurity strategy is not an easy feat. A complex technological system works when designed correctly. However, adding the human factor as an element to this system is an ever-escalating paradox and a potential cyberthreat.

—Ludmila Morozova-Buss

Internet services are the lifeblood of covered entities and are obviously critical to IoMT services. The internet quite literally is the electronic conduit for sharing information. Without it, there is no IoMT story. But it is important to secure these services, and not securing them is one of the major oversights of organizations. Not all organizations are perfect at protecting the internet services, which affects the security ecosystem of IoMT devices and the associated data.

But what are internet services, and why are they important? Internet services are either used for the back end of covered entities or the front end. They provide the connectivity for the internal (or external) IT teams, related business functions, insurance, RHIO connectivity, and so on. They also act as the connectivity for IoMT, related services, and even customer information. Most of these services sit on top of the internal network (or cloud services) of the organizations they help. In this chapter, we will take a look at these services, how cybersecurity fits into that picture, what the major faux pas are, and a few options for how cybersecurity can help protect covered entities and IoMT devices from cyberattacks.

Internet Services

In many ways, internet services are the doorways to the covered entity and its data. They are absolutely critical to modern healthcare organizations, but they come with a host of challenges that organizations meet with varying degrees of success. Not being robust in the approach to protect them can be detrimental to the continual operations of the services that are offered—not to mention being a risk to data being compromised.

Network Services

The network really is the backbone of any organization, whether you are talking about traditional corporate infrastructure or cloud infrastructure, which has a logical simulation of network infrastructure. What you put into the network helps determine what you get out of it. Most of us are familiar with basic home networking where you can get an internet feed into your home. Larger organizations do not feel comfortable with just one feed, so they have multiple feeds from internet service providers (ISPs). Cloud services often have a range of different connections that feed into their services for maximum redundancy. In both cases, if one feed goes down, companies have a backup to work with. This is referred to as *high availability*. High availability provides an additional layer of resiliency for organizations.

Availability is critical for covered entities, as is the confidentiality and integrity of IoMT and data. We have already discussed firewalls and the flat network. While we touched on VPN tunnels in the previous chapter, we have not spent a great deal of time discussing individual VPN connections from working machines. VPN tunnels have become all the more critical since COVID-19 caused many companies to change their work strategies from in-house to working from home—at least to some extent.

This may seem like a minor change, but from the perspective of many companies, the VPN has become a critical—especially with the work from home model. Unfortunately, that adaption was less than smooth. Some companies adapted by moving to cloud-based VPNs. The advantage here is they could adapt quickly to the increased demand. Other companies stuck with traditional physical VPNs that they needed to quickly upgrade to adapt to the increased demand. Still others used software-based VPNs.

From an IoMT perspective, they represent yet another link in the chain where something can go wrong. They are, in many cases, a weak point in the architecture of organizations as they literally are the connection to the internal network of organizations. A weakness here could represent access to a covered entity's internal network—often to the extremely vulnerable IoMT devices. Extra care must be used to set up, monitor, and protect these devices—including using strong authentication.

Websites

In Chapter 2, we touched on the challenges related to websites and the importance of having strong security baked into an SDLC process. Obviously, not having strong security can ultimately mean that the system can be compromised. This is true for IoMT systems and associated technology, and also any software that can be developed (also known as coding), including websites that can be either purchased as an off-the-shelf product or developed by internal team. As also discussed in Chapter 2, many of the challenges related to software are due to not having security in the SDLC process at all. Reasons like this create the challenges that we are facing today. But what are some of the base disciplines within a secure SDLC? What does it comprise, and how can companies best become secure?

The first step in our journey is having standards for developing applications. What is immediately relatable for the non-technically inclined are items like how to handle forgotten password changes. From a programming perspective, any process can be created for handling forgotten passwords. For example, one can create a list of all users on the system and allow an end user to click on an end user and simply change the password—no authentication required. Most people would say this is an egregious security violation on many levels. While it would be easy for people to change (anyone's) password in this situation, it would not be very secure. Anyone could gain access to the site under anyone's account. A more secure practice would to create a lost password function and require strong authentication with specific password requirements.

While this is an easily relatable example, most secure programming practices are not too unlike these requirements. They think about common fallacies in software development and institute development practices that prevent the software or system from being hacked. One such standard that many companies follow is the OWASP top 10 requirements. We touched on OWASP in Chapter 2 in relation to IoT vulnerabilities, but it is better known for application security. One of the requirements from OWASP is to have input validation for what characters can be added to an input field in a dialog box—such as on a website. Not doing this basic input validation means that the system can be hacked relatively easily by those who know how. It is one of the most important things programmers can do to protect websites.

While we did not get into the weeds concerning the OWASP top 10 requirements, you can get the general idea of what should be done to best protect the organization from a standards perspective—having a standard that includes, at the very minimum, security requirements from a reputable source such as OWASP. Large organizations have very large manuals, filled with requirements. Some even develop training programs around learning the corporate requirements as a means of ensuring not only security, but conformity to internal coding practices within the organization.

But coding standards are not the only consideration for a secure SDLC process. There are a number of tools on the market to help achieve better coding. These are referred to as Static Code Analysis tools. Essentially, they scan through code looking for both bugs and security problems as a proactive way of finding issues. This combined with peer reviews and security reviews of software is one of the best ways to catch problems within the code itself. Doing this in a development environment without real data is the safest way to develop software.

We will explore some other methods in Chapter 14, but other considerations include using separate tools that can compensate for some of the problems. The most prominent tool is the Web Application Firewall (WAF). A WAF is similar to a normal firewall except that it specifically focuses on application security. It filters traffic to the website from incoming attacks. They can even filter OWASP top 10 attacks—to varying degrees of success. Today, WAFs, like many technologies, often utilize machine learning to help protect the software they are defending. In fact, PCI-DSS allows organizations to choose between a secure SDLC and a WAF though this is not always advisable as WAFs can go down. If the WAF goes down and traffic is still permitted to go to the website, how then do organizations protect themselves? Either they lock down the website or they operate insecurely in those cases. Neither is an ideal business outcome—covered entity or not.

In the end, a secure SDLC, as opposed to developing any way a developer may desire, is absolutely critical for organizations. A poor SDLC process is often one of the causes of poor security in IoMT devices. There are many different options and strategies for protecting websites, software in general, and IoMT interconnections. Doing things like hardcoding passwords into a website is almost assurance that a website will be hacked. Either the code will be recognized and on the website or hackers will figure out what the password is through a variety of different hacking techniques. Including secure SDLC requirements into corporate software development processes makes for better security across the board for IoMT and covered entities. Having an extra layer such as WAF adds to the overall security of organizations.

IoMT Services

For most readers, it should go without saying by now that most IoMT devices should not be exposed to the open internet from a security perspective. A few of you may be thinking that if they meet UL 2900 and they can be patched and have protective software on them, they should be safe, right? The answer is that it is safer, but it still is not a good idea without being more specific about the context. We spoke about the perils of a flat network. The flat network applies to web services as well. In a properly secured environment, the DMZ (ideally where a web server would sit) should only fleetingly have data in it. Anything else fits into the faux pas category.

Unfortunately, IoMT devices can be found exposed directly to the internet occasionally—even ones without the UL 2900 seal of approval. With organizations, if they do not understand the importance of the UL 2900 seal, often they will miss some other key cybersecurity considerations. Having the right knowledge, leadership, and open communication in place is absolutely critical for an organization. Basic considerations for cybersecurity are among the most critical to protect organizations.

Other Operating System Services

While any number of additional services can be installed on operating systems, the two that are perhaps the most common for organizations to have facing the internet (other than web servers) are Secure Shell (SSH) and Remote Desktop Protocol (RDP). Both have very different roots, but have similar kinds of risks, and RDP tends to have more vulnerabilities associated with it. The one other strong differentiator is that RDP provides greater access to full systems (typically speaking), which enhances the impact associated with a breach of the protocol. RDP was originally designed to allow Windows operating systems to connect to one another within a network. SSH, on the other hand, was designed as a secure replacement to two relatively insecure protocols—Telnet and

File Transfer Protocol (FTP)—both of which allow passwords in plain text. As an FTP replacement, the access can be limited to a small subset of folders and not a full operating system. Many of the exposed SSH systems have a reduced risk compared to RDP.[1]

RDP has also been the subject of a number of attacks. In fact, a report from Vectra, a cybersecurity company, demonstrated that 90% of the organizations that used one of their products had RDP cyberattack behavior within their organization. Throughout their RDP report, they cite how RDP is used by APT attackers—something serious enough to have an FBI warning concerning RDP.[2]

The plain-text protocols of FTP and Telnet make it imperative to switch to SSH (or another secure method) as a means of accessing servers from the internet. Both SSH and RDP are good substitutes, but by themselves, both protocols have risks associated with them—especially if they are not patched right away. If either is absolutely required for business purposes, there are some options for those services. First, if possible, ensure the access to those services are within a VPN tunnel. If a VPN tunnel is not a viable option, limit the access to those services to an IP address range of the companies that need access. Hackers can work their way around such a limitation, so multi-factor authentication should also be used. Finally, RDP and SSH do have configuration parameters for the servers, which should be carefully considered before making these protocols available on the open internet.

Open-Source Tools Are Safe, Right?

It may be helpful for some of you to understand the different options for legal software. If you have a home computer that you purchased through a company, the associated software is free and completely legal. That is paid software. There are also tools that can be downloaded for free from various companies. These are called *freeware*. A number of tools are also available that are open source. Open-source software is free, but anyone who can access the software can see source code when they download it. Legally, they can even modify and/or upgrade the

---

[1] Students of risk assessments will be right to point out here that the reduced risk depends on the context. If there are millions of records available, this could put a covered entity out of business.

[2] Vectra AI, An inside look at RDP cyberattacker behaviors and targeted industries, 2019

software in any way they so desire. It can then be uploaded for anyone to copy and use. There are many people who feel that this software is safer and more secure.

Eric S. Raymond wrote a brilliant book called *The Cathedral and the Bazaar* back in 1999. In the book, he talks about two fundamentally different approaches to software security. One method is the cathedral, which represents companies like Microsoft that wrote software within their own metaphorical walls. In these walls, the software was written by their own people, but it was not reviewed by other people coding the software, so it was bound to have many vulnerabilities. Having a hundred thousand people pouring over the source code that comprises an application means that bugs in the code could be worked out. The cathedral just does not have that many people perfecting a product. The bazaar is the model of Linux, which is largely open source, where a hundred thousand people could go through the code, find problems, and resolve them. As a result, in Ramond's view, the end product is far safer if it was created and reviewed in the bazaar and not within the cathedral.

That was fairly sound reasoning in 1999. At the time of this writing, it is close to the end of 2020, and the number of vulnerabilities very much depends on the type of Linux (referred to as *flavors* in the Linux community) and what year you are comparing. Different versions of Linux are more secure than others—especially if you are talking about raw numbers of vulnerabilities. Debian Linux, for example, had more vulnerabilities than any other operating system between 1999 and 2019—topping out at more than 3,067 vulnerabilities. It was beaten out by Android in 2019, which had 414 vulnerabilities compared to Debian's 360.[3]

The number of vulnerabilities, by far, does not tell anywhere near the full story. There are a number of other factors like how severe each vulnerability is, what other packages are installed, how quickly the system is patched, and so on. One big difference between Windows and Linux is how software is installed for Linux. Linux, as an operating system, is far more modular than Windows. While Windows has a few modular components, a large portion of Linux can be removed to create a base install of the operating system. In this state, assuming nothing is installed, Linux can be more secure than Windows. Unfortunately, quite often, when you want to install a specific application, there are other

---

[3] Surur, "Analysis shows over the last decade Windows 10 had fewer vulnerabilities than Linux, Mac OS X, and Android," March 8, 2020, https://mspoweruser.com/analysis-shows-over-the-last-decade-windows-10-had-fewer-vulnerabilities-than-linux-mac-os-x-and-android/.

applications that the primary application is dependent on that must also be installed. A system that had 500 applications installed on it can easily balloon out to thousands of applications. These additional applications can very much affect the vulnerability of the overall system.

But there are a host of other challenges that affect the security of open-source software. Many APT actors are infiltrating open-source software development projects that are freely available on the open internet and adding their own malicious code. Many organizations, covered entities or not, install these applications and then become infected. The cascading application requirements for Linux systems can mean hundreds of different packages can be installed, for just one piece of software. Any of these packages could be infected, and it is a real nightmare to protect organizational security in those cases. It is a very common problem as an estimated 95% of companies use open-source software within their organization.[4] Healthcare companies in particular typically use at least 65% open-source software in their organizations.[5]

The end results today are that the open-source movement is rife with problems. This should not be all that surprising to many of you. If you think back to Chapter 1, very few schools are teaching security as part of their curriculum. This means many software developers are creating software without a thought for security. Seventy-five percent of the freely available software development projects on the open internet contained vulnerabilities, with 49 percent containing high-risk vulnerabilities. This can mean very significant vulnerabilities for covered entities. As an example, there is a web server called Apache that is commonly used on Linux systems. It has taken a metaphorical beating over the years with 70 vulnerabilities, as of this writing, related to Apache Struts—14 of which allow for a complete compromise of confidentiality, integrity, and availability. Apache Struts is accessible from the internet if the system is internet facing.

From a cybersecurity perspective, open-source software should be vetted prior to installation on a production site. There are many ways to vet that software. Software composition analysis tools are designed specifically to look at the raw code of open-source software to detect vulnerabilities. Another option is to take the time to analyze the tools by performing a code review of the software prior to using it in production. Yet another option is to isolate the machine on the network

---

[4]Curtis Franklin, Jr., "How Hackers Infiltrate Open Source Projects," 2019, https://www.darkreading.com/application-security/how-hackers-infiltrate-open-source-projects-/d/d-id/1335072.
[5]Synopsys 2020 Open Source Security and Risk Analysis

and use tools to observe its behavior. If there are anomalies, then there is a good chance that one of the packages contained software that was compromised in some way.

Another way that many covered entities can protect themselves is to purchase a flavor of Linux that automatically vets the software prior to allowing implementation. In this way companies are in a position to have an additional layer of protection prior to installation. It is a much easier and safer way to ensure that the software has a reasonable level of assurance that it is not compromised compared to random open-source code on the internet.

Open-source software can be used safely, but there are a lot of concerns that covered entities should have related to the source code. From an IoMT perspective, oftentimes Linux is used as the base operating system. Sometimes it is very pared down to include only the minimal requirements. The challenge is, if that software is on the internet, it will have vulnerabilities just as Windows-based systems will. Like Windows-based IoMT, sometimes the manufacturer does not permit updates to the software, leaving it open to being compromised. Both strategies have their value in organizations, but being extra thoughtful about the approach related to open-source software is certainly warranted—especially if it is being used in conjunction with IoMT.

Cloud Services

Cloud services are an integral part of larger covered entities today. Using cloud services makes logical sense for many organizations, whether one is talking about the servers and network that make up a custom environment in PaaS or IaaS or a more fully built cloud solution such as SaaS offers. The one thing that all of the solutions have in common is a custom portal. Not looking at the specifics of each portal and the capabilities that correspond to it is a major oversite—especially when the potential damage can be so catastrophic. In many instances, everything in the cloud can be completely compromised. Today, most external actors either silently steal information and/or add ransomware. Insider attacks, if they are from disgruntled employees, may be more likely to remove the software.

That said, there can be multiple strategies to protect infrastructures. For example, allowing different groups of people access to different clouds and having failover to alternative clouds is a really strong option for protecting organizations from both insider risks and ransomware risks.

From a problem detection standpoint, we spoke about the importance of monitoring in the previous chapter. Many log monitoring solutions can also monitor a large array of cloud services including IaaS, PaaS, the cloud portal, and many SaaS solutions. Where applicable, many of these log monitoring solutions can monitor the operating systems and/or applications within the environment. We'll discuss more about these solutions in Chapter 16, but they remain a very critical component to detecting the problems related to the cloud.

Today's cloud solutions usually have logs associated with them that can be read by SIEM solutions, an array of managed log/security solutions (explored in Chapter 16), or even Cloud Access Security Broker (CASB)/Secure Access Secure Edge (SASE) solutions.

SASE solutions, also referred to as CASB, are the Swiss Army knives for the cloud. They are capable of far more than detection, and they remain an excellent way of not only monitoring logs, but also for how systems interact with various cloud environments. This is on multiple levels. For example, some SASE solutions can monitor the communications between a computer and cloud environment. Not only can they evaluate the cloud's security level, but they can determine if it is a corporate instance of the cloud (and block if appropriate) and perform some data loss prevention in the cloud itself.

SASE solutions also have the ability to block malware in the cloud—in many cases using antivirus solutions from other vendors. This is extremely useful for any kind of file sharing—especially for the corporate instances of cloud sharing tools such as Dropbox, Office 365, Box, and so on. If someone shares an infected file, the antivirus solution might delete it prior to someone else getting their computer exposed.

Cloud services, like all other services, need to be protected—often more so because quite often anyone on the open internet can gain access. Not giving serious attention to cloud security means that if that cloud is controlling IoMT, the IoMT is at risk from the cloud. It may also mean that data sent to the cloud may be at risk. Today, the cloud really is part of many IT ecosystems, including IoMT. How we protect the cloud needs to be given serious attention in order to protect IoMT.

Internet-Related Services Challenges

Even though a number of internet services are older technologies, they are still very relevant today. These services can have a profound impact on the security of IoMT, even if some of those effects are indirect. They can provide either information or an inadvertent conduit to the organization and/or help reduce lateral movement time once a hacker is inside. Either way, taking the time to really understand how these related services affect an organization is absolutely critical.

Domain Name Services

Domain Name Service (DNS) is the key to making the internet a friendly place to surf for the average user, but many threat-ridden web sites are available through DNS, and there are numerous attacks on DNS itself. But let us take a look at how effective DNS protection can be. Cisco has a product called Umbrella, which can greatly reduce the number of viruses in an environment. Based purely on the DNS layer, it was 51.8% effective at detecting malware, while if Umbrella was used with a selective proxy, the detection rate jumped to 72.6%. The numbers are even higher when considering Umbrella against secure Web Gateway capabilities with the detection rate above 90%.[6] What is not mentioned here is the Umbrella also blocks malware, but well before that malware hits enterprise environments. This means that DNS is extremely effective for blocking certain types of malware.

DNS is so critical for other reasons. Internal DNS, which is DNS within an organization, should, at all times, be separate from external DNS, which is generally available on the whole internet. Sometimes companies make the mistake of making their internal DNS identical with external DNS. This exposes the naming convention and IP addresses of the whole internal network—essentially making things easier for the hackers to find what they are looking for.

An innocent mistake that amplifies that specific risk is a poor naming convention for computer names. For example, naming a server "database server" (assuming it is a database server) informs potential attackers that this is a system that is key to gaining access to within organizations. Many organizations go a step further and use the brand name of the server as the server name. These mistakes inform potential hackers not only what ports to focus on, but also what vulnerabilities can exist on a particular system if patching is not up-to-date. It makes hacking organizations all that much easier. If the naming convention

---

[6] Taymourian Negisa AV-TEST Places Cisco Umbrella First in Security Efficacy, 2020, https://umbrella.cisco.com/blog/av-test-places-cisco-umbrella-first-in-security-efficacy#:~:text=Cisco%20 Umbrella%20performed%20significantly%20better,the%20blocking %20rate%20to%2072%25.

is made public through having internal DNS exposed to external DNS, cybercriminals can more easily plan their attack without having to be inside of an organization. Once inside, their activities can more easily remain hidden.

Looking at DNS-related issues from another angle, many cyber-criminals use a technique called typosquatting. Typosquatting is the practice of purchasing a domain name that may be easily mistyped. For example, instead of `wiley.com`, a typosquatter may buy `qiley.com` because q is next to w on a keyboard. An unsuspecting victim may type `quily.com` rather than `wiley.com`. If cybercriminals had purchased `qiley.com`, they could do anything they want. They could add malware on the web server thus infecting the victim's machine. According to *SecurityWeek*, researchers had obtained 120,000 corporate emails by typosquatting. Monitoring and subsequently blocking similar domain names can help organizations protect against these kinds of attacks. In some cases these are sites used by cybercriminals, while in other cases, they may be competitors with a similar name—either way, it is good for organizations to stay on top of these kinds of threats so they can respond appropriately.

Related to DDOS attacks is the DNS amplification attack. Long ago, hackers figured out that DNS servers with recursive capabilities could be used to amplify the effects of a DDOS attack. A simple configuration change can turn off this kind of capability, thus better protecting a covered entity.

There are a number of other attacks on DNS that are important to consider. But protecting DNS is absolutely critical. There are DNS Security (called DNSSEC) guidelines that can be used to harden DNS servers from problems such as cache poisoning. There are also a number of solutions on the market related to protecting DNS—many of them using divergent strategies including the utilization of machine learning to protect organizations from DNS-based attacks.

It may seem a bit much to focus so much on one protocol, but it is a foundational protocol for the internet, and most companies face at least one DNS-based attack over a period of a year. In fact, according to the 2019 *Global DNS Threat Report*, the average company had over nine attacks per year.[7]

---

[7] Romain Fouchereau, Konstantin Rychkov, 2019, "Global DNS Threat Report," June 2019. https://www.efficientip.com/wp-content/uploads/IDC-EUR145072419-EfficientIP-Infobrief-final.pdf.

In the end, DNS can have a tremendous impact on the security of IoMT devices and the associated covered entities and data, so it's important to consider how insecure DNS can amplify the problems related to IoMT.

Deprecated Services

While TCP/IP is the central protocol today, there used to be a number of protocols that were used within organizations. Examples include everything from WINS, NetBEUI, AppleTalk, IPX, and others. We are not going to take the space here to go through each one, because the technology is old and seriously outdated, but there are probably a few covered entities that need to keep some of these protocols around because of old technologies. Suffice it to say that they should not be exposed to the open internet if at all possible.

Internal Server as an Internet Servers

Because of COVID-19, many corporations have sent their employees home to work. As a result, businesses that relied on internal corporate systems such as firewalls and NIDPS to protect systems suddenly found that those protections were largely missing for home workers. Further, in some cases, updates were available only if the system was connected to the internal corporate network. Many of the legacy antivirus servers are set up this way—as is patching. What this often meant was that individual workstations were neither protected by traditional network protections nor able to protect the machines while working from home.

There are obviously many different strategies companies can take to remediate this. In some cases, the uplift to implement a more powerful VPN that can handle a greater amount of traffic was relatively small, so few changes were required to protect systems. In other cases, this was not a reasonable business expense, so internal servers were placed facing the internet. For example, the antivirus servers, which were originally designed to be internal update servers, were now placed where everyone can get their updates—the internet.

On a certain level, this is an innovative approach to handling the extreme impact of the work from home model, but these kinds of innovations can come with their own set of challenges. In some cases, the internal servers (and sometimes the associated software agents) were not patched because the risk was considered low. Placing the server on the open internet oftentimes meant that cybercriminals could easily gain access to the server—thus reducing the security of the environment. On the other hand, some servers could not be upgraded quickly because people were working from home. From a cybersecurity perspective, some companies were caught between a rock and a hard place.

This same type of challenge also appears when working with IoMT. Most IoMT devices were never designed to face the constant perils of the open internet. That said, some companies choose to have IoMT devices on the open internet. This can be done for ease of access or other business purposes. At this point, it should go without saying that it is extremely risky to put an IoMT device on the open internet. It should not be done. It is a cybercriminal's dream to have these devices connected to the open internet because they are often very easy to compromise.

In the end, if it is deemed necessary to have internal servers that are externally facing, ensure that appropriate protections are put in place for the software. In some cases compensating controls can be used to help protect software that cannot be updated appropriately. Many of the network tools mentioned in the previous chapter can be used to help protect these kinds of services. Firewalls, Network Intrusion Detection Systems, and so on are only some of the options available to covered entities.

There are other options available in many of these cases. Forcing end users to log in to a centralized corporate network can resolve many of these issues equitably, but that is not the only option. Many of the internal services either are available via the cloud today or there are alternate solutions borne in the cloud. While the cloud can be compromised, quite often that risk can be lessened because the system is not connected to any of the internal corporate networks. Either way, thinking about the strategy will have an indirect impact on the security of IoMT, and all options should be weighed carefully.

The Evolving Enterprise

From an IT perspective, much of what we have been talking about is part of the enterprise infrastructure. This includes servers, workstations, network devices, and so on. That almost antiquated view, which was held until the early 2000s, had a lot of corresponding assumptions. It harkens back to a time when antivirus and firewalls were reasonably sufficient to protect most businesses. IT and security were, generally speaking, not separate disciplines. The standard metaphor to describe how to protect the enterprise is that of a castle and moat. Nothing more was required. From an IT perspective, as long as things worked, you were good to go. Email messages would occasionally have some bad stuff, but thumb drives and CDs were also primary ways of distributing malware. The few occasions where that would occur, old-school antiviruses were sufficient to stop most of the threats.

Expectedly, though, things changed. Businesses began to outsource their connectivity all over the world. They began to intermix with other businesses as different companies had products that could save them time and resources. They started to rely on cloud services for their infrastructure. In Chapter 2 we spoke about PaaS, SaaS, and IaaS, which are part of more modern enterprises—part of what is now considered the extended enterprise—the traditional perimeter is not the same as it once was. Mobile phones became more sophisticated and now are an aspect of the IT umbrella. This began the rise of the extended enterprise—it included devices that were part of the organization, but not part of the old moat methodology. As COVID-19 forced businesses to rethink their work-from-home strategy, the quickly evolving paradigm is the perimeterless model where the line between personal and corporate systems has become more blurred. One evidence of this is the bring your own device movement where personal phones are permitted to access corporate resources. Those phones can have any software, compromised or not, with access to internal systems, emails, or other kinds of sensitive data.

With this evolving enterprise comes a radically different approach and skill set. With each new vulnerability, each new permutation of the attack vector means that covered entities need to develop more and more unique ways of defending themselves. It may seem simplistic to say, "Let us add a new device type," but it takes due diligence and thoughtfulness to come up with a strategy for defending it.

In Summary

Internet services are among the most important services for business reasons, but they bring with them a whole host of problems for organizations. Anything connected to the internet represents a large risk that cybersecurity and IT teams must put their heads around in order to determine the best strategy for protecting those services. There is no simple one-size-fits-all approach when it comes to cybersecurity—especially when protecting IoMT systems. The best cybersecurity approach is dependent, in part, on the IT strategy of the organization and looking at those challenges holistically. Making a decision to put what was an internal system on the internet requires a thoughtful and considerate approach, carefully weighing the pros and cons of that decision. Maybe the best thing is to go back to the business and state, we need a better approach to solve the business challenges.

What we have presented throughout this chapter are a wide variety of different context and challenges. The tools and recommendations here are radically different from one another and require very different skill sets to set up and monitor the system securely. With each change in the overall service, you almost need to add a new person to the team to support that change or give internal people the time and resources to manage the enterprise more thoughtfully. Please keep in mind that we are just touching the tip of the iceberg when it comes to protecting IoMT and covered entities. It is far from simple, and many more layers of protection need to be taken into account.

In our next chapter we will be touching on IT hygiene and everything that entails. It is yet a new direction, a new way of looking at IT and ensuring the security of IoMT is certainly part of that process. The solutions are not always clean or perfect, but they do point to a positive direction in which companies can go to better protect IoMT.

IT Hygiene and Cybersecurity

One single vulnerability is all an attacker needs.
—Window Snyder

In the cybersecurity world, IT hygiene can take on slightly different meanings depending on who you talk to. At a high level, IT hygiene is no different from personal hygiene. You don't want COVID-19, so you wear a mask, wash your hands and clothes, and sanitize your house. The parallel in the IT world relates to topics like IoMT devices, updating (patching) systems, configuration management, and installed tools to protect the system. What we will be omitting from the discussion here is password hygiene as that will be discussed in Chapter 13, "Identity and Access Management."

IT hygiene is not just about the operating systems, though. It applies to virtually everything in the IT world. We have spent a considerable amount of time talking about networking, and IT hygiene applies to the network, too. Cybersecurity is about looking at the same systems that IT looks at, but in a slightly different way. In this chapter, we'll talk about networking from an IT hygiene perspective, but the same concept can apply to monitoring, identity and access management, forensics, and so on. That is one of the things that distinguishes cybersecurity from IT. The cybersecurity practitioner will look at a system differently depending on where it is on the network, the type and amount of data on a specific system, and how important that system is to the business. In short, cybersecurity cares about functionality, but it also cares about patching, configurations, identity, forensics, and so on. Cybersecurity is about the layers of the various systems systems. IT hygiene covers a few of those layers.

However, that's easier said than done—especially with the current security state of many IoMT devices—many of which do not meet HIPAA or other privacy regulations and/or frameworks. As a result, sometimes alternate strategies should be used to protect insecure IoMT devices, which we will explore here.

The IoMT Blues

Given that IoMT is such a challenge and that doing the right thing like patching a system can invalidate a warranty, alternate strategies must sometimes be utilized to protect both the devices and the hospitals from harm. That said, there are many interesting challenges that organizations face related to IT hygiene and the unique challenges that IoMT has.

IoMT and IT Hygiene

It should come as no surprise to you that the IT hygiene of IoMT can be really good or really poor depending on the specific device and the manufacturer. UL 2900 device compliance generally means that the systems can both be patched and updated and, where relevant, security software can be installed on specific systems. Non-UL 2900–certified devices are dependent on the whims of the manufacturer and the specifics of the device to determine whether or not systems can be patched, have antivirus installed, or be configured to protect themselves.

We will touch on some of the specifics of solutions in the following sections, but these kinds of business decisions by the manufacturers are part of the reason that covered entities are experiencing a high number of breaches. Not permitting patching, antivirus, or stronger configurations essentially leaves IoMT defenseless in the face of even the most inexperienced cybercriminal—even those systems that are behind firewalls. Remember, for APT actors, the most common vector of attack is email.

Past Their Prime

All technology has a limited life span. Every IoMT manufacturer can only support the upkeep of devices for a few years before it becomes cost prohibitive to maintain. Many of those manufacturers are also dependent on the companies that develop the base operating systems. As pointed out in Chapter 2, many covered entities typically rotate systems every three to five years, but IoMT can be kept as long as fifteen years—much longer than they were designed for. What this means is that many of the vulnerabilities that either the devices develop or the underlying operating system simply have no hope of ever being patched—even if they wanted to go against the manufacturer's requirements.

The reality is, purchasing fancy new IoMT technology is not free. While much of it saves money in the long run, changing devices on a regular basis can be expensive. It is costly in terms of the equipment, configuring systems, training the staff to use the technology, having the IT teams to support the technology, and so on. While it makes logical sense to replace the equipment as soon as there is a known risk, this philosophy poses a challenge, practically speaking. Some things are easier to say than do. As a result of the complexities behind all of the factors, devices have far more vulnerabilities than they would have otherwise had. To be fair, some of these devices have exorbitant price tags, which means that keeping them a few extra years makes perfect business sense. It does, however, add to the overall risk of healthcare organizations.

Selecting IoMT

There is a lot of history within organizations about which processes are governed by what individuals. Ten years ago, a random IoMT device here and there was not a big challenge from a security perspective. As IoMT devices became more numerous, the risks also grew. Unfortunately, as pointed out in Chapter 1, it was over a relatively short period of time that the number and use of IoMT devices spiked. On its own, that is a positive thing for hospitals, but a negative from a security standpoint. In the past, cybersecurity practitioners were not involved in the selection process of IoMT devices. The attitude at many organizations is, why would cybersecurity get involved? They have not done so in the past, so why would they now? Whose needs are more important? The needs of a doctor who is saving human lives and requires the latest tool, or cybersecurity's needs because of some abstract risk about data being stolen?

The positive about the ransomware and all the breaches is that there will be a tipping point for organizations where they have to include security in the selection process, or protections (controls for the security fans) must be put into place to protect the devices. From a security standpoint validating the security of devices can be a time-consuming process. Often, security programs are strapped for resources and don't have time to investigate. Astute readers are probably already thinking that the organizations should just purchase UL 2900–certified devices. As stated in Chapter 4, that is what the VA is doing, but all hospitals are not. It makes sense in many cases to follow UL 2900, but maybe not in all cases because innovation happens faster than the UL 2900 certification process. It is a balancing act that hospitals need to make—determining whether it is more important to have the latest devices that save lives, or security. This is when alternate protection strategies (also known as compensating controls) must be utilized to protect the devices, hospitals, and our data.

IoMT as Workstations

It should not surprise anyone by now that IoMT devices can be very easy to log in to. Sometimes this is related to the device itself, while in other cases hospitals allow staff to log in to the devices in order to use the devices with only their usernames and passwords, the same way they would log in to any other station. As a result, they have access to all the software and applications on the system—so what do people do? They surf the web. They check social media. They check their email. They do what people would do anywhere else. An accidental click (or mouseover) on malvertising, and the system can be quickly owned by a group of cybercriminals—unbeknownst to the IoMT operator.

Mixing IoMT with IoT

As mentioned in Chapter 2, IoT technology has many of the same weaknesses as IoMT technologies. In fact, IoT may be a little worse overall because it does not have PHI data to protect. The impetus for security is just not there. There are a few places where IoT devices may be used within an environment—cameras (which are notorious for their security flaws), IoT beds and similar devices, and personal assistant devices such as Amazon Echo, etc. Cell phones could be included in this category too, but they can be added to IoMT as well because they contain PHI data.

But let us start with Amazon Alexa–enabled Echo devices. As voice services are still imperfect, companies like Amazon pull in the data from these devices in order to improve their responses to voice commands.[1] Imagine something like that in a hospital setting—even a breakroom. These innocent-looking devices could pick up on PHI that others at Amazon may listen to. In a recent case, a court ordered Amazon to turn over two days of recordings in a murder investigation.[2] Now Amazon does have limits on what they can do, but accidents do happen. For example, a couple in Oregon accidently sent recordings of their conversations to one of the husband's employees—apparently because Alexa heard a background conversation during which it woke up when it heard its name and then interpreted another name as a name in the contact list.[3] Amazon does have quite a few security and privacy features built into Alexa such as a way to turn off the sound recording, but it takes diligence to ensure these protections are in place.[4]

While listening to music on your Amazon Alexa device is very innocent, there are privacy risks that have to be considered. There are people listening to the input to these devices in order to improve the overall service. In theory, they do not capture information until you say Alexa, but there are always mistakes, and information can remain unprotected (from a HIPAA standpoint) when those mistakes occur. Amazon is really striving to do the right thing by improving their service, but healthcare organizations using it in their environment always brings legal challenges. Since that time, Amazon has developed a cousin to Alexa-Lex, which is HIPAA compliant, but the focus is on the voice-to-text translation.[5]

---

[1] Matt Day, Giles Turner, and Natalia Drozdiak, "Amazon Workers Are Listening To What You Tell Alexa." April 10, 2019, `https://www.bloomberg.com/news/articles/2019-04-10/is-anyone-listening-to-you-on-alexa-a-global-team-reviews-audio`.

[2] Minyvonne Burke, "Amazon's Alexa may have witnessed alleged Florida murder, authorities say." November 2, 2019, `https://www.nbcnews.com/news/us-news/amazon-s-alexa-may-have-witnessed-alleged-florida-murder-authorities-n1075621`.

[3] TrigTent, "Amazon Echo Murder Case Confirms Fears, But Upside Hard to Deny," 2018, `https://trigtent.medium.com/amazon-echo-murder-case-confirms-fears-but-upside-hard-to-deny-76c3f5c482f3`.

[4] Amazon Alexa and Echo devices are designed to protect your privacy Accessed December 17, 2020, `https://www.amazon.com/b/?node=19149155011`

[5] "Amazon Lex Achieves HIPAA Compliance" December 11, 2019, `https://aws.amazon.com/about-aws/whats-new/2019/12/amazon-lex-achieves-hipaa-eligibility/`.

As mentioned in Chapter 2, IoT technology is largely in the same boat as IoMT technology in terms of its security. The impetus to be secure is not the same. The IoT bed is a good example to demonstrate this. It is a non-medical device that is often in a hospital environment and can still be connected to a network. The insecurities of such a device can pose a similar risk to hospitals as other IoMT devices, but they are sometimes less secure (especially when compared to an environment that only uses UL 2900 IoMT devices. In short, it adds to the overall vulnerabilities of an environment.

From a Wi-Fi perspective, another challenge with bringing non-HIPAA compliant devices into an environment is that they may have vulnerabilities like any other device. They can bring down the security posture of an organization in a similar fashion as the bed—especially if they are connected to the same network as other devices. Cybercriminals or malware may propagate from one device to the next.

The Drudgery of Patching

Patching, or applying updates to systems, is a time-honored part of the IT process. If you only work on computers at home, it may seem like a fairly easy task. Either the system takes care of itself or it is centralized through an app store that makes the system easy to update. Now imagine having to do that to 500 systems. Imagine that many apps are not part of a centralized catalog for easy updating and that there are interdependencies between the different kinds of applications. Now you are starting to understand the challenges that IT teams have when updating systems. IoMT adds new wrinkles as some systems cannot be updated and some can. They may have further disparate update mechanisms. Another added wrinkle is that many systems are critical for human life. Having a system down because a system needs a patch or a system not being available because of a glitch in a patching process when someone's life is at stake is simply not reasonable. Human life always comes first.

Patching is not always as simple as it may seem on the surface. There is a reason why companies pay for programs and/or services to help them with their patching processes. By itself, the scope of work is simply too large. Quite often an army of people would be needed to do the work by hand, which is not a reasonable business decision by anyone's standards. The further that organizations can move toward automation, especially in the realm of patching, the better off they will be.

Unfortunately, many of the cybercriminals are aware that organizations need to use tools for patching. For example, a Russian APT actor compromised SolarWinds, an IT management company, through an automated patching tool; specifically, their Orion product. That tool was deployed on fewer than 18,000 environments. Surprisingly, Russia has probably been in the SolarWinds product since March of 2020. To make matters worse, a security researcher warned SolarWinds that their update server could be accessed by using the password "solarwinds123"—which is definitely not a secure password.[6]

The total fallout of this hack may not be known for quite some time, but it does illustrate the challenges that nation-state actors pose to organizations. They can be very difficult to catch. FireEye, a well-known and respected cybersecurity company, was also affected by this breach. In fact, after they determined they were hacked, they ultimately reported that it was a nation-state actor and that the breach happened through SolarWinds.[7] In the end, it does point out that companies, even when using a trusted partner, should not fully trust those partners—even if they have good intentions.

Mature Patching Process

Testing is a critical function in a mature enterprise patching process. Part of the reason it is done is to determine if any serious problems can be fixed prior to implementation. This usually requires a reasonable copy of a production environment to be created. Depending on many variables, this can be referred to as a number of different things, but I'll refer to it here as a Quality Assurance (QA) environment. It's distinguishable from a production environment in that it usually does not have the full set of data that is found in other environments. There can be a list of other differentiators depending on the covered entity, but the goal here is to work out bugs in QA while minimizing interruptions to production.

In light of the SolarWinds hack it may be a good idea to get two separate products for patching—one to implement patching and one to validate the integrity of the patches. That may sound extreme, but utilizing two different companies for implementation and validation may be the best way to protect organizations from these kinds of threats.

---

[6]Kari Paul, "What you need to know about the biggest hack of the US government in years," https://www.theguardian.com/technology/2020/dec/15/orion-hack-solar-winds-explained-us-treasury-commerce-department.
[7]Ibid.

IoMT Patching

Assuming that the manufacturer permits patching of devices, patching IoMT systems can bring its own set of challenges. In most cases, there is no QA environment; everything is a production environment. Should covered entities purchase a $2 million IoMT device to test prior to going in production if it will never be used for any other purpose than to test patches? Probably not. But if you had two $2 million devices, you might test on one before the other. Companies need to compromise all the time for legitimate reasons. The same is true of workstations—test a few workstations of non-essential workers prior to an organization-wide rollout to ensure that there will be as few snags as possible.

Testing patches for IoMT devices, when they can be patched, sometimes brings special challenges. In some cases, the monitor must be patched before or after the IoMT device. Sometimes the transitions between cloud services must happen for device functionality. There are many different options that must be considered as part of that patching process—many of them involve less than perfect circumstances from a testing perspective.

Windows Patching

Windows is probably the most common software used in most organizations. It can be set up to perform individual patch updates, but there are also centralized patch mechanisms included with Windows. However, tools included with Windows do not cover the wide range of other applications often installed on systems. There are many options on the market for patching not only Windows, but the various applications that are installed on top of Windows—which may be easier said than done.

Many organizations are not necessarily aware of all of the applications residing on their systems. Windows comes with a plethora of software that can be installed. Some covered entities are really good at monitoring the software installations across their organization, while others are not, which is a critical faux pas. How do you update software if you do not know it is installed? Smart organizations monitor and/or control the software in their environment so they know how to respond if any issues arise.

The reality is that employees can do just about anything from a software perspective—especially if they are just out of school. Some do not understand the intricacies of software licenses and may download their own personal versions, or use file-sharing utilities to download their favorite music and inadvertently end up with infected files that can affect the entire system. In other cases, they may install black-market versions of the software, which can create enormous problems for covered entities for many of the same reasons.

For Windows systems that are IoMT devices and, by contract cannot have software installed, what do you do when people install unauthorized software? How does the IT and/or security staff even know if the software is installed? People can install just about anything without anyone other than the user being aware. To add insult to injury, that software may have vulnerabilities or bring legal issues on a company because the software is unauthorized. Assuming it is legal, how do you get it patched? Not permitting software on IoMT-related systems is like walking into a fight blindfolded. You don't even know what or how you should protect those systems for applications, which may or may not be in place. It is not just malware and data, but also licensing considerations that can blindside organizations.

Linux Patching

In the last chapter we spoke a great deal about open-source software, which is more common on Linux systems than Windows systems, but can be found for almost anywhere. All of those considerations are extremely important to consider. That said, the patching process for Linux is not terribly unlike the process for Windows in many cases except that the end result is that multiple applications are affected instead of a more monumental operating system. One unique challenge that Linux offers is that sometimes the dependencies upon other software can shift, which can leave Linux with another set of challenges. What happens after the patching is that, in some cases, further work may need to be performed in order to further secure the device from the new applications.

Mobile Device Patching

Mobile devices, like everything else, should be patched on a regular basis. Mobile device management (MDM) tools can help with that process, but they are not always perfect in patching applications on the device—especially when those applications are not from a well-known application store. In many instances controlling the applications to a limited number of authorized applications is the best way to govern those tools.

When considering the BYOD trend, how far can a company manage the end user's phone? Can the company deny the installation of applications? Can they install the MDM solution mentioned earlier? How are staff going to feel when every phone call can potentially be monitored by internal systems? In some cases, parents allow their kids to have games on their phones—perhaps inadvertently accessing corporate data. A worse situation would be that malware infects the phone allowing sensitive data to be compromised. Should the organization mandate the corporate antivirus be on the phone? All of these issues need to be thought about in depth.

Final Patching Thoughts

Patching systems sounds like an easy task, but when you consider all the different types of patching that goes on within an organization—especially with the IoMT challenges—it is not. Complex organizations have project managers that work with teams to coordinate outages to ensure they do not occur at unplanned times or affect equipment not related to the outage. This can sometimes make patching difficult. In fact, most organizations have patching issues, especially in 24/7 environments. These issues mean that cybercriminals and nation-states have additional avenues to take in their assault on covered entities.

The right thing to do from a patching perspective is only purchase systems that allow continual patching and updates. It is the only way to truly protect the systems from cybercriminals. Yes, it costs our healthcare companies more, but the question is, do organizations want to pay more up front for a critical capability, or do they want to pay when they are compromised? All of these factors should be carefully considered when selecting IoMT devices.

Antivirus Is Enough, Right?

As pointed out in Chapter 8, Symantec estimated that traditional signature-based antivirus is only 45% effective according to 2014 data. Traditional antivirus today is even less effective today due the explosion of malware and continued innovation from cybercriminals and nation-state actors. Even next-generation antivirus, which uses machine learning, has been less effective than its proponents would like, but it is more effective than antivirus by itself. There are a still significant number of breaches happening to covered entities due, in part, to challenges with IoMT devices. Given the relative insecurity of many IoMT devices, a good malware defense strategy is absolutely critical—not only for IoMT, but for other systems in the environment as well.

Antivirus Evolution

To defend systems against today's threats, clearly something needed to change. As a result, a new technology has been developed—Endpoint Detection and Response (EDR). EDR is a significant shift from traditional antivirus. Antivirus was originally designed as a protective control—it blocks malware from getting on the system when it detects a signature. EDR is largely a detective control—it detects malware that gets onto the system. Automated responses can be set up for many instances, but not in all use cases. Instead of being a proactive tool to stop the malware, it is largely a reactive tool to detect the malware with some protective functionality. That said, its detection rate is far higher than the detections of traditional signature-based antivirus. The strength and capabilities of the response depends on the specifics of the particular vendor. One review gave SentinalOne a top product pick specifically for response capabilities with a score of 4.8 (out of 5).[8]

Most of the vendors know that the response capabilities of EDR solutions are less than perfect, so they have developed a Managed Detection and Response (MDR) solution that allows them to gain access to the system and remove any potential malware. For many companies this is a huge win because they do not need to have their staff involved in incident response activities the way they used to. The MDR service works with the company to develop a set of rules called a *playbook* for how the company wishes to respond to different kinds of incidents.

Solution Interconnectivity

While antivirus, EDR, and MDR solutions are a fantastic win for organizations today, they can always be better—especially if they can interconnect with other security tools on the market. That is exactly what many MDR services are moving toward today. In fact, they can be tied into EDR or MSSP (as defined in Chapter 16) solutions. Some MDR solutions can take feeds or alerts from logging or SIEM solutions to create a more holistic practice for their customers. Part of the reason they do this, aside from aiding the customer, is that EDR does not have a 100%

---

[8] Paul Shread, "Top Endpoint Detection and Response (EDR) Solutions" 2020, https://www.esecurityplanet.com/products/edr-solutions/.

detection rate. The reality is that APT threats are constantly being re-created to work around existing solutions on the market. As a result, today's antivirus (and associated) solutions are in that "innovate or die" category we spoke about in Chapter 1.

But these are not the only kinds of interconnectivity tools that are on the market. There is another set of tools known as Security Orchestration Automation and Response (SOAR) that more advanced companies are utilizing. SOAR tools are designed to automate actions from several sources, but more often than not from SIEM. If they detect an alert, they can automate responses from a SIEM to antivirus to block threats.

Antivirus in Nooks and Crannies

So far, we have been talking about antivirus as if it is something for individual devices such as computers, servers, phones, and so on. While those are excellent use cases, antivirus also has a place in many other situations as well. With no solution being 100% effective, many threat actors are playing a numbers game to see what slips through the defenses of organizations. As a result, applying antivirus to a range of other solutions makes perfect sense.

Two obvious use cases for email antivirus are around phishing attacks—emails that have a malware in them (such as a file) or a URL embedded within in email that links to a website that has malware. Adding additional capabilities to protect against both of these kinds of phishing attacks is yet another set of features within Secure Email Gateways (SEGs). They rely on many of the same capabilities (and often the same companies as antivirus companies) for these protective capabilities. In fact, oftentimes many SEGs employ a virtual host to detonate the attack so they can see exactly what the effects of the malware are (or if a file has malware in it) prior to letting it hit the host. Not all SEGs employ web filtering. Some rewrite the URL so that if the URL is malicious, the provided link will be rendered inert. There are other web filtering tools, such as Secure Web Gateways (SWGs), that often include an anti-malware component to help protect systems from harm.

Aside from that, it is useful to scan corporate instances of file-sharing tools such as Office365, Box, Dropbox, and so on. One vector of attack is for a malicious actor (or an insider who does not know a file is infected) to put a piece of malware in a corporate file. This in turn can be downloaded by someone in a company, thus infecting one or more computers. We mentioned using SASE tools, which often contain antivirus tools (some can add multiple tools to maximize effectiveness), to eliminate threats prior to hitting someone's workstation.

From a network perspective, antivirus and associated signatures can also be found. Tools such as NIDPS, some firewalls, especially those considered Unified Threat Management (UTM), often have antivirus signatures built in. UTM firewalls have a range of different capabilities, but have multiple strategies for stopping malware on the network (as opposed to local machines). Amongst those strategies is often antivirus. This way if any known (or often unknown) malware is traversing the network, it can be blocked prior to hitting multiple machines. There are also some antivirus signatures in some deep packet inspection systems.

This is not intended to be a complete list of all the places where antivirus is found in today's modern enterprise, but it does start to demonstrate the flavor of how pervasive it is amongst many of the technology vendors. In the end, understanding these nooks and crannies where malware may show up makes a great deal of sense—which is why we are seeing antivirus show up in so many places. All things considered, all of these different avenues where antivirus can reside provide organizations with additional protection.

Alternate Solutions

As antivirus becomes less and less effective, some companies are switching up their overall strategy. Some are even dropping antivirus altogether. While some strive to rely on EDR/MDR solutions without the antivirus, others are taking a whitelisting approach—essentially using a compensating control to replace antivirus. Whitelisting involves allowing only certain files to execute by permission, and no others. Blacklisting, by contrast, is just the opposite—denying certain files to execute. Blacklisting is a parallel to traditional antivirus as it relies on knowing what bad software is out there and blocking it. While it can offer some protection, its value is diminishing with each passing day. On the other hand, whitelisting offers a great deal of protection. If a piece of malware gets onto a system, it may not be able to execute—thus rendering it inert. This is probably one of the better strategies for protecting systems today.

Such wonderous potential is not without its drawbacks, however. Knowing each and every action on each and every system is extremely time-consuming. It also means that a strategy has to be devised for operating such a tool. For example, if there are different groups operating the tools and implementing changes on the systems, the two tools need to coordinate with one another to get anything done. This arrangement means that things will be much slower, but every change on the system should, in theory, be accounted for, which not only helps against malware, but also significantly reduces insider threats. It does mean that more work needs to be done between the two teams to coordinate. This becomes a cost-benefit analysis to determine if it is worthwhile or not for an organization. Given the rising costs of breaches, it might be an option for companies to think of. For IoMT devices that are permitted to have software installed, it is probably a really intelligent way to go.

For IoMT devices that are permited to have protective software installed, there are other options that may be better. In the IoT world, there is a new breed of software to block any and all activity except a very narrowly permitted set of activities. It is only good for systems that do not change much—perfect for many IoMT systems. Typically, they take some time to learn the system, but once they see all the activity, they can shut down any other extraneous activity, thus securing the system from future malware outbreaks.

Yet another strategy for protecting organizations from malware is called Content Disarm and Reconstruction (CDR). The technology behind CDR takes a very different approach, and it is focused on files. It takes an incoming file, copies the content, and puts it into a new file without transferring any malware the file might contain. This way, if the file contained with malware, the recipient will not even know the file was infected. This is a brilliant strategy for stopping malware and there are variations for email and web browsing. Through API integration, this can even be applied to individual systems. While not perfect, it is one of the more foolproof mechanisms for protecting organizations today, but is often overlooked by organizations hoping to strengthen their security posture.

IoMT and Antivirus

Whether or not IoMT can have antivirus installed depends very much on the specific device. Some IoMT devices are little more than firmware and clearly cannot have antivirus or other security tools installed. In these cases, taking a more network-centric approach to antivirus can make a lot of sense. Those devices that can have antivirus installed should have everything installed on them that they possibly can—follow the full standards of the organizations if at all possible.

The Future of Antivirus

Antivirus solutions continue to innovate and change. Many of them are built off of machine learning capabilities in order to find and/or block different kinds of attacks. Given that some APT actors have seemingly unlimited resources, it will not be too long before machine learning and artificial intelligence start to show up as part of the attacks against organizations. MalwareBytes, an antivirus company, wrote an article in 2019 stating that they believe artificial intelligence will start to show up in the next one to three years in minimal ways, but will grow more sophisticated over time.[9] In the end, we may need to have artificial intelligence battling artificial intelligence; whichever side has better computing power and better AI will win that battle.

Antivirus Summary

Antivirus and the various augmentations and/or alternate strategies are clearly needed to protect today's covered entities. As the number of insecure IoMT devices continue to escalate, stronger compensating controls are required. In fact, even without IoMT, stronger solutions against malware are required. It is no wonder that so many innovative techniques are used to stop this general malware menace afflicting our covered entities and IoMT. It is a veritable arms race that our healthcare systems are in against organized crime and nation-state actors. Our healthcare systems are quickly losing the battle. The poor security in IoMT is like strapping an arm behind your back before entering the arena.

Misconfigurations Galore

It is quite apropos that a discussion of misconfigurations comes just after a discussion of malware. Quite often malware propagates itself over poorly configured services. While this is largely a patching issue, it is also about secure configurations, which are absolutely critical for defending systems, not just from malware, but also from hackers and other miscreants who may be searching for proverbial low-hanging fruit—data they can steal or a system that is easy to compromise.

---

[9] Pieter Arntz, Wendy Zamora, Jerome Segura, and Adam Kujawa, 2019, `https://resources.malwarebytes.com/files/2019/06/Labs-Report-AI-gone-awry.pdf`.

Another good example of why configurations are so important was discussed in Chapter 2, where we explored in depth the challenges with S3 buckets in AWS. But this issue is not exclusively an AWS problem. In fact, it is a problem with almost any technology—including IoMT. If careful consideration and attention are not given to the configuration of every system within an organization, any of them can be part of a greater problem. Innocent configuration mistakes can lead to covered entities—or worse, IoMT devices—being compromised.

Sadly, configuration management in many covered entities is sometimes an overlooked discipline—both for IT and for cybersecurity. From an IT perspective it is not sexy to dive through pages and pages about how to configure something securely. It takes countless hours to learn how to configure something right. It also does not have the "magic" of making something work. It is about being very diligent about the overall processes for configuring systems. In a hospital environment, where often things need to be up and running yesterday, the discipline of secure configurations can be lost—the "we'll get to it later" mentality. Typically speaking, later never comes and the configuration management challenge looms even larger because doctors require 100% uptime for the systems they use. For many companies, configuration management is a huge challenge to stay on top of that ends up hurting security posture of organizations and often data within an organization.

To make matters worse, with aging IoMT systems, oftentimes trained technicians have to come out and reset the systems to factory specifications. These basic configurations are far from secure. Since the technician is primarily focused on getting the IoMT functioning again, there is a good chance that they may not make the settings secure-only adding to the overall challenges relating to IoMT security.

The Process for Making Changes

In the IT world, there are numerous ways of making changes, but it is generally acceptable that changes should not be ad hoc. People should not be wandering around making whatever changes they want whenever they want to make them. There should be a definitive process within an organization for making changes. That process is typically known as change management.

Change management defines who can make changes in an environment. This is usually tied to roles within an organization. The janitor should not be making configurations on a Windows server; a Windows administrator should typically be making those changes. The composition of those roles depends on a number of factors, which we will discuss in the next chapter. What is important here is that roles are designated to make changes in change management.

When changes are made is also typically specified within the change management process—sometimes as dictated by business needs. Quite frequently, there may be different windows of time for different systems. Sometimes changes may depend on the severity of the incident. For example, maybe on Fridays changes are not permitted in production, but if a production system goes down on Friday, that becomes an emergency incident, and changes are permitted under those circumstances. While organizations can devise a large number of rules concerning how to request changes what the change management processes are, and when, changes can take place.

A number of different changes can occur for a variety reasons. The business may want a new feature on a website. That entails making a change to that site. Security may want some changes to ensure the appropriate security configurations of that site. That may be a different kind of change. There may be a new connection to a business partner; that too is a change and should be part of standard change management process.

Approvals are also a part of change management process. In theory, there should be a quorum (a group of people that approve a change across an organization), and it should include the appropriate IT and security leaders.

In short, change management is the process of aligning and approving changes within an organization so they are not ad hoc. It is a process of modifying changes in an orderly fashion. Some organizations have architectural groups that may have pre-meetings to define what changes will go into a change management process. Others do not. In the end, organizations need to define the process that works best for them. That said, it is important for organizations to develop a strategy for changes—including a configuration strategy.

Have a Configuration Strategy

In theory, new projects should not reduce the security of an organization. There are, however, exceptions. Sometimes a piece of software may conflict with the best configuration, but overall, it improves security so there is a net reduction in risk. Sometimes there is no other way to accomplish a goal. That said, having configuration goals is critical to the success of a configuration management program. From a configuration standpoint, there are numerous standards to work from, but from a commercial/healthcare standpoint, the Center for Internet Security (CIS) has benchmarks that provide a great place to start.

The CIS benchmarks are configuration guidelines for organizations to protect their systems. They have everything from operating systems, databases, cloud portals, mobile devices, virtualization technologies, Zoom—everything you can think of except for IoMT. In short, they are a great place to start a configuration management journey for an organization. Essentially, each benchmark contains a list of configurations for securing the individual devices. Many of these guides are more than 100 pages long and contain hundreds of recommendations along with a how-to guide for making those configurations. They are very technical and not for the layperson, but even a non-technical person should be glad that these configuration guides exist.

These guides can be the basis of a configuration strategy across organizations. IT teams that have access to their respective benchmarks (they are freely downloadable) can start to secure their systems (as approved by the organization). Plans can be made, exceptions can be documented, and organizations are a little more secure just from using these standards. If we take the case of the insecure AWS S3 bucket discussed in Chapter 2, CIS has a benchmark for that which can help diligent engineers and administrators avoid costly mistakes and better protect their organizations.

IoMT Configurations

Obviously, some of the CIS benchmarks can be applied to parts of some IoMT systems. For example, if the IoMT system has operating systems or cell phones, those benchmarks can be applied—if permitted by the manufacturer. Some manufacturers will apply their own standards to IoMT devices to make them a bit more secure. This said, this still leaves us with the development of independent configurations of specific IoMT devices. Having a security expert look through the individual settings of the individual devices is probably a good place to start. It will not solve all of the challenges that IoMT brings to the table, but it may be enough to reduce some of the risks. For better designed IoMT devices, risks can be reduced quite significantly through this process.

Windows System Configurations

Windows configurations, at least for the last several years, tend to be fairly straightforward. The only consideration other than what we just discussed is what will be installed on the Windows systems. In general, only the parts that are required for that specific server should be installed. For example, if the server is not going to be a DNS server, do not install DNS services. Overall, this is not very difficult because of the way that Windows is designed. The greater challenge with Windows are the applications. Those challenges are defined later in "Application Configurations."

Linux Configurations

In the previous chapter we covered a number of challenges with Linux configurations that are important to remember here. The minimal build and trusting the range of software that comes with Linux are among the largest challenges. One thing that was not brought up was what do you do to secure those needed 500 applications that come with a Linux system? In some cases the applications can be disabled or permissions added to nullify access, but that creates a whole new problem that makes tying those packages together extremely challenging. Do you think those 500 subapplications are secure? In many cases, those subapplications can bring extra security headaches for the Linux administrator. These are some additional considerations when purchasing applications as well. There becomes a reasonableness limit for how much effort goes into configuring the systems. At a certain point, it is just easier to use a compensating control to protect Linux. Each organization will have to look at the specific requirements for themselves.

Application Configurations

Whether Windows, Linux, or phone, making applications secure sometimes involves configuring them to ensure that they are set up properly. IIS and Apache, for example, have very specific guidelines that CIS provides. In many other cases secure configuration guidelines have to be created by the vendor or by the organization that uses the applications. The process is not unlike the recommendation for creating IoMT standards. Looking at other CIS baselines can really help point the way for application configurations. Of course, knowledge of encryption standards, ACL configurations, identity (which is covered in the next chapter), and so on are all very critical to creating application configuration standards.

The real challenge here is, how do you configure all of these applications? Organizations can have thousands of them. It simply is not reasonable to configure them all, so a general strategy needs to be formed.

From a security standpoint, it is important to focus on the most critical systems first. One reasonable strategy is to follow the data. What systems have access to the data? How much data do those systems have access to? The more you can set up strong security configurations on those systems, the better off you are.

A few of you may be thinking that IT has access to all of those systems. You would be right to point that out. In fact, most compliance frameworks mandate that how IT teams access the environments be part of the scope of the assessment. If IT teams have access to the data, that access is very important from both a risk perspective and a compliance perspective.

There is no way for any organization to be 100% perfect with their applications, but striving to be as close to perfect as possible is a critical part of IT hygiene. Sometimes just creating gates to let only certain software in is a mechanism to reduce the risk posed not only by the applications, but also to IoMT devices and covered entities.

Firewall Configurations

Many of the major vendors have CIS standards that organizations can follow. There are two other challenging parts of firewall configurations—reading the basic firewall configurations and the associated ACLs. If you remember from Chapter 10, ACLs are the central key to the firewalls, and there can be a small or large number of ACLs. What makes monitoring them a bit more challenging is that what ought to be in the ACLs will be different depending on the environment—especially if a portion of the firewall is used to block of VLANs with IoMT. Many of the powerful tools have been discussed in Chapter 10.

Mobile Device Misconfigurations

Mobile devices are an interesting from a configuration management standpoint for multiple reasons, some of which have been covered in previous chapters, but important to emphasize here because they can have a direct impact on the configuration management strategy. For example, we touched on applications that listen in on conversations. Knowing that, would you want those applications as part of the overall IoMT strategy for a hospital? How would that impact the BYOD strategy that some covered entities utilize? Surely organizations that employ BYOD would not want to prevent someone from having Facebook on their personal devices?

But the concerns are not just about that. Multiple types of malware may be on personal devices that can make mobile devices a likely location for loss of information. With BYOD, companies need to accept that possibility. Organizations need to perform a risk assessment about the likelihood of data being lost and what the potential impacts can be—especially if mobile devices are part of the IoMT ecosystem or if data is being accessed through a mobile device. It is important to keep in mind that the HIPAA requirements are not designed for specific systems, but systems in general. One oversight of organizations is to bypass requirements for mobile devices because they seem less consequential.

From a legal standpoint, though, the configuration requirements are quite important. For example, the University of Rochester Medical Center was fined $3 million for failure to encrypt laptops and thumb drives.[10] These requirements apply to mobile phones every bit as much as other devices. If the same PHI was on a cell phone, the results may have been very similar for the University of Rochester Medical Center (or any covered entity).

Fortunately for covered entities, CIS does have configuration benchmarks for most major cell phone manufacturers. The benchmarks include encrypting mobile devices and are therefore sufficient. In a way, the real challenge when it comes to mobile devices are all of those extra applications, just as the ACLs are a major challenge for firewalls.

In the end, MDM solutions can handle all these kinds of challenges from a technical perspective. That said, mobile devices are a bit challenging because compensating controls are not possible—everything needs to be on the device in order to protect it.

Database Configurations

Most of the major databases have CIS configurations, so on a certain level it is a bit easier to follow the guidelines to set up the database securely. It is important to note that there is a distinction between a database server and a database. A database server can have hundreds of databases on it—each one needing to be encrypted. This particular need may be based on the type of data in the database. If it is sensitive data such as PHI, obviously it needs to be encrypted. Distinguishing which

---

[10] "Failure to Encrypt Mobile Devices Leads to $3 Million HIPAA Settlement," Health and Human Services Press Release, 2016, https://www.hhs.gov/about/news/2019/11/05/failure-to-encrypt-mobile-devices-leads-to-3-million-dollar-hipaa-settlement.html.

databases need to be encrypted and which cannot can sometimes be a challenge and requires working closely with the IT teams.

The other consideration is that databases are connected to other tools—quite often with a website front end (which may or may not be internet facing). Ensuring that the connection between the website front end (or comparable) and the database server is also encrypted is critical to setting the system up securely.

Configuration Drift

Anyone who has ever been through an audit that looks at configurations in detail will tell you that configurations change over time—even in the best environment. This is change is called configuration drift. Administrators or engineers deal with emergency situations, and they make changes in order to get their work done more efficiently. Maybe they made 40 different changes—trying things to get something to work over the course of hours. Striving to remember every change in situations like this can be challenging to say the least.

The end result is that configurations change over time—even in highly secure environments. All it takes is one engineer failing to recognize the importance of a security configuration when making a change to allow a system to be compromised. These innocent mistakes happen all the time. People make mistakes, or they are unaware of how closely IT and cybersecurity are related. This goes back to the lack of security training in schools, which we've discussed several times in this book.

Configuration Tools

If it isn't clear, configuration management can be overwhelming—even if the covered entity is only monitoring the security settings. Clearly, because of configuration drift, the "set it and forget it" mentality is not the right approach. Even if a covered entity had only 100 systems to monitor (a very small number for hospitals), this would be an impossible feat to keep up with manually. As a result, tools should be used to monitor those configurations on a periodic basis.

There are configuration management tools built into vulnerability management systems. These tend to focus on minimal configurations within operating systems, but they are an excellent place to start when building a configuration management program. Most cover the operating systems and the standard web servers for the operating systems. They also tend to focus on CIS. The obvious drawback is that they cannot scan network devices, components of some kinds of IoMT, and mobile devices. They also cannot holistically monitor changes beyond the security configurations.

Some companies utilize MDM tools, which have the advantage of being good at monitoring and configuring mobile devices at the same time. They can also be very selective about the specific applications they allow on the systems.

File Integrity Monitoring (FIM) is another strategy, which, depending on the vendor, has some huge advantages on vulnerability management tools. FIM tools basically monitor systems for changes in files—an excellent way of determining if unauthorized changes are being made to systems if compared against change management. They tend to be much broader in scope in that they can monitor not only CIS configurations, but a range of different options, so other changes that are made within change control system can be monitored against the changes that are actually made. FIM systems can also monitor network device configurations and many types of IoMT. This makes FIM tools the natural fit for more mature configuration management programs.

Some firewall vendors have configuration management capabilities as an addon component to the core firewall, which is useful for those that do not have a corresponding CIS standard. This simplifies many of the more complex aspects of managing firewall configurations. There are also tools designed specifically to look at network security systems for CIS and other standards. Depending on the compatibility with the vendors, this is another good mechanism for defending organizations. Of course, those tools typically do not look at IoMT configurations.

IT automation tools are sometimes used to validate configurations, but the challenge with this approach is that many of those tools are great at implementing changes, but do not have the best monitoring validation mechanisms—sometimes only supplying a set of logs. Logs are great for incident response, but poring through thousands of logs to determine gaps can eat up countless hours, and they are not necessarily the best tools for validating and demonstrating changes.

Exception Management

If mistakes are not uncommon, how should organizations handle configuration drift? The way to handle it is through an exception management process and to monitor. For each configuration item, think about how the organization relates to that configuration. How do they monitor that a configuration is off? People may forget if they have to perform an extra level of due diligence. For example, when dealing with a time-out on access to a network device, 10 minutes might seem like a long time to not make any changes, but administrators can be hopping from device to device making network connections. Ten minutes is not such a long time in that situation. As a result, network administrators may change the time to infinite or disable the function so they can do their jobs. Because of these and other reasons, configuration management can be a little more complex as the systems change over time. Oftentimes changes like these are not captured in the change management system.

Organizations will have to decide how they proceed. Do they change the logon time for devices to be longer than 10 minutes, or do they continue to push for the 10 minutes? The answer might be that it depends on the context. Maybe the best way to handle the situation is allow an exception for a few minutes, but then change it back. Then again, if you allow for an exception, how do you know the change will be reverted? These exceptions are a small part of what leads to configuration drift. Having the right oversite related to exceptions is crucial.

Enterprise Considerations

In the past several years companies have been buying up many of the smaller companies in an attempt to grow into juggernaut organizations. Such centralization means in the long run greater centralization and to some degree standardization, in that while there are numerous types of IoMT systems, companies tend to standardize on one type of vendor for one type of IoMT to simplify the overall environment for organizations in the long run. The obvious challenge here is that the longevity of IoMT devices can mean that the standardization can take years to achieve. But it also means that, more often than not, security will increase over a period of time because the concerns of security are amplified across environments.

In Summary

On the surface, IT hygiene seems like it is a very simple proposition—just do the right thing. For many organizations, however, wanting to do the right thing and actually doing the right thing are metaphorical oceans to cross. Outside considerations such as doctor preferences for specific IoMT devices, budget constraints, etc., can lead to additional pressures preventing companies from doing the right thing.

All considered, IT hygiene is a way of greatly reducing vulnerabilities and is a very critical part of protecting organizations. Without at least some semblance of IT hygiene, hackers have almost free reign, which means more theft of data and more ransomware. Even if there are exceptions to the overall processes due to manufacturer requirements, the more organizations can do to protect themselves, the better off they will be in the long run.

Basic hygiene also includes looking at accounts that IT administrators may use, password hygiene, and a host of other identity-related considerations. Due to the volume of information on the topic, identity and access management are covered in the next chapter.

CHAPTER 13

Identity and Access Management

If you reveal your secrets to the wind, you should not
blame the wind for revealing them to the trees.
—Kahlil Gibran

Identity and Access Management (I&AM) is a critical aspect of cybersecurity in general, but also for protecting IoMT. Part of what attackers do is compromise accounts. Once they have done that, they can move virtually invisibly within organizations because the behavior comes from a known and/or authorized account. The attackers then can then determine the whole layout of the organization, see all the server names, and make modifications with impunity. While the goal might be to compromise an administrative user (one with higher privileges), often hackers will escalate the privilege of existing accounts to accomplish their nefarious goals.

Understanding why I&AM is so important does not really explain how to protect these various accounts. For some, it is a full-time profession, but essentially it is the practice of managing account life cycles and access including the various authentication functions. In short, it is the totality of the governance of accounts related to identity. It includes everything from password management, authentication mechanisms, setting up and removing accounts, and the various technical measures to interconnect accounts over a broad range of systems.

Today's IT systems are much broader than they were 20 years ago with the advent of cloud technologies, IoT (including IoMT), and others. They now require a layering of technologies to appropriately administer and access. The proliferation of these technologies also creates a slew of challenges for the end user. As a result, many new technologies have been developed to compensate for this critical, but partially disparate technical world. But let's start with an understanding of how minimal identity practices can affect the security of covered entities and IoMT devices.

Minimal Identity Practices

Most of us are familiar with usernames (referred to as accounts in the IT world) and passwords from having to log in to our home or work computers, mobile devices, websites, and so on. It seems very straightforward, but behind the scenes in the IT and security space, there is much more to it than that. There are many different kinds of accounts—local computer accounts, directory (also referred to as domain) accounts, application accounts, physical access accounts, IoMT accounts, service accounts, and identity-related technologies such as single sign-on. What most people are aware of is only the tip of the iceberg, and not having strong identity-related practices regarding accounts can lead to serious problems. As mentioned in Chapter 5, hackers will try to compromise accounts as part of their strategy to steal data and/or utilize ransomware against a covered entity—mostly because once an attacker has an account, the actions from that account seems more legitimate.

In a perfect world, as soon as someone leaves an organization, the account associated with that person is disabled so they cannot gain any further access. However, people may have access to a range of different accounts—not just the login to their corporate computer and phone. Many organizations (covered entities or not) have a plethora of cloud systems that they may utilize, which can also be a large risk (depending on the system). If a specific person has access to 20 clouds, that requires 20-plus systems to log in to in order to remove their access— assuming that an organization knows about all the access an individual may have. The same can be said for internal systems that covered entities utilize. The bigger the covered entity, the more systems there may be in use, and not all of them connect into internal authentication systems. The disparate nature of identity makes it, in many large organizations, a tremendous challenge to handle effectively.

But so far, we have only been skimming the surface of access. People in organizations are given access rights based on their roles in the company, from normal user rights to administrator privileges, where they can make whatever changes they want to the system. For example, a Windows Administrator may have full administrative access to Windows servers. However, people can have multiple roles within an organization, with varying levels of access privileges, which can make monitoring them very complicated. Position's change, people are transferred, or people may leave the company, all of which can make identity management difficult. Let's explore some of the options related to different accounts.

Local Accounts

Local accounts are probably the easiest to understand for most people. A local account is an account that is on the device you are working on. So, the account that you made on your home computer is a local account. The account you have to log in to your phone is a local account. Easy, right?

While easy to understand, local accounts are both good and bad from a corporate security perspective. The local accounts are good for two reasons. First, local accounts can be used as emergency accounts in case a domain is not available. They can also have specific machine privileges that are tied only to a user and the machine that is configured to that specific user. Both are good for special situations. They are bad because tracking them can be tricky and disabling accounts in the case of hostile termination can be problematic. It is much better to do this on a domain level because it only needs to be done once to terminate access across the board.

Unfortunately, some IoMT systems require local accounts and not domain accounts. That can create a great number of challenges. If someone with multiple IoMT passwords leaves, either the organization will need to use an automated system to change access to those accounts or someone will need to change each account manually—a time-consuming, painstaking, error-prone process. Some organizations also only use local accounts, which can be problematic from an administration standpoint.

Domain/Directory Accounts

Domain or directory accounts are very different from local accounts. Think of them as a set of accounts that can be used across multiple connected machines. If one machine goes down, the user need only log in to another machine on the domain (using the same credentials) in order to access resources. This would not be possible with local accounts. Further, if someone leaves the company or is fired, domain accounts can be disabled centrally, which makes them some of the easiest accounts to manage.

Service Accounts

Service accounts are somewhat similar to user accounts, but they are primarily used by applications and not people. The privileges and purpose should be different to reflect those needs. Unfortunately, in some organizations, user accounts are used as service accounts without modifying privileges. Since many people have service account passwords, that can be a real challenge for organizations unless they purchase a special tool to rotate those passwords. Additionally, changing those passwords can be detrimental to system stability as it takes a great deal of coordination to change passwords—especially for always-on accounts. Years ago, before modern tools, those accounts used to keep the same password for years, which is risky because a former employee may remember or keep service account passwords and maintain access to company resources long after they leave the organization.

IoMT Accounts

IoMT devices have a range of identity challenges depending on the device or the overall system. Some IoMT have no accounts and anyone can use the system. This type of IoMT device typically has no security, but occasionally there are important settings that anyone can modify. In other cases, the IoMT accounts are hard-coded into the system along with the password. This means that the password does not and cannot change. Anyone can search for the password online and then use the system. This is a huge security issue that makes protecting the device almost impossible. Still other devices do have configurable usernames and passwords, but someone needs to log into the device and configure each device manually—sometimes physically and sometimes by connecting to the device over the network. Either way, the impracticality often means that organizations do not want to take the time to change the passwords, which presents yet another challenge to adequately protecting IoMT. The IoMT devices that connect into Active Directory are actually a dream because in these situations, the accounts can be managed centrally—along with the passwords.

Physical Access Accounts

Physical access accounts are accounts that provide physical access to an environment. There are a while range of options for how this is accomplished. In some cases there is a physical access card with RFID that registers the owner of the card and provides the appropriate level of access. Hotels often use physical access cards, but often organizations do the same thing. Unfortunately, many organizations do not take the time to review the physical access in depth. Physical access accounts are just as critical as other account to review. Physical access to a device usually means you can completely control it—IoMT or not. Reviewing the physical access to a location is a critical part of cybersecurity, especially to data centers or other locations that may have infrastructure that is critical to the well-being of an organization.

From a physical security perspective, IoMT accounts are in a unique situation because almost anyone can walk into a hospital claiming to be visiting a patient and then literally walk up to a device and start using it. Of course, the extent to which this is true is completely dependent on the access controls of the device. In some cases, a simple internet search is enough for a cybercriminal to gain access. In other cases, they may have to reset the specifications back to factory default, but then can gain access. In the end, the physicality of the devices and the other characteristics makes protecting IoMT systems from harm that much more difficult. Luckily, most people enter the hospital for benevolent purposes, so the likelihood of someone doing this is low, but certainly present. As a result, staying on top of the security of IoMT is all the more critical.

Cloud Accounts

The cloud, like every other system, has accounts that are tied to their use. The critical cloud accounts are the portal accounts. Those accounts, especially for PaaS and IaaS, almost literally have the power of a full data center in them in many cases. Those accounts should be monitored and protected as much as humanly possible. SaaS accounts, while typically less impactful, can also be a big concern for the organization. As a result, monitoring these accounts is dependent on the specific business purpose, but monitored the cloud accounts and ensuring that only authorized people have access is extremely critical.

Consultants, Contractors, and Vendor Accounts

Consultant, contractor, and vendor accounts are often among the most challenging to work with for a variety of reasons. First, the work is often short term or ad hoc, and these accounts are often not tracked the way other accounts are in a centralized fashion. For example, an IT consultant may have their account set up by the IT team. The only team that may know what they have access to is the person who set up the account for that consultant. In some organizations, human resources is the go-to location for employees (and thus accounts). But what happens if there is no centralized authority and a distributed model is used to "manage" accounts? This is how accounts become forgotten or overlooked within organizations. In these cases, the accounts can stay active well after a person has left the organization, which can be a cybersecurity nightmare. In the end, these kinds of accounts affect the identity governance process (discussed next).

Identity Governance

It is important to distinguish between administration and governance of accounts. In simple terms, administration includes account creation, account modification, and account removal. Governance includes all of the validation activities—the reviews of accounts that take place to ensure that they do not have excess privileges and should not be disabled and/ or removed (per company policy). This may sound easy, but in many cases, because of the complexities of IoMT and the disparate nature of systems, identity governance can be an absolute nightmare to do the proper way. The centralized systems are easy to pull data from, but by the time you consider IoMT, various cloud services, unique independent systems, old operating systems, and the different kinds of accounts, it can be an almost impossible task.

Getting the most current information is only a small part of the challenge. How do you know what role people are in and what access rights you should measure against to ensure appropriate access? What are the sources you need to visit to know what consultants and contractors should have access? There can be a large range of people who are able to authorize access to resources, but they do not necessarily look at the big picture when doing so. That can make security assessments of those access rights egregiously imperfect in many cases. Oftentimes organizations accept the imperfect assessments because of resource limitations.

Just because the assessments are imperfect doesn't mean that strategy cannot be applied to those assessments. Maybe account reviews are not done appropriately every quarter, but over the course of a year, a full review can be performed. Maybe only privileged accounts, the most sensitive accounts in an organization are reviewed on a regular basis. Sadly, many organizations do not even go this far in their processes, which leaves them more vulnerable than they need to be.

Assessments are just the first step in the governance part of the process, though. You find some problems, but then those problems need to be remediated. The highest priority in a hospital is human life. Quite often there isn't enough staff to do more than deal with the high-priority problems, which can make it difficult to take care of a seemingly small need like disabling that account of someone who no longer works there. In these cases, authentication is where we have to look to help defend the modern hospital.

Authentication

At its most basic, authentication is the process of validating a particular user. Typically, this is done through passwords, and in today's world, it is a critical part of cybersecurity. As discussed previously, the recent Solar Winds hack may be partially the result of a poor password.[1] If authentication is done right, it can be used to protect people's accounts from being taken over, hackers from getting into systems, and so on. There are mistakes that organizations make along the way related to authentication. Some of them are a result of the older operating systems that IoMT devices use. We'll explore these issues together.

Password Pain

Although imperfect, passwords are here to stay. Everyone uses them for most devices and every cybersecurity professional has an opinion on them. Most work environments have policies that require a minimum of eight-character passwords, with least one of each of the following: one uppercase letter, one lowercase letter, one special character, and one number. These minimal requirements are echoed by many compliance

---

[1] Brian Fung, Geneva Sands, "Former SolarWinds CEO blames intern for 'solarwinds123' password leak," February 26, 2021, https://www.cnn.com/2021/02/26/politics/solarwinds123-password-intern/index.html.

frameworks today—some do have more stringent password require-ments, especially for servers as opposed to workstations.

But this is just the beginning of most password policies. Usually, pass-words need to be changed periodically—90 days is a standard time frame—but many users actively dislike having to do that. Some people change their password to follow the policy, but then just change it back again to the original password. To combat this, most requirements make it impos-sible for users to reuse the same password until after a certain number of iterations, or don't allow them to be changed more than once a day.

Failed logins are also a consideration for passwords. Oftentimes an account will be set to lock after a number of failed logon attempts. While this can be annoying for the end user, it does prevent hackers from exe-cuting a large number of password-based attacks against an account. This methodology is referred to as a *brute-force attack*, where hackers use a piece of software to force their way into accounts by using lists of passwords. If an account has a weak password and few other protective measures in place, it can be hacked over time. Sometimes hackers will use a low and slow methodology to hack into accounts, meaning they will only try a few passwords a day in order to avoid detection or trip-ping some of the controls in place. This usually is the hallmark of a good hacker, because brute-forcing accounts as quickly and noisily as possible can attract a lot of attention from security systems.

Hackers have other password-cracking tools at their disposal. For example, many people reuse passwords between work and home accounts, and the passwords on home accounts can often remain in place indef-initely. By using a combination of stolen passwords (often sold on the dark web) and looking at social media to see where people work, hackers can effectively buy access to a corporate environment

Before we talk about the next tool, it may be helpful to talk a bit about password storage. On systems, passwords are stored for a variety of different reasons. In a properly set up Windows environment, Win-dows passwords are stored in Active Directory—essentially on a server. In today's mobile age, this is not reasonable. If someone is on a plane with their laptop, the password has to also be stored not only in Active Directory, but also on the laptop—otherwise an end user cannot log in. This is a configurable setting that, for most users, happens automatically, and they do not need to think about it.

These passwords are reasonably protected. Windows both salts (adds one or more extra characters) and hashes (electronically fingerprints) the password with the hash. The hash value is then stored. When someone logs in, Windows adds the salt, creates a hash, and matches the hash against the hash for that username. If they match, the user is permitted to log in. While ingenious, this system is not impervious to hackers. If a hacker hacks into a system, one of the common things they do is go after accounts and passwords. They want that hash value. Toward that end, there are a number of password crackers that hackers can use to crack that account. These password crackers go through possible passwords creating and matching a hash. This can be time-consuming, but the shorter the password, the faster it is to crack the password. For example, the 7-character password of "abcdefg" would take less than a millisecond to crack. The 12-character password of "abcdefghikjl" would take upwards of 2 centuries. The longer the password, the more difficult they are to compromise. Adding complexity into the password (uppercase, lowercase, numbers, and special characters) also increases the time it takes to compromise an account. For example, if "Password" was a password, it would take a few seconds to crack. If the password is "P@ssw0rD," that can take 14 years to crack.[2]

To speed the process, hackers use something called rainbow tables. Rainbow tables are simply lists of computed hash values and the associated password. If the hash matches the hash within Windows, that can provide an attacker with the password. It can speed up the compromise time of an account immeasurably. Of course, the larger the salt value, the more rainbow tables will be required to crack the password. The number of tables depends on the size and complexity of the password and the size of the salt added to the password. In short, though, if enough hash values are kept on the hacker's system, all they have to do is find the corresponding hash within their tables, and they have the password for the system.

It should not be a surprise that IoMT devices may or may not meet these password requirements. In fact, many of them do not. As pointed out in Chapter 2, many IoMT devices have hard-coded passwords. Hackers, in those cases, do not even need to hack them. They can just look on the manufacturer's site and log in. In Windows, there is a setting to lock accounts if someone fails to type their password correctly after a few tries—thus limiting brute-force password logins. Once an account is locked, even the person with the correct password cannot log into the systems. IoMT often do not have nuanced approaches to password security that other systems have. These oversights represent greater risks

---

[2]https://www.betterbuys.com/estimating-password-cracking-
times/#:~:text=Nine-character%20passwords%20take%20
five,bad%20for%20one%20little%20letter.

to covered entities. If you have a front door with a lock but the key is in the door, that lock does not do much good.

Passwords still have value in today's world, but that value is diminishing, especially with key loggers that steal usernames and passwords. As a result, alternate technologies were developed to help mitigate these threats to authentication-mainly multi-factor authentication, which we will explore next.

Multi-factor Authentication

Multi-factor authentication (MFA) is security's answer to the compromises from using usernames and passwords alone. As any cybersecurity expert will tell you, when it comes to MFA, there are three general factors for authentication—something you have, something you know, and something you are. Something you have is a security token, bank card, key, etc. A good example of something you know is a password or a PIN. Something you are refers to your biology—fingerprint, retinal pattern, and so on. Using two or more of these factors to authenticate to a device greatly reduces the risk of an attacker gaining unauthorized access.

But let us dive a bit deeper into the specifics of MFA because those specifics matter. For the purposes of this discussion, we'll assume that a standard password is in place. Any of the factors we will discuss can be used by themselves as a single factor. In fact, many covered entities only use a second factor as an authentication mechanism, which certainly violates the purpose of having MFA to begin with. This is not intended to be a complete list nor anything close. The National Institute of Standards and Technology (NIST) has done a reasonable job at that.[3] The purpose here is to explore a few of the more popular MFA technologies and relate them to basic security considerations.

Hard Tokens

Starting with the most secure tokens first, the hard token comes in several different forms, but generally speaking it is a physical token that demonstrates that you have that physical device. Sometimes it is a USB key fob that must be plugged into a computer in order to allow authentication. In other cases it is a simple device that shows a series of numbers on the screen for a one-minute period of time that are often used in conjunction

---

[3] The National Institute of Standards and Technology, https://pages.nist.gov/800-63-3/sp800-63b.html.

with a password in order to log in. After that one-minute period of time, the numbers change, and the old numbers are no longer valuable.

In all cases, hard tokens must be mailed or physically handed to someone. They are not software to be installed (see "Soft Tokens"). They are more secure because they are usually not connected to a device and cannot be hacked in most instances. The only thing a hacker can do is hack the MFA server for something called a seed file, which provides the mechanism to determine what the MFA codes will be. If that is compromised, the only thing that can be done to protect yourself is create a new seed file and physically send the user a new hard token.

The challenge with hard tokens is administration. The hard tokens need to be aligned to a specific user account and physically handed to someone or physical mailed to them through the post office. While reasonably secure, this is a heavy administrative burden. If a company had thousands of people needing MFA, a project like that can take months or more to just send out the tokens. It just is not feasible in many cases. Further, hard tokens can be lost or run out of power, which means there is a high total cost of ownership to maintain the program.

Soft Tokens

Soft tokens are very similar to hard tokens except that they are software based and are installed on a computer or a cell phone. They do not have the administrative burden that hard tokens have because the end user can do the installation. They often offer a series of numbers that can be typed in, the same as a hard token.

From an administrative perspective, soft tokens are much easier to manage that hard tokens. First of all, depending on the solution, the end user can set up the account, which means administrative staff do not need to go through the process of setting up the accounts. If the solution does need to be set up, the tokens do not need to be mailed out to the individual as is required for hard tokens. This makes the process much more palatable to IT staff.

Soft tokens, as they are more connected to computers, are more easily hacked. If a laptop or cell phone is compromised, there is a high degree of probability that the second factor on that device is also compromised. More often than not, it is the laptop that is compromised, so many cybersecurity professionals recommend having the second factor on a separate device such as a cell phone.

Authenticator Applications

Like the soft token, the authenticator application can be installed on a computer or a cell phone, but they are considered a little less secure because they involve a bit more human interaction (someone clicking a button). In the authentication process, the system will send an alert to an end user. The end user must accept or reject that authentication attempt. An attacker, who has one set of account credentials, can trip the system into making a secondary alert that the end user can accept or reject. If a user is caught off guard, they may think the system is being glitchy and accept the authentication attempt—not realizing they are letting in a cybercriminal onto the network.

Short Message Service

Short Message Service (SMS) is essentially a text message you get with the second factor that you need to type into a website in order to gain access. In reality it is turning something you have into something that is sent over to you—unlike soft or hard tokens. SMS is far less secure than any of the other forms for a variety of reasons. Since the code is sent to you, it can be intercepted. Codes for cell phones can be bounced all over the world and read by a large number of organizations. There are a host of other attacks against cell phones that companies are concerned with where a determined hacker can go after specific cell phones. While these attacks are far less common, they do point to further concerns with cell phone usage for MFA.

QR Codes

A QR code is a machine-readable code that has a series of black and white squares on a square background that is scanned by cell phones. QR codes are not unlike barcodes except that they contain far more information. COVID-19 has accelerated the use of QR codes by creating a link to a menu. Instead of having a physical menu that may pass COVID-19, many people can just scan the QR code to link them to a website that has the menu. Unfortunately, hackers have added their own QR codes in order to redirect unknowing victims to malicious websites. That said, QR codes can also be used as a second factor in authentication. After adding a username and passwords, a QR code will show up on the screen and require that the user scan the code with a phone in order to log in to a website. Overall, they are a fairly secure second factor because they require a pre-registered secondary device to authenticate against them.

Other Authentication Considerations

Authentication tools are becoming far more sophisticated than they were years ago—even including machine learning in their algorithms. One example is that this can lead to step-up or contextual authentication. For example, systems can recognize the specific laptop that someone uses. They might only need a username or password to log in if they are working at a familiar location. But let's say they travel to a new country; the system may require that they include a second factor in their authentication. After a while, systems may recognize that new location. But if the user logs in from somewhere 5000 miles away from that location within a five-minute period of time, the system can be configured to send an alert to an SOC and require heightened authentication in order for the user to gain access. Similarly, systems can become familiar with times that users log in to various systems. Anything that is out of the behavioral norm for a specific user can require extra authentication. There are a whole host of considerations that can be fed into today's systems that greatly increase the authentication security. Companies should evaluate all of these as part of their overall authentication strategy.

Dealing with Password Pain

As the web has grown, so too has the number of passwords; in many cases there can be hundreds of internal and external connections. Further, many organizations are using SaaS-based offerings. From 2017 statistics, an employee needed to have an average of 191 passwords for their work environment.[4] This causes people to use the same password across multiple systems (a cybersecurity challenge that no CISO would blame the worker for), or write them down, which brings up a whole list of other business issues, such as lost time as a result of needing to change passwords, calling various help desks to reset passwords, and so on. The costs can be staggering to organizations. As a result, new technologies were developed to help offset these challenges, such as password managers and single sign-on (SSO).

Password managers are exactly as the name suggests—they manage passwords. They can also help people create passwords so they can gain access to the systems more easily without having to memorize

---

[4] "Average Business User Has 191 Passwords," November 6, 2017, https://www.securitymagazine.com/articles/88475-average-business-user-has-191-passwords.

191 different ones. In fact, many password managers will generate a long unique password that hackers would be hard-pressed to crack in a reasonable amount of time. They also include links to websites you might commonly use as part of the service—you are just automatically logged in with your complex password.

For many organizations this is not the direction they want users to go. They want to have people automatically log in to resources without the hassle of using a password manager or creating individual passwords. In these cases, SSO is the way to reduce the time it takes to connect into various systems. The short story behind SSO is that it essentially creates a token (which is invisible to the end user), which validates who a user is and allows them to log in automatically. For many organizations, this makes so much sense. It takes passwords out of the equation entirely for end users.

MFA Applicability

MFA is not a direct HIPAA requirement, but it is a powerful tool for reducing authentication and identity-based attacks. In essence, it helps to validate the accounts of people. As HIPAA is not a direct requirement, the next best approach is a risk-based approach. Focusing on the systems that are most exposed and the people who have access to HIPAA data is a great place to start.

Aging Systems

There are quite a few other considerations regarding authentication. Older systems have more vulnerabilities, which give hackers a better chance of getting through poorly developed authentication mechanisms. While this has been stated previously, it is also true within the realm of identity. Older systems just don't have the ability to protect accounts from being compromised. Where possible, upgrades should be made to patch and/or upgrade systems where appropriate.

Privileged Access Management

Privileged Access Management (PAM) is something of a revolution in the I&AM space. If used properly, it has the ability to sharply reduce risk as it is a holistic platform that affects many different aspects of identity. It has become such a powerful part of the identity landscape that identity governance tools integrate PAM into their assessment capabilities. The key thing to note about PAM is the first word—privileged. While many of the technology companies that have a PAM tool have branched out into other identity related technologies, the core of PAM is around privileged accounts. Privileged accounts are generally the accounts that IT teams utilize for doing their day-to-day work—often referred to as administrative accounts.

From a use case perspective, PAM is typically used in the same site as servers and/or other equipment. Users will typically log in to a PAM portal and access the servers they need to use to do their jobs. The permitted access is generally through telnet, SSH, RDP, and HTTP/S, as discussed in other chapters. We'll define some of the backend considerations in this section.

From an IoMT perspective, PAM can be a huge benefit, as often it can be used to set up access to IoMT systems. If the only way to gain access from the network is through PAM, PAM becomes a huge barrier for hackers and an overall win for IoMT security.

Roles

Setting up roles in a PAM environment can save a tremendous amount of work, especially in large organizations. For example, if you have several people with the role Windows Administrator, you could give them all the same access to the Windows servers. If a server is added or removed, it is a simple change to ensure all administrators have access added to or removed from specific servers simultaneously. From an administrative perspective, it is a huge win.

The challenge is that there is a trade-off with some of the PAM technologies. In order to get that role identical, everyone in a specified role must use the same account, not for logging into the PAM servers, but for access from the PAM server to the server the administrator is gaining access to. When looking at the logs on the local server, those logs will show "Windows Administrator" rather than the specific person doing the action. That can add a level of concern from an attribution perspective, but PAM solutions often have compensation mechanisms for this drawback—they can log every action a person takes thus creating attribution to the specific Windows administrator. Many PAM solutions also have the option of recording everything that someone does on a server, which goes much deeper than a log so people can watch what is happening on the backend.

Password Rotation

One of the key capabilities of PAM is the rotation of passwords for accessing a system. For those who think changing a password every 90 days is not sufficient to stop attackers, PAM is the answer. The password can be configured but can change on a daily basis or sometimes with every login. This is a way to thwart the low and slow password attack mechanisms—especially if that password changes with every logon. Another advantage of letting the system rotate the password is that the passwords will probably be more secure as they are created by the randomization function of a machine rather than a person. People are not great at creating passwords because they need to have a password they can remember, which is, more often than not, a little less secure.

MFA Access

There are a few ways to set up MFA access within PAM, depending on the product. First, the web portal that people log in to can have MFA on it. If this is a gateway to systems that cannot have MFA, it is a strong compensating control for lack of MFA on a specific system. Once a user is inside the web portal, MFA can be required to access a specific system. This means that the administrator will have to type a username, password, and MFA credentials in order to access the target system. Alternatively, administrators can click on the system they are accessing, and the password and MFA can be used to automatically log in to the local system. Whatever organizations choose, it is a win from a multi-factor authentication perspective.

Adding Network Security

In part, PAM can be thought of as an access gateway because it can be used for others to gain access, but in combination with network considerations, it can be a powerful means of keeping hackers out of important parts of the network. If you think back a couple of chapters on the flat network, think about the benefit if the only way to access IoMT from an administrative perspective is to access the IoMT devices through PAM. Of course, not all IoMT devices can be set up this way, but for those that can, it can greatly reduce risk.

Other I&AM Technologies

There are a range of technologies to help organizations cope with all aspects of the identity process. They can help with everything from the basic administration of accounts through the full governance process—including cloud accounts and sometimes IoMT accounts. The technologies can also tie together a range of disparate systems to reduce the administrative burden.

Identity Centralization

One of the most critical functions of identity management is centralization. This is especially important in cases of hostile termination. Let's go back to that 191-passwords per employee example. If 100 of those accounts are cloud passwords and there is a hostile termination, that leaves 100+ systems that may be subject to an attack by a disgruntled employee. The teams disabling the accounts related to that employee would need to access a hundred cloud accounts—and that is assuming they are even aware of what could accounts are in place. At a certain point, decentralization is just not the best way of handling these identity related risks. The more systems that can be centralized, the better off organizations will be.

A whole range of technologies are available on the market for centralization. Windows and Linux have centralized directories, and Microsoft also has AzureAD, which helps with cloud-based connections. There are also solutions that connect those identity centralization capabilities. SSO, for its part, is also considered a mechanism for centralization because it helps to interconnect those various environments, whether internal or external systems such as cloud. There are also a host of other possibilities such as LDAP integration, Federation, and so on. The point here is that there are a range of solutions that can be used alone or in concert to help bring accounts and identities together. The more organizations can do to interconnect the systems, the less overall work the organization will need to do.

It's important to keep in mind that, especially with IoMT, everything you can do to increase the security will slow potential hackers down a little and help reduce the risks related to IoMT, hospital environments, and the associated data.

Identity Management

In many ways, identity management tools really help to simplify the work of setting up accounts. For example, say an IoMT engineer is starting at a company. Ordinarily, this person might need access to 200+ different systems. Using one of these tools, the administrator would simply have to click a button and the work would be done—all the connections for the IoMT engineer would be set up on the backend automatically. While this might be a slight exaggeration of how clean and efficient most operations are, the point is that identity management tools save companies a tremendous amount of time setting up accounts.

They do not make sense for every covered entity, however. There is a cost-benefit analysis that organizations should make to see if they would be worthwhile. A small doctor's office with two computers is not a good candidate in most circumstances for these kinds of tools. The larger the organization, the better fit they typically are.

Identity Governance Tools

Identity governance tools are often tied into identity management tools, but not always. Essentially, identity governance tools are designed to be a check against the identity management process. They too can be a huge help to IT teams even though they are not involved in the direct administration. They can be used to pull information automatically out of accounts and match them against the level of access they ought to have, terminated users, and so on. Without an identity governance tool, the IT teams may need to collect information from an array of different sources and send that information back to another team for analysis, which is a painful process. Analyzing that information can also mean hours of work that could be better spent on other activities. In the end, for many organizations, these kinds of tools make perfect sense.

Password Tools

There is currently a great deal of innovation in the identity technology space. Passwords are no exception. There are tools on the market that can block an array of different habits that standard users make. For example, some solutions can block leet. Some password tools can capture the different variations of leet to make it harder for people to use common passwords. Other tools help with the basic dictionary, but they may also import names as well in order to prevent people from using names they have heard around the world. Better yet, other tools capture stolen passwords that are found on the dark web and prevent people from reusing them. The list goes on for various features, but all of them are good for helping to protect organizations.

In Summary

For those who are outside of IT, I&AM probably seems like a very simple subject—usernames and passwords. Mature places will include MFA. The reality, though, is far from simple. With a heavy shift toward cloud-based systems and a proliferation of a variety of different options, I&AM has become a very critical part of both the IT and security departments. Without mature identity practices, covered entities are far more likely to be compromised.

There is a tremendous amount of knowledge about what works and what does not in the industry. Reading the right reports or communicating with others in the industry is a critical part of deciding on what strategy to use to protect organizations. Further, practicing due diligence and due care within the I&AM space can help organizations significantly reduce their footprint in regards to I&AM vulnerabilities.

This leads us to our next topic—threat and vulnerability. I&AM represents only one such area of threat—a critical one, but it is far from complete when understanding the complexities of risk. Threats and vulnerabilities deserve special attention and are the subject of our next chapter.

Threat and Vulnerability

Even the bravest cyber defense will experience defeat
when weaknesses are neglected.

—Stephane Nappo

We have spent a great deal of time discussing how IoMT devices are vulnerable, how they do not meet HIPAA or other privacy regulations, how they can be used to compromise other systems, the challenges related to anonymized data, and so on. While these are fairly recent issues, the problems center more around the sheer volume of IoMT devices, which has had a tremendous impact from a threat and vulnerability perspective.

What exactly are vulnerabilities beyond a technical flaw that allows hackers to attack organizations? What can organizations do about vulnerabilities, and how do they relate to IoMT? Are there any special challenges related to IoMT? How do covered entities manage vulnerabilities? These and many more questions will be answered in this chapter.

Part of managing vulnerabilities is about more than the vulnerabilities themselves. It is about managing the corresponding risks. This can mean many different things to different people. For some it is about the techniques, while for others it is about the various kinds of threats that may come from the threat actors. In this chapter we will explore some of the technologies that help organizations identify and reduce vulnerabilities and how those technologies and processes fit together to help companies reduce their overall risk.

247

Vulnerability Management

Throughout this book we have talked about the challenges that organizations face due to highly vulnerable IoMT devices. In short, they make organizations much more susceptable to cyberattacks. As IoMT devices that cannot be updated keep piling on the vulnerabilities, how do you handle that as an organization? How important are 100 critical vulnerabilities versus 200 critical vulnerabilities? In both hypothetical cases, a hacker can gain control of the device. If there is nothing you can do, what good is analyzing the problem? It becomes a metaphorical sinkhole within the organization. This is yet another challenge that healthcare organizations are facing today because of IoMT devices.

Traditional Infrastructure Vulnerability Scans

When most people talk about vulnerability scanning, they are referring to infrastructure—scanning specific systems for vulnerabilities, such as operating systems, network devices, servers, and often the applications on these devices. Twenty years ago, the central approach was to use a tool that performed an agentless scan. Essentially, these tools would "scan" a range of IP addresses that had been configured for a particular system and send out a modified attack to see if the system would detect a vulnerability. An agentless scan is a scan without agent (modern scanners all utilize agents). They scanned over the open internet to detect vulnerabilities. These early scanners were very "noisy," meaning that anyone monitoring the logs could see these attacks taking place because thousands of ports were being scanned.

In those days, the scans were full of false positives—the result would show that the system appeared to be vulnerable, but it was not. In many cases, the analyst looking at the results would have to resort to other methods to determine if it was a true positive (the finding was real) or if the finding was false. To make that determination, analysts needed to validate the patch level or download another tool. It was a time-intensive and painful process.

Today, the systems are much better than they were 20 years ago. They utilize an agent, which is basically a program that connects back to a vulnerability scanner to report on the issue. It validates if something is a true positive or a false positive, which is a huge advantage over agentless scanners. The work that analysts had to do by hand 20 years ago is done automatically today. That does not mean that there are no false positives, however. On the contrary, if a patch is deployed on a system and it skips a minor step (which does happen), the vulnerability management system may report a false positive. These are more the exceptions than the rule, which is a vast improvement.

There are also tools that use a *dissolvable* agent, which is an agent that temporarily installs itself on a computer, performs a scan, sends the information back to a central console, and then deletes itself. When it comes to some types of IoMT devices, this is a huge advantage because it gets around the "no installation" rule on a specific system. Again, this does not work with all IoMT devices, but it can be a way of determining the vulnerabilities for some of them—especially operating systems.

One of the other advantages of modern vulnerability management products is that they usually describe how to remediate them. This is extremely helpful to both the IT and the security teams for knowing what to do as a result. Twenty years ago, this was not always the case.

Traditional Application Vulnerability Scans

Application vulnerability scanning primarily applies to web applications. Dynamic Application Security Testing (DAST) scanning tools can be used to scan live websites to determine vulnerabilities. The scans themselves are very different from their infrastructure cousins. The infrastructure applications can perform a scan within a few minutes, while DAST solutions can run anywhere from a few minutes to hours, or even days, depending on the size of the application. Usually, very large applications are broken down into bite-sized pieces so they do not run more than several hours. DAST is not agent-based; it is typically performed with a username and password for a website (they can be performed without a username and password, but they would be much less effective).

IoMT Vulnerability Challenges

The fact that many IoMT devices cannot have agents installed on them is a challenge for vulnerability management, but what is more challenging is that many IoMT devices cannot be scanned at all. To make matters worse, some IoMT cannot handle the traditional vulnerability scanning—in some cases they can prevent the system from functioning if scanned. As a result, completely new strategies need to be devised.

As covered entities face greater IoMT vulnerability challenges, they are turning to products on the market to fill that void. That market is in the process of maturing, but the central strategy for monitoring IoMT vulnerabilities stems around monitoring packets in the network. We touched on packets in Chapter 10, but the idea behind packet monitoring is that a network monitoring device sits passively inline and monitors the information flow but pays a little closer attention to IoMT. Some of the network monitoring devices will recognize the software versions of the IoMT systems and recommend upgrades. Others are more about specifying the vulnerabilities. Both have merits.

Nonetheless, these alternate strategies for monitoring IoMT are critical for forming action plans to handle IoMT vulnerabilities. Some network monitoring tools will not have viable solutions to the problems they pose. For example, if the vulnerabilities are related to a Windows 7 operating system that cannot be updated because of manufacturer's warrantee requirements, all they can do is recommend an upgrade. In that sense, an organization can void the warrantee and update the device (if there are no technical limitations), install unauthorized software to protect the device, or try some of the strategies discussed in Chapter 10.

Rating Vulnerabilities

The primary rating system for vulnerabilities is called the Common Vulnerability Scoring System (CVSS). CVSS rates the risks based on confidentiality, integrity, and availability, taking into account the attack vector, complexity, the privileges required, and user interaction.

CVSS has undergone many changes over the years, but as of this writing it is on version 3.1. Version 3.1 identifies the risk levels on a scale from 0 to 10, as depicted in Table 14-1.

Table 14-1: CVSS v3.0 Ratings

CVSS V3.0 RATINGS	
None	0.0
Low	0.1–3.9
Medium	4.0–6.9
High	7.0–8.9
Critical	9.0–10.0

Source: National Institute of Standards and Technology, https://nvd.nist.gov/vuln-metrics/cvss

It should be noted that the way that these are scored is by testing, but sometimes the vendors do not provide the transparency required to fully understand the vulnerabilities, so the score is based on the worst-case scenario. Further, the CVSS score does not reflect the risks of a real-world environment. Cybersecurity practitioners should use their judgment based on the context of the vulnerabilities.

It is important to sometimes do a deeper dive into the scores. The scores detailed in Table 14-1 may indicate a huge confidentiality risk, but not necessarily a data integrity risk. A little extra care can help organizations to prioritize the risks, and not just base them on the CVSS score alone.

Vulnerability Management Strategies

Most covered entities do not strive to mitigate all vulnerabilities in their organization. It is not a reasonable business strategy in most cases and can often be a huge waste of resources. Covered entities need to develop strategies for handling these vulnerabilities or face being overwhelmed. The first thing they tend to do is determine how much risk they are willing to absorb. This is a business decision based on their risk appetite—are they willing to take any risk, or just a little risk? Once this is determined, it can be used to provide guidance on what vulnerabilities to remediate and what can be tolerated by the business.

Asset Exposure

One way to strategize around the volume of vulnerabilities is to think about the exposure of the asset. Does a system exposed to the open internet have the same level of risk as an asset buried three levels down in the organization? I am not here to answer that question for a specific organization, as there can be additional considerations. One way to tell is by utilizing the firewall management tools mentioned a couple of chapters ago, but this kind of information is starting to show up in vulnerability management tools as well.

Another way is to check if there are active exploits on the dark web. If there are, the likelihood of the system being exploited naturally increases. Modern vulnerability management tools some add-on solutions can take the feeds from vulnerability management tools and provide this kind of information. Other tools help to focus the output based on modern hacking techniques, to help organizations focus on the most relevant scores.

But the dark web is also important because there may be a known campaign against a specific organization by an APT actor. Knowing that can help organizations determine the likelihood that a specific vulnerability can be compromised. There are companies that specialize in dark-web information that can help along these lines. The best defense is to be aware of all of these vectors and plan accordingly.

Importance

Knowing the importance of assets from a business perspective can also be extremely useful. For example, a particular website may not contain information that can be hacked, but it is the face of the covered entity. The business unit might make the determination that a website without sensitive data may be more important than a website that contains valuable data. In that case maybe similar protections and considerations should be taken into account for that organization.

Websites that contain PHI and PII data are more important from a compliance perspective. The goal of HIPAA and other security and compliance laws is the protection of information. This should be standard for any covered entity as it is built into HIPAA and HITECH.

Both cases can be built into the overall program as variables to consider when selecting what vulnerabilities to remediate and what vulnerabilities to tolerate.

Compensating Controls

Another factor when looking at vulnerabilities are the compensating controls for the weaknesses. For example, some systems have alternate means of accomplish a primary control objective. This may mean that while a specific control may not be in place, such as a patch, hackers cannot exploit the vulnerabilities related to that patch. Understanding the overall environment—with many of the recommendations we have discussed so far, along with programs we have yet to cover—enables organizations to keep in line with not only the vulnerability management strategy, but also the risk management strategy of the organization.

Zero-Day Vulnerabilities

We touched on zero-day vulnerabilities when we spoke about Spectre and Meltdown. In most cases, these kinds of vulnerabilities are simply unknown and cannot be scanned for—nor is there a resolution in many cases. The advantage to knowing about the vulnerability is that there may be compensating controls that can eliminate it. It can also be a separately created ticket—not necessarily managed by a vulnerability management platform. In that sense zero-day vulnerabilities are something of a misnomer—they existed prior to identification, but an attacker (or researcher) found a problem, and the former took advantage of the zero day to the detriment of the covered entity.

In the case of zero-day attacks, it is important to research the particularities of the zero-day as much as possible to figure out how to defend the covered entity and to assess the various risks. Sometimes the risks can be devastating, and sometimes they are not. The strategy for defending against each type of zero-day can be different depending on the specifics.

Less-Documented Vulnerabilities

The vulnerabilities that are published via CVSS scores are far from the only ones. Many pieces of software are not large enough or distributed widely enough to make it into the CVSS scores. There are simply too many different pieces of software and too many small vendors to catch everything. Many of them have not taken the time to enter the CVSS process. Some small IoMT manufacturers may fit into this category and may not even be aware of the vulnerabilities in their products.

For the IoMT and other software products that do not have CVSS scores, sometimes the best way of becoming aware of the vulnerabilities is to sign up for their appropriate mailing lists or make it a habit of reading their website for patching updates. While this will not provide the rich details that the CVSS score provides, cybersecurity experts can make their own estimations about the severity of the risks related to the products.

This is yet another reason why IoMT devices are so challenging to deal with. They may have undocumented vulnerabilities, which makes reporting the vulnerability information to senior management more challenging. It is also another weakness in the managing scheme of things because it is difficult to challenge what is tested by CVSS scores, but if a cybersecurity specialist makes a claim, that claim may need to be supported with specific details—if those details are even available. In the end it may be the difference between doing something about a vulnerable IoMT device or not doing something, as credible information is key and people are fighting for their budgets.

Putting It All Together

Not all these details are important for all covered entities; they are simply options to consider. Sometimes simple is better when it comes to vulnerability remediation. It just depends on the context. It takes some extra care and feeding to properly integrate the information into security programs because of the added complexities of needing to work with IoMT that does not permit standard methods for detecting vulnerabilities.

An important factor related to a mature vulnerability management program is automation of change management tickets. Not all vulnerability management tools are created the same in this capacity. For example, one patch across multiple systems could remediate ten vulnerabilities. Would it make more sense to have one ticket or ten tickets? With exceptions, most organizations would rather have one ticket focused on how to remediate than 10 tickets focused on the same remediation. Some vulnerability management tools can do this, while others cannot. Paying attention to these kinds of details are factors that everyone should take into account when building a vulnerability management program.

Additional Vulnerability Management Uses

An additional use case for vulnerability management tools is to use them as part of an IT hygiene program to validate systems prior to them going live. With IoMT, this is particularly important because some of the systems cannot be scanned or upgraded and it may be the only time a system can be validated. Given that IoMT systems can be modified over time by end users for a variety of reasons, but not by IT/security teams, it creates a lot of additional challenges for organizations—none of them positive from a cybersecurity perspective. Doing everything you can to measure the differential over time can help to support ongoing challenges with the existing systems and is important for long-term system changes in covered entities.

Penetration Testing

Penetration testing also falls under the threat and vulnerability umbrella. It is a little bit like the black-hat hacking except that it is done with authorization so that organizations can figure out what the vulnerabilities are before the black-hat hackers do. Unlike a vulnerability assessment that validates for the existence of vulnerabilities, a penetration test actually exploits those vulnerabilities. But penetration testing is much more than this because it not only takes the results of a vulnerability assessment, but it goes a few steps further looking for human logic flaws and other vulnerabilities that are not found as a result of a vulnerability management scan. The scope and the processes are also much more detailed than what is found in vulnerability assessment. As a result, penetration testing is a critical part of a threat and vulnerability management program.

What Color Box?

When performing penetration testing, the context is important. To that end, there are three types of testing—black box, gray box, and white box. Black-box testing means that the penetration tester is essentially running blind and must discover everything about the organization the way a normal hacker would. In gray-box testing, the penetration tester has some information about the organization. It may include the types of systems, key IP addresses, a network diagram, and so on. It isn't complete information. A white-box test is a test where the penetration tester is given reasonably complete information about the environment. The advantage here is that white-box testing tends to be less expensive because time is not spent learning about the environment and then choosing targets. In many cases, the targets are provided ahead of time.

The box colors and the related effects all have their strengths and weaknesses depending on the context of the penetration test. The black-box test, especially if it is time bound, provides the perspective of a real-world attacker, but because it takes more time to research the organization, the penetration tester often does not have the time to test the number of vulnerabilities that exist within the scope. As the boxes move to gray, then white, the real-world-attacker scenario significantly reduces, but more vulnerabilities are often discovered.

What Color Team?

Penetration testing is traditionally done by a red team—people who perform the attacks against organizations. They follow their attack playbooks and try to get past the defenses of the organizations. On the opposite side of the house are the defenders. They use their existing tools, techniques, and practices to try to detect the attackers. Some organizations choose just to focus on specific attack methodologies for the purpose of tuning their SIEM and/or SOC to detect those methodologies. In these cases they are working as a cohesive unit and not operationally separate; this is referred to as purple teaming.

Penetration Testing Phases

There are many schools of thought regarding penetration testing, but most of them follow a similar pattern for a specific type of attack. Of course, there are always exceptions depending on the scope. Here we explore some of the key aspects of penetration testing.

Scope

Scope is important for both internal and external penetration tests. Remember that the difference between a black-hat hacker and a white-hat hacker is authorization. Determining the scope helps to determine the authorization. It also helps to determine the time frame.

Organizations can choose multiple types of penetration testing. There are physical penetration tests where the tester tries to get past the physical security of an organization in order to compromise it, and social engineering tests, where testers attempt to manipulate people by calling them with the intent of gaining access to the system. There are external penetration tests where the tester attacks the external network to try to gain access. Internal penetration testing involves a scenario where the tester is on the inside of an organization trying to take over resources.

There are also other kinds of penetration tests that organizations perform depending on their needs and/or concerns. Companies can be as creative about this process as possible—even using blended attacks that utilize multiple strategies to attain their goals.

Reconnaissance

Reconnaissance is a very critical phase in the penetration testing process as the penetration tester will use a variety of methods for collecting information about the organization, such as open-source intelligence (OSINT). Information can be gathered simply by using a search engine in creative ways or by checking sites like LinkedIn to see who works at the company and what projects they are working on. Shodan is a tool that aggregates information about an organization and can enable pen testers to view that information from a hacking perspective. There are literally hundreds of OSINT sources, including a company's own website.

Reconnaissance is much more than OSINT tools, however. It can include running scans against organizations. These can be vulnerability scans against machines, but most hackers will initially decide to use a port-mapping tool such as NMAP. NMAP happens to be the most powerful tool, and it is free to download for anyone. It has a large number of settings so that penetration testers can be as loud or as stealthy as they like when performing active reconnaissance against organizations.

Vulnerability Assessments

Vulnerability assessments are another tool that hackers often use when profiling the vulnerabilities of an organization. The key difference in this case is that oftentimes the vulnerability assessment is unauthenticated, which means that it is often more prone to false positives. In fact, some compliance frameworks require organizations to perform an unauthenticated vulnerability assessment against their own external websites so that they can focus on the vulnerabilities from an attacker's point of view.

There are numerous other tools on the market that a penetration tester might use. There is a version of Linux that aggregates many of these tools—Kali Linux. Essentially it is a combination of tool types that include reconnaissance, vulnerability analysis, penetration testing, stress testing, and forensic utilities, which can be used by penetration testers in the course of an authorized attack.[1]

The Actual Penetration Test

The next phase of the penetration test typically is the active exploitation of systems. This is where the attacker gains access to the individual systems in order to exploit them. In some cases, data can be gathered right away from the web application without compromising the operating system itself. For example, if an organization does not use appropriate input validation on various fields on the web page and the server is connected to database server, data can be gathered from the database server through the web page. In other cases, the penetration tester will gain access to the server itself and then use that as a jump point to attack other servers. This is known as lateral movement and is also a very common methodology for black-hat hackers.

There are a few tools on the market for performing penetration testing, but there is an open-source tool known as Metasploit that provides pen testers with active exploitation for many kinds of attacks. The open-source project is now managed by the cybersecurity company Rapid7.

---

[1]https://tools.kali.org/tools-listing.

Reporting

Reporting is one of the most important parts of penetration testing. If there is no report detailing what happened or how it happened, the penetration test has limited value to organizations. The more information in the report about the vulnerabilities discovered during the penetration test, the more valuable the report becomes. As stated previously, the point of doing a penetration test is to be remediate vulnerabilities before a cybercriminal or nation-state finds them.

Penetration Testing Strategies

For those outside of IT or cybersecurity, it may be surprising to learn that penetration tests are almost never performed throughout the whole organization on every single machine. They are focused on key systems—often the ones with the greatest internet exposure or the ones that hold the greatest amount of data. Sampling of machines is another tried-and-true method to detect problems in organizations. Oftentimes, especially with internally developed software, lessons learned from one system can be applied to other systems. Organizations can learn from the mistakes they have made and improve upon them in the future.

Of course, penetration testing should be performed against IoMT systems as well—especially using sampling if there are a lot of machines. Reporting these findings back to the manufacturer can be helpful, even if they don't immediately do anything to address the issues. Eventually, though, with enough pressure, the manufacturers may do the right thing in the long run. It is also a good way to illustrate to senior management just how vulnerable the systems may be. Stating that the passwords could be hacked and actually having them hacked can have a dramatically different impact on how senior management responds—especially if those passwords are connected into a medical system.

Cloud Considerations

Cloud providers, often by design, create challenges when it comes to vulnerability assessments and penetration testing—depending on the vendor and the context. When selecting a vendor, determining how penetration tests and vulnerability assessments are performed is a critical part of the process. Many SaaS vendors, for example, will not permit penetration testing against their site. Those that do may put limitations on them in order to prevent their organization from being continually hit by penetration tests. This may seem a bit extreme, but cloud providers may have thousands of clients. Performing a penetration test from each client every year could quickly overwhelm an organization's resources. So for IoMT manufacturers that have websites, covered entities should not expect to test the security of that provider.

IaaS and PaaS are a different matter. In both cases the cloud provider does not perform an application penetration test of the web applications on the site. It is simply outside of their purview. The company using IaaS or PaaS must perform a penetration test of their own site to maintain compliance.

New Tools of an Old Trade

The threat and vulnerability world is maturing and expanding very rapidly as the need for cybersecurity grows. Both the vulnerability management and penetration tools are becoming more sophisticated, but so is the discipline. These are some of the new innovations occurring in the market today, and as the attackers continue to evolve their strategy, the market will continue to evolve as well.

MITRE ATT&CK Framework

MITRE, a company that focuses on cybersecurity and many other disciplines, has put together the MITRE ATT&CK framework. It is a comprehensive listing of the adversarial tactics and techniques that attackers use to gain access to organizations. This type of systematic, comprehensive approach to categorizing the attack techniques provides defenders with information about how they can best protect organizations from the various kinds of attacks.

As a result of this, there have been many new kinds of software that have either incorporated the MITRE ATT&CK techniques into their products or created new products to help organizations defend themselves. Some of the products are strictly on the defensive side of the house doing what they can to protect organizations. Breach and Attack Simulation (BAS) is one such product set.

Breach and Attack Simulation

BAS products are designed to perform continual automated attacks against organizations. The advantage of BAS is that penetration tests are expensive to perform manually, and this new type of product automates many of the features of a penetration test. From an organizational perspective, they are continually aware of their cybersecurity posture as the MITRE ATT&CK framework defines it—much broader than the information from a vulnerability management program alone. While BAS is not quite as effective as a human penetration tester against human logic flaws, it does represent a large step toward the continual monitoring goals. Many organizations consider BAS as yet another part of IT hygiene. Although it is relatively new, it is quickly becoming a staple among more advanced organizations.

Crowd Source Penetration Testing

What has also been an interesting change is the crowd sourcing of penetration testing, around which a few companies have created a business model. This entails allowing a number of penetration testers access to a covered entity. They will search websites on a regular basis looking for vulnerabilities, and like a standard penetration test, the tester needs to provide a repeatable process for performing the attack. The difference is that crowd-sourced penetration testing is an "always-on" function, but a penetration test is usually done during a defined period. That always-on functionality can give organizations the heads up when it has a new vulnerability, whereas the once-per-year penetration test has a limited time frame in which to catch vulnerabilities.

The challenge with the crowd-sourced penetration testing is getting them to sign business associate agreements (BAAs). BAAs are legal agreements between entities to ensure that HIPAA is covered. Quite often the back end of the organization signs contracts with individual members who do the penetration testing on their own time. While it is common for these solutions to limit the country from which the penetration test happens, it is quite a different story for each member to sign a BAA who might want to pen test a specific site. Mileage may vary depending on the vendor and the organization.

Calculating Threats

Whether for vulnerability management or penetration testing, understanding the threats against covered entities is becoming more important—especially as those threats continue to escalate over time and as cybercrime often rewards the attackers in terms of payouts. As vulnerabilities are discovered through old technologies or new, organizations need to prioritize them to focus on the greatest risk. It is important to balance the threats against the vulnerabilities in order to gain a better understanding of the risk and where IT teams should focus their resources.

Some threat and vulnerability management programs are oriented toward vulnerability management only. Many programs only do the vulnerability management side of the house and do not take the time to prioritize and think about the risks to organizations. Cybersecurity is hard. Today's tools have much maturing to do, but there is tremendous progress being made to create better and stronger programs where the threats are automatically being taken into account as part of the risk calculus.

In Summary

Threat and vulnerability management is an important part of protecting organizations. Despite some IoMT device manufacturers not being the most cooperative in this area of cybersecurity, it is critical for organizations to strive to measure the vulnerabilities to the best of their ability, even if alternate mechanisms need to be used.

But also understanding how the attackers operate ultimately helps to educate others and can help cybersecurity professionals determine the right strategy to best protect their organizations given the available resources. The information from vulnerability management tools can directly help some vulnerable IoMT, but not others. Covered entities, especially hospitals, need to understand the risks, and a threat and vulnerability management program is a must. Any improvement in the overall cybersecurity posture is a win for covered entities.

Data Protection

Master data management is a discipline that goes hand in hand with information governance. Forward thinking organizations are instituting processes to gain agreement on roles, responsibilities, policies, and procedures surrounding the maintenance of a single view of the entities needed for conducting business and measuring its performance.

—Henry Morris

Technically everything that we have spoken about in this book to protect IoMT is a form of data protection, but that's not the focus of this chapter. This chapter will focus specifically on techniques for protecting the data itself. Many of these techniques are not a direct requirement of some compliance frameworks, but they are tried-and-true methods of protecting data within covered entities.

Twenty years ago, the primary location for data was within a database or on a corporate computer. Sometimes that data would be placed on a thumb drive or burned onto a CD, or possibly printed. Today, that data is also placed in a number of platforms online, which have become a primary means for organizations to share large volumes of information or use collaborative workspaces while focusing on a project. This has made data security more complicated than it was in the past.

That said, despite the changes, a whole host of solutions have been created to better protect that data. The basics of data security are still just as critical as they were before, and having new solutions to focus on those new technologies is more important than ever—doubly true for email, as PHI lost through email is the number-one concern for most hospitals. What is important from this perspective is the human element and how the mistakes people make sending lost email can easily apply to any number of the data collaboration tools that are on the market.

Data Governance

Data governance is the set of rules that permeate an organization regarding the creation, acquisition, and sharing of data, including the people, processes, and technology surrounding that data. In today's world, IoMT is part of the ecosystem of data collection and therefore a consideration within data governance. As pointed out in Chapter 4, all of the data collected by IoMT devices (so long as it comes from a health professional) is in scope for HIPAA, and the associated risks to the data should be the primary considerations from a data governance perspective. Remember, too, that many states have data requirements related to PII and PHI—most notably CCPA. Those should be factored into the data governance equation as well. Companies are always free to go above and beyond the law to protect the devices—in fact, it is highly advisable to do so.

Data Governance: Ownership

It may seem a bit odd to the uninitiated to talk about data ownership, but it is actually a very critical issue—especially with HIPAA and some of the privacy regulations that are coming out. How we approach these concerns affects the overall approach to the data as a whole. Stepping outside the HIPAA realm for a moment, some of the modern privacy rules state that any person whose data is being accessed is the data owner. Think about the discussions around CCPA from Chapter 3. People have a right to know what information is available about them, and if they choose, they can request that data be corrected or even deleted. That is a very powerful right. It means that any corporation that holds that data is merely a steward—it can't distribute or sell that data without the knowledge or consent of the data owner. The repercussions of this are huge. HIPAA regulations are beginning to follow suit from a legal perspective. Data collected on a patient, for example, belongs to the patient, not the entity that collected it. They are simply "borrowing" it, and the onus is on them to protect it.

Being very careful about questions like data ownership can have a huge impact on organizations. IT, for example, should not be the data owners. They are simply the custodians within an organization. It is their job to manage the data and take care of it. The responsibility of actually protecting the data and all of its associated risks belongs to the business.

Establishing clear directives within organizations about data ownership is a critical part of overall data governance. So establishing clear directives within organizations about data ownership is a critical part of the overall data governance strategy within an organization.

Data Governance: Lifecycle

Having a well-defined data lifecycle is critical to the governance process and can affect many other tools, techniques, and practices within organizations. It just makes logical sense. How long should an organization keep data? As long as HIPAA requires is a good answer, but what about other parts of the business? What are the long-term business strategies? Answering these kinds of questions is really important to determining how long the data is kept.

It isn't just about the data being stored within the organization. What are the sharing agreements with other organizations? How are they impacted by the governance lifecycle? Do those agreements need to be modified as a result of the overall data strategy? Looking at the business holistically is a critical part of creating a data governance standard. Maybe the covered entity stores data from other organizations, but different organizations have different data termination requirements. How does that impact the policy? In these cases, can IT meet those requirements? What do they need to know ahead of time to plan for these kinds of efforts?

Finally, how are these policies going to be implemented? IT usually needs to have a strong voice in this process to talk about what the options are for removing data, and handling data throughout the data lifecycle. If they do not, that can create challenges down the road for business and ultimately for the real data owners: people whose data the business stewards.

Data Governance: Encryption

One of the key things to take into account when it comes to data governance is how that information is stored, transmitted, and used. For the most part, that data should be encrypted except when in use. There are often a few noted exceptions, however, that should be spelled out as part of the data governance policies. For example, sometimes security tools need to unencrypt the data in order to protect the data. Some of the network security tools discussed in Chapter 10 are a good example.

Generally speaking, the larger the covered entity, the stronger the tie to technology. This means those organizations input the data into systems rather than use printed material (although there are many exceptions). In this case, examining the technological processes to ensure that all privacy and security requirements are built into them is a critical step—especially when it comes to encryption. This means that there should be an end-to-end encryption for all data and systems with only a few exceptions.

But what does end-to-end encryption mean? It means doing an in-depth review of the technology to validate that it is being protected. We'll start with the database. The database itself must be encrypted. This makes it more difficult for hackers, because even if they were to get access to the database, they would have to devise a means of decrypting it in order to use the data. For many cybersecurity practitioners, encryption simply part of configuration management or IT hygiene. It is important to choose the right database (and possible compensating control) because some databases do not have the ability to encrypt data. If the database does not have encryption, sometimes a product can be chosen to encrypt databases despite the database not having the inherent capability to encrypt data.

Another consideration is database connectivity to a web server. That connection should also be encrypted, although it is not technically required by HIPAA. It is a best practice, however, because there is some risk that a hacker could gain access to the data if the server is compromised.

The next step in encryption is knowing how that information is shared both internally and externally. For example, websites that use HTTP instead of HTTPS are not encrypted, which means that data flows unencrypted across a network. From a HIPAA standpoint, this is acceptable when internal to an organization, but the moment that HTTP connection faces the internet, that is a HIPAA violation. The reason that is so important is multifold but revolves around the man-in-the-middle attack—essentially someone can steal not only the data, but also the login credentials because the data is traversing the internet in clear text. It should be noted that just because it is permissible to not encrypt data internally to an organization does not make it a best practice from a cybersecurity perspective. Encrypting traffic, whether internal or external, is a best practice to protect organizations. Another important consideration is Secure Sockets Layer (SSL) offload. Without going too far into the technology, SSL is related to digital certificates that encrypt a website.

In some cases, it makes perfect business sense to offload the certificate prior to hitting the website. This improves performance at the website level and is typically done on a device known as a load balancer, which is a system used to balance loads (that is, traffic to web servers). Among other things, it can decrypt the connection and allow the traffic to go to multiple web servers to prevent too much traffic from going to any one site. The key here is that traffic between the load balancer and the web server is unencrypted, and this is acceptable from most compliance frameworks despite that the traffic is not encrypted for a very short distance. Most reasonable cybersecurity practitioners would say this is an acceptable risk and worthwhile risk. The man-in-the-middle attack risk is so low as to be a major risk. These are the kinds of decisions that IT and cybersecurity practitioners must make when handling sensitive data.

Data Governance: Data Access

One of the items that was purposefully left out of the discussion of I&AM in Chapter 13 was the data governance angle. Part of the reason that identity governance is in place is to focus on the access to data. Not everyone should have full access to all data. For many states, consent is required to gain access to PHI. Although there are emergency cases that allow medical professionals to access the data legally, they are exceptions to the rule. Those cases should be investigated to validate that they were performed under lawful conditions.

The challenge here for organizations is to determine where their data is. If all of the data was carefully placed inside of a database and never appeared anywhere else, data access would be extremely easy. That kind of data is referred to as structured data. The flip side of structured data is unstructured data, which is data that is anywhere else in the organization. Often that data is there for legitimate purposes. Maybe the organization is performing an incident response, and some of the data is required to be in evidence. It does mean, however, that the data may be spread throughout the organization. Once it is loose, in theory, it can end up anywhere—even in the hands of people who really should not have access to that data.

But how do organizations know where that data is located? That is where data discovery tools are useful. They can scan an organization's technological assets and determine where the data is located. Data discovery tools have different capabilities, but they can look at databases, server shares, PDFs, office documents, and so on. The output from these tools can provide organizations with information so they respond appropriately. But maybe there are minor permissions issues that need to be corrected. Perhaps someone changes the role within an organization and they no longer need access to their previous permissions. Standard identity governance tactics are not always the most effective. Instead, identity governance tools might be a better approach. These tools not only map the access that people have, but also map their access to different types of data. This can make a huge difference in organizational security—the difference between authorized or unauthorized access to PHI. We'll take a look at those tools a bit more deeply later in this chapter.

Closing Thoughts

Although we skimmed the surface of data governance, we touched on enough of the subject for you to understand why it is so important. From an IoMT perspective, each device may offer an alternate means of protecting associated data. For example, some IoMT devices can have accounts that send information, but not read information. In other IoMT devices, all account types will have the same type of access, and there is no option to provide alternate access. Using thought patterns like these and understanding why certain access is required for some users but not others will allow covered entities to think more clearly about the access to data and possibly even the IT mechanisms required to help protect organizations. There is no silver bullet when it comes to identity governance because the privacy and risk landscape changes on such a frequent basis that determining the exact place to land may pose challenges. Reviewing the policy and the practices on a regular basis can help organizations gain better insight and create better paths forward to protect our data. Data governance is also the foundation for determining what data loss prevention (DLP) products should be used to protect organizations as we will discuss next.

Data Loss Prevention

DLP, also known as data leak prevention, is a critical part of an information security strategy. There are a range of tools on the market from installed servers with agents, to network devices, to cloud-based solutions. All of them have the ability to detect or prevent data from leaving an organization. Surprisingly, it is not required as part of many cybersecurity and legal frameworks—including HIPAA. It is considered a data protection tool because it specifically focuses on protecting data—including PHI and PII. It monitors for specific data types within organizations. DLP solutions can be used purely as a detection capability, but many organizations prefer to set it up to block data from leaving an organization. Depending on the solution, these tools can monitor a range of different types of data, including everything from the aforementioned PHI and PII to drivers' licenses, credit cards, and even less structured data. Many solutions can pattern-match information of almost any kind to detect or prevent data from leaving organizations.

Traditional DLP covers all modes of data entering and leaving a computer. For example, DLP tools can block data from being sent to websites, but can allow sending data to thumb drives, CDs, and other external drives. Most solutions cover both workstations and servers, and some even cover mobile devices.

Fragmented DLP Solutions

DLP solutions have become extremely fragmented. They are built into a whole range of products. Traditionally DLP was an endpoint solution that sits on workstations, but the old DLP solutions from the workstation are no longer as effective because of the number of storage options available today. If the data is sitting in a shared drive on the cloud and someone adds a new user within the cloud, traditional DLP will not detect that new user. If covered entities allow the uploading of PHI to the cloud for business purposes, where that data goes from there is unknown.

The way to combat this particular concern is with a cloud DLP solution, a data governance solution, or our old friend SASE (previously CASB). These solutions utilize an API interface to the cloud to detect data. If a particular file contains PHI, it can be blocked from sharing, or sharing can be permitted on a very specific basis as authorized by the covered entity. This is why taking the time to understand the various access rights is so important. It can lead to unintended data loss. Thinking through and analyzing that access really is that important to protecting the data.

As mentioned in Chapter 6, email is another location where data can be lost easily. While some of the desktop solutions will block data to an email account, they do not block within the web versions of that email. As a result, having DLP within email solutions—especially within cloud solutions—is important to comprehensively prevent data from leaving organizations.

Network DLP is yet another option, but it is slightly less common. The goal of network DLP is to analyze traffic by looking for any types of files that may have been missed by local desktop or server DLP. This can be extremely useful for IoMT devices—often because of the flaws that those devices may have. For example, if data is in clear text, the network DLP solution can detect where the traffic from IoMT is going. If it is going to an unauthorized location, network DLP can block it.

DLP Challenges

All this said, DLP solutions are far from perfect. In many cases these disparate solutions come with different levels of capabilities. Just because something is blocked from one avenue doesn't mean that another solution on another device will do the same thing. This can lead to challenges within organizations for having a holistic DLP program; covered entities need to make choices about what solutions work best for them.

But these are not the only challenges that DLP has. In a way, encryption is one of the enemies of DLP. If files are encrypted, some DLP tools can get past some types of authorized encryption (such as TLS). However, if the data within that file is also encrypted, there is no way for DLP tools to detect what kind of data it is. For example, if someone emails a file containing encrypted PHI, the DLP detection mechanism may not block it.

Steganography is another challenge for DLP. At its roots, steganography is the art of hiding information. It has broad capabilities, but it can be as simple as using a white font on white email. It is invisible to the eye, but someone can highlight the font and see what is written. DLP tools can easily pick up on information hidden this way. However, other forms of steganography are more sophisticated and can get by DLP tools undetected. A common technique is to hide files within files; for example, what appears to be just a simple web graphic may have a Word document buried in it. In that case, a steganography or forensic tool would be required to detect that information, but this is often not included within DLP tools.

Enterprise Encryption

Enterprise-level encryption is a big topic and covers a range of technologies. We have touched on some in this book (and even in this chapter), but there are three more types of encryption we'll mention as part of that data strategy.

File Encryption

There is more than one type of file encryption tool available on the market. First, there are individual file encryption solutions where a modicum of automation can be put into place to ensure that individual files are encrypted. These types of solutions are fantastic for small sections of operating systems such as SFTP servers.

What is a bit more interesting are file encryption mechanisms that are based on roles. For example, someone in finance cannot read documents from human resources and vice versa if that is the way the product is set up. The only way to read the files in an organization like that is to get the password to access them or masquerade as another user. These solutions are relatively new over the past few years, but more and more companies are starting to test these kinds of solutions.

In a sense, these solutions are a brilliant way to handle unstructured data throughout an organization—all of the files are automatically encrypted. It adds an additional level of complexity for hackers to deal with and is a great way to protect data.

Encryption Gateways

Less common in the industry are encryption gateways, but they can be a very powerful way of protecting data within organizations—especially if they are in the cloud. Encryption gateways, in short, are gateways that encrypt information as data passes through them. Encrypted information sits on one side of the gateway, while unencrypted information sits on the other side. When unencrypted data is sent through the gateway, it is encrypted when it goes through the gateway. When the data moves from the unencrypted side of the encryption gateway, it is decrypted. On the encrypted side, that data cannot be read by people or machines. If someone tries to access the data, but not access the data through the encryption gateway, they would only get the encrypted information, and not information in its unencrypted format. This can obviously be very frustrating for cybercriminals, but secure for organizations.

Of course, if data needs to be processed (enhanced, modified, read, etc.) on the encrypted side of the encryption gateway, this creates some challenges. To get around these challenges, the systems on the encrypted side of the gateway need some way of reading the encrypted information prior to processing that information. Once processed, that data would have to be re-encrypted. As a result, encryption gateways do have some limitations. In addition, some cloud providers require unencrypted data, which also limits the usefulness of the encryption gateway.

Encryption gateways are a great way to encrypt data, but they require some logistics and strategic thinking. Some logistical challenges may be insurmountable, especially for those organizations that use a cloud-first strategy and have employees working from home.

Data Tokenization

Data tokenization is probably one of the most powerful ways of protecting data within an organization, but it's not commonly used in healthcare organizations. Some cybersecurity professionals are not aware of it. Very simply, data tokenization is about replacing data with a token of the data. A token can be used to retrieve the data, but it is not data in and of itself. If a cybercriminal stole tokens from a database, no data would be lost—only tokens of the data. In short, tokenization is about replacing data with tokens. By doing so, the risks related to data are drastically reduced.

But tokenization is as much about identity as it is about data protection. If data were tokenized and that was the end of the story, tokenization would be a worthless process. Authorized users need access to data. Different roles may need different levels of access. One role may need complete access to the data while another role may need access to only a small portion of the data. What is important here is that access rights to that data need to be clearly identified and set up within a tokenization solution. This takes a level of identity maturity that many covered entities are not ready for.

The end result is a very secure system. If someone did not have the appropriate level of access within the tokenization solution, all they would see is a meaningless token. From a cybersecurity perspective, this renders several vectors of attack useless. The key vectors of attack are either concerned about ransomware or they are concerned about identity-based vectors. This represents a drastic reduction in risk. Even if a particular identity were compromised, the level of access to the data is reduced to the access level of the compromised user.

Tokenization is often used to protect credit card data. The same principle applies to credit card data as it does to healthcare data. There is one huge value add in the credit card compliance world compared to the HIPAA world. If data is tokenized from a credit card perspective, it can help to significantly reduce the scope of a credit card audit.

Strategically it is of vital importance for reducing risk—not only from a cybersecurity perspective, but also a legal compliance and privacy perspective.

It is not easy to set up and maintain, however. The various roles need to be set up appropriately for each user, which means that a very mature identity program needs to be set up from both an IT perspective and a governance perspective. Not all organizations are mature in their identity processes—or worse, they are too mature, and they have too many identities. Either way can spell disaster for building and/or maintaining a data tokenization program.

In a mature environment, data tokenization initiatives are also part of the identity governance program—they are just focused on the data, but in a different way than most identity governance solutions. Those are primarily focused on unstructured data, whereas data tokenization is almost exclusively focused on structured data. The reviews have to take into account all the access levels of the tokenization solutions. In this way tokenization really adds to both data protection and identity governance, in that if there were major oversights in the identity governance process, they would become crystal clear if people did not have the right level of access.

That said, tokenization is probably one of the best ways to protect organizations from data theft. That protection helps organizations to maintain control of the data (with some exceptions such as emailing data), in that it significantly reduces the risks from data hacking, but unfortunately not ransomware. Reducing the risk also means that the fines OCR dispenses are reduced because materially there is less data. In turn this also reduces the risks associated with privacy fines such as found with CCPA or HIPAA.

In Summary

Data protection is a bit more specialized for many organizations than is typically found in some covered entities, but represents a really important part of protecting that data. It is far from simple, however, and involves upping the identity and access management game for organizations. Done right, it can help with many kinds of risks that covered entities face, but it's typically not something that small doctor's offices would engage in.

That said, data aggregators are very keen to gain data. It would behoove covered entities to gain a better understanding of the protections discussed in this chapter from a legal, IT, and cybersecurity perspective.

The impacts can be very profound—especially with CPRA, which makes deanonymized HIPAA data count as HIPAA data for California residents.

From an IoMT perspective, this chapter is incredibly important because IoMT tends to increase the number of records a covered entity may have. It drastically changes the impact of the risk that regulators may leverage against them. Sometimes the simple application of thoughtful discussions and getting the opinion of general council (or a lawyer for companies without a general council) can do companies a world of good for protecting organizations.

CHAPTER

16

Incident Response and Forensics

We discovered in our research that insider threats are not viewed as seriously as external threats, like a cyberattack. But when companies had an insider threat, in general, they were much more costly than external incidents. This was largely because the insider that is smart has the skills to hide the crime, for months, for years, sometimes forever.

—Dr. Larry Ponemon

For those without a cybersecurity background, it may seem odd to talk about incident response and forensics as a means of protecting IoMT, but it is actually a very important part of a sometimes-forgotten key consideration—lessons learned. Every breach that covered entities go through is an opportunity to learn about an environment. What controls failed? What controls worked? What needs to be improved? Incidents are an excellent place to learn how to do better before the next attack.

With the high-level incidents that hit the news on a regular basis, it is easy to get swept up in thinking that attacks are extremely sophisticated and require the power of a nation-state, a criminal organization, or a kid in the basement that happens to be a computer genius. While these are concerns of every cybersecurity professional, sometimes it is the middle-of-the-road incidents that are the most important to think about.

Loss via email is one of the most common problems with healthcare breaches. These involve someone sending emails to the wrong recipients.

Maybe a better process needs to be defined for sending out emails, or maybe it would be better to send the information by another means—one that adds more steps to the process but could help covered entities avoid hefty fines.

These are not the only cases. The AWS S3 bucket discussed in Chapter 2 is an excellent example. Changing the setting from internet facing to internal facing is not complicated. One just has to know about it and configure it appropriately.

People make mistakes all the time. Oftentimes it is these small faux pas that can lead to serious incidents, but looking at the small things can prompt organizations to make large, systemic changes. For this reason, it is really critical to have a mature incident response and forensics team—if only for continual improvement.

Having a strong incident response team also means responses to incidents will be faster, and more than likely the amount of data that is stolen will be reduced. Whether it's IoMT or a system in the healthcare ecosystem, ultimately the result will be a reduction of loss—all things being equal.

Defining the Context

Before diving deep into what incident response and forensics actually entails, we'll explore some of the key terminology. This will help you understand a few of the complexities of the whole incident response and forensics process. One of the ways that analysts determine if there is a breach is to look at logs from Windows, network devices, IoMT devices, and other cybersecurity tools. In turn, the logs can trigger an alert from a detective system, which experts use to define an incident. Analysts use that information from that log to start an incident investigation. They may use information within an alert to search more deeply through the larger set of logs for important information and/or clues not found in the original alert. Based on the information, a cybersecurity expert may determine that a breach took place.

Of course, this is not the only way to determine if there was a breach. Many breaches can be discovered without an associated log. For example, if someone loses a laptop with HIPAA data and that laptop was not encrypted, there may be no logs to determine that there was a breach; however, from a legal standpoint, this is usually considered a breach. While there are certainly other breaches without associated logs, a log is an excellent place to start exploring how breaches and other incidents are detected.

Logs

We will do a deeper dive into log management, but almost all systems have logs. As mentioned in Chapter 9, a log is a record of what happens on a system. From a cybersecurity perspective, most logs are relatively benign—a laptop was powered on, a service was started while the system was powering up, a user logged in to a system, and so on. Nothing here is overly surprising. But let's say a user logs in from San Francisco and five minutes later they log in from New York City. Both events are fairly standard log events, but the tie-in between them is obviously unusual and could be the indicator of an attack. Which one depends on many factors. Maybe both of them are attacks. Without context or additional information, it is hard to say that either of them represents a potential threat. Still, it is an indicator that something is wrong.

Just because a log is created, that is a long way away from an alert. A mechanism has to be in place to note the discrepancy. Maybe the systems recorded the login, but did not alert on that log? Maybe the logins were recorded on disparate systems. How does an individual system "know" that information could be related or that there is an issue? This gap is a small part of the reason why centralized identity and/or logging systems are so important. If there were disparate systems for the login and nothing was analyzing the information, there would never be an alert and the incident would be completely invisible to an organization (without additional detective capabilities). The first step to handling logs is aggregating them from as many different sources as possible. Traditionally, due to speed (bandwidth for the technophiles) limitations on the network, only server logs were sent to central SIEM tools. Even sending all logs from servers could take down some internal networks, so quite often specific log sources needed to be selected. The network had to be designed to handle all of the traffic—which in the early days was not always possible. This is why server logs were the most typical to focus on years ago. Recall from Chapter 5, though, that most of the successful attacks from APT actors start with a phishing email. The first line of defense is the workstation and not the servers. This left many companies virtually blind to workstation compromise. Knowing and understanding what is happening on the endpoints is more critical than ever. Now monitoring the logs on workstations is an absolutely critical part of the defensive strategy of most organizations.

Keep in mind that we are not just talking about operating system logs. The more sources of logs, especially from cybersecurity software such as next-generation antivirus and EDR and so on, the better visibility the organization may have into potential attacks against the covered entity. Adding in disparate systems such as networking equipment, firewalls, applications, and even the logs from IoMT devices is par for the course. Knowing when changes take place to those devices or when those devices are under attack is critical.

As mentioned in Chapter 9, a SIEM tool is the best place to aggregate all these logs. Years ago a SIEM tool had to be on-premise, but today's SIEM tools are often in the cloud as a SaaS solution. Some store logs locally, and some store them in the cloud. Whatever the model, a covered entity may choose to use a SIEM tool as a centralized way to aggregate these logs from all kinds of sources.

Alerts

Aggregation is only one part of what a SIEM tool can do. Aggregation by itself for its own sake may help meet some compliance requirements, but it does not help detect problems within organizations. The process of determining what is and is not an alert within an organization is also another aspect of SIEM solutions, but these must be set up and tuned to create alerts. To do that, there are several important factors for organizations. These include thresholds, dependencies, threat intelligence, machine learning, and so on. We will touch on only a few basics to get the general idea for casual readers.

Thresholds are important because not every "bad" event is something to be concerned about. A failed login attempt is not a cause for alarm. It could be someone who fat fingered a password. Creating an alert based on that event would mean an incident response team would be wasting time looking for events that are not worth consideration. A threshold is where organizations decide that if a "bad" event occurs enough times, it is worth investigating. That number of thresholds may be different for different systems within a covered entity, depending on the context.

Context is also very important for SIEM systems. Maybe there were 200 attempts to log in to a machine before there was a successful event. It could just be a legitimate user failing a login 200 times and succeeding on the 201st try. Even though there could be an innocent reason for this occurring, it is of relevant interest to an alert and is worth investigating.

Threat intelligence can include anything from known APT attacker locations (IP addresses, for example) or information about a known bad piece of malware. Today, threat intelligence can be aggregated from a number of different sources including commercial sources, open source, and even threat intelligence sharing services. There are even sources that focus on IoMT devices.

Finally, there are other considerations like machine learning (discussed in Chapter 3) and User Endpoint Behavior Analytics (UEBA). These kinds of tools look for abnormalities in the behavior of systems and users to send alerts. As these are based on behavior, they can provide additional value to alerts that were based on other factors.

SIEM tools are a great way to search for problems within organizations, which can then take the necessary actions. Ultimately the goal is to create actionable alerts and help responders deal with incidents within organizations. The goal here is to right size alerts for the organization. For example, if a particular system is sending out too many false positives, a alerting strategy should be designed to work around that issue. A one-to-one ratio of alerts to events means that responders waste too much time sifting through alerts to determine what is important and what is not. With today's threats, it is hypercritical to use a multitude of technologies within SIEM to keep on top of alerts and prevent wasted time. Wasted time can discourage employees from responding to alerts and allow potential threat actors to accomplish their goals unseen. While this is far from complete for the security-oriented perspective of managing a SIEM tool, it provides a glimpse into what that realm looks like for creating alerts.

SIEM Alternatives

In discussing SIEM, we did not go into everything that needs to be set up. SIEM is the basis for something called a security operations center (SOC). The SOC is where the alerts from the SIEM become actionable and a new set of people, processes, and technologies can really enable organizations to do a fantastic job. For many covered entities, however, this is not a viable option. As a result, they may go with one of any number of different options to support them—sometimes those services overlap with one another. Options for organizations include everything from partial SIEM utilizations to managed SIEM options where incident response teams are added on top of SIEM solutions.

Covered entities can also use a Managed Security Services Provider (MSSP). MSSPs provide everything from the logs to working with EDR and MDR providers (see Chapter 12 for a refresher) and have started to become MDR providers themselves, but these solutions often have challenges because they handle a limited number of log sources. As a result, there is a new breed of providers called Extended Detection and Response (XDR) that are able to handle a broader range of inputs than traditional MSSPs.

From an IoMT perspective, some MSSP services cater specifically to logs related to IoMT services and threats that typically accompany other hospital equipment and systems. For many covered entities, this is the most reasonable option.

We quickly covered the alternatives. Entire books can be written around SIEM, SOC, and the various kinds of management solutions. All of them are useful for protecting data and IoMT devices. Right-sizing the options that best suit covered entities is the trickier part of the process. Nevertheless, utilizing a monitoring tool of some kind is an important step to detecting and stopping a cybercriminal or nation-state attacker.

Incidents

Aside from the challenge of right sizing alerts is the challenge that the alerting process itself is imperfect. Some attacks may take place that are never alerted on—essentially, they remain undetected. This could be from the lack of available monitoring (such as is common with IoMT) to attacks that are too subtle to detect with traditional monitoring tools (such as we saw with the Solar Winds debacle). Any event that happens, whether detected or not, is an incident. A false positive is also an incident, but incident responders need to determine if the event truly is a false positive as part of an incident investigation.

In either case, it is the alert that triggers that incident investigation. The incident handlers take information from the variety of different sources to piece together what is happening or what has happened. From there, they can determine the next step in order to respond to the incident. For example, say an SSH server is exposed to the open internet and attackers are hitting it with usernames and passwords. A prudent response would be to block the attackers' IP address so they have no chance of compromising the server. That is essentially what happens during an incident response process.

But SIEM/MSSP/XDR are not the only sources of incident investigations. Incident information can come from anywhere. Oftentimes companies become aware of problems only when law enforcement first approaches the covered entity about the issue. In this case, based on the information, an investigation needs to take place related to the incident—even if nothing was detected internally. In other cases, such as with ransomware, the first indication may be from the attacker emailing notification about a ransom. In the end, incident responders are not just relying information from their internal systems, but also sometimes word of mouth or a number of other potential sources.

Breaches

From the CEO of covered entities to the shareholders (if applicable), a breach is one of the scariest situations that covered entities have to come to terms with. It can mean anything from potential ransoms, HIPAA fines, continued OCR oversight, and potential loss of business from systems being down. When it comes to healthcare, especially during a crisis such as dealing with a global pandemic, no covered entity wants to deal with a breach. It takes a bad situation and makes it measurably worse.

But what a breach is and when it is reportable requires a bit of nuance because it depends on the context. For example, if a nurse inadvertently receives PHI about another nurse's patient within the same facility, that is not a breach, and it is not a reportable condition. There is little risk that the data will be exposed further. However, if that PHI were stolen or emailed to someone who had no authority to see it, that is a considered a breach and must be reported. Not all cases are this cut and dried, so it's always safer to submit a report if there is any uncertainty about what happened to the data. Otherwise, there is a risk of being seen as willfully negligent in the eyes of the law.

Incident Response

Obviously, there is a great deal more when it comes to incident response than what we have discussed so far. It is a discipline as important as any other in IT or cybersecurity. While many incidents are not breaches and never end up under legal scrutiny, it is important to create a standardized process that captures the elements of the incident. Some key considerations include the following:

- Who is the incident responder?
- How was the incident detected?
- When did the incident start?
- What are the affected systems?
- Was data exfiltrated?
- What were the responses to the incident?

While these are extremely basic questions, they give an overall picture of the kinds of details that an incident responder would need to determine the severity of an incident. In certain cases, working with a vendor who might provide additional details or getting law enforcement involved to help with the overall incident may be valuable, especially if the case may go to court. The details are everything.

The amount of detail is really dependent on the situation. Some key questions to ask are: Is human life at risk? Was there a reasonable chance that the data was lost? How many records were lost? Remember that an incident does not necessarily mean that data was lost. It could be that an attacker was trying to gain entry into an organization, but they never made it. That is a genuine incident, but not a reportable condition from a HIPAA perspective.

From an IoMT perspective, it is important to do a deep dive into the incidents. Maybe an attacker managed to infiltrate an organization on a flat network and then easily accessed the IoMT devices. Seeing that IoMT devices were compromised fairly quickly is an indicator that something should be done to bolster their security, or better protect them by taking actions such as unflattening the network (or any of the other recommendations in the book). Remember that there is a huge difference in the eyes of senior management between the theoretical possibility that something could be hacked and the reality that they actually have been attacked. That distinction is absolutely critical for making changes within organization.

Evidence Handling

Incident responders need to collect information and store it in a forensically sound manner, which requires a hash to be made of the individual files (for example) to ensure data integrity down the road. If the evidence is relevant to a specific case, an investigator may use special tools to quickly sift through the data logs (grep is a good example from the Linux world for the technophiles) and pick out the specific lines of interest (these are referred to as *cuttings*). A hash would be made of the cuttings to ensure the forensic validity of the information by the evidence custodian. In this way, forensic investigators can keep information indefinitely. It also makes it forensically sound evidence if there is a need to take that evidence to court.

The art of writing incidents in a forensically sound fashion is also important for incidents that may go to court. These reports should include dates and times and other details of an incident, such as the actions performed, when the evidence was placed in storage, where it was stored overnight, the security around the storage, and so on. Each piece of evidence can potentially lead to more pieces, so properly documenting and storing them is critical. Even where the information is written can be important. For instance, a spiral-bound notebook is not sufficient because a page can be torn out without anyone being aware. By contrast, a notebook that has a smyth-sewn binding, where a number of pages are folded together and sewn through the length of the book, is forensically acceptable because it is much more difficult to tear out a single page without affecting other pages. If one page is torn out, it is obvious.

How the evidence was handled is also very critical. Was the evidence pulled from tools on a compromised machine? Attackers are known to compromise local files in order to hide their tracks, so this is not a forensically sound practice. Files separate from the potentially compromised system should be used—otherwise there is a reason to doubt the overall findings within an investigation. Of course, with many types of cloud environments, this is simply not possible because the evidence may relate to the portal itself, in which case the logs from the portal are what matter. Pulling those logs off of the portal such as through a SIEM tool is vitally important in those cases.

Forensic Tools

Forensic tools can be a huge aid to organizations performing forensic investigations. Oftentimes the best thing to do during an investigation is to make a full forensic backup of the machine prior to taking it offline. These tools can perform a bit-by-bit copy of every single sector on a hard drive—this means every piece of information, every item in memory, and every hidden file on the system. From a forensic perspective, it helps with everything from chain of custody to lessening the risk of altering the compromised machine because you are looking at an exact replica. It really is one of the more intelligent ways to approach incident investigations.

Automation

While services like MDR are lifesavers for organizations, there are other options. One is to include automation into the incident response process. Security Orchestration Automation and Response (SOAR) is one of the key technologies that has reached the spotlight in recent years. It is primarily used by more mature organizations, but it is not well integrated into MSSP technologies. However, it integrates really well with many SIEM tools. SOAR has the capability to automate the entire alert-response process, cutting out all the manual steps usually done by human responders. For example, if the SIEM tool has an alert, the SOAR tool can read it, tell where the attack is coming from (the IP address), and then respond to it in a variety of ways. It can be set up on an endpoint product to automatically respond and block the attacker. The same could be done to a firewall. SOAR can monitor inbound and outbound traffic to a possibly infected machine and automatically pull data up from the SIEM solution. This would lessen the time it normally takes to manually search through the information. The automated response can potentially stop an attack soon after it starts by blocking hackers or creating setbacks for them—without using up the minimal resources of internal teams.

Of course, these tools take time and energy to set up so they do not make sense for all organizations. For those who have the resources, though, they can be invaluable in reducing the impact of a breach. According to a recent IBM study, fully implemented security automation tools reduced the cost of a breach by an average of $3.58 million, and having even some automation reduced the cost of a breach by 1.92 million.[1]

EDR and MDR

We spoke about EDR and MDR solutions previously as part of the additional tools added on top of today's antivirus. In a sense, they take the place of the automation that SOAR tools put into place. They can respond to an incident at 3 a.m. without having to wake up the IT and/or security teams. EDR and MDR really are incident response. Typically, they do not do the full forensics required by mature incident response processes, but they are extremely effective at stopping many forms of attacks and doing much of what SOAR tools do automatically. This is part of what makes EDR and MDR solutions so valuable for organizations and why they have their place in the incident response processes.

IoMT Challenges

Predictably, IoMT brings to the table many challenges with incident response and forensics. Some of the devices have no or very poor logging. In those cases, even knowing when a device has been hacked can be a tremendous challenge. Not permitting installation of any software on devices means that many of the triggers that may be on a workstation

---

[1] Ponemon Institute, July 2020, IBM, "Security Cost of a Data Breach Report 2020."

or server are absent; some of these devices simply lack the best tools for detecting problems IoMT devices (certainly not all of them).

What is interesting is how a handful of challenges in IoMT can spread across a range of disciplines in cybersecurity. Incident response and forensics are no different. In some cases, the best "forensic" tools within an organization may be the configuration management tools for monitoring changes within an environment. This is yet another reason why it is so important to set up the appropriate level of monitoring and why all of those compensating controls within organizations are needed when dealing with the enormous drag factor of many IoMT devices.

Lessons Learned

After any kind of incident, one of the most important things to do is review the lessons learned. Where were the controls failing? How and why were the devices attacked? What controls worked, and what could have been improved in the overall process? It is vitally important that the business understand what took place and what investments will better protect the covered entity. Maybe more strategic decisions need to take place within the organizations. The lessons learned help everyone to get on the same page when it comes to events; they can help organizations to better understand the big picture.

In Summary

Incident response and forensics are absolutely critical for far more reasons than just governing the issues surrounding IoMT, but they can significantly help tell a story to make changes within organizations. These connected disciplines are also about protecting covered entities from hackers who will often both steal data and demand ransoms. It is an ugly business, and covered entities—particularly now—are under massive strain to try to protect themselves. As the COVID-19 pandemic continues to be an issue, the challenges to the healthcare system continue to escalate.

Determining how to address these challenges and which tools to use are the kinds of decisions that covered entities are facing. How much should be invested in IT and/or cybersecurity? How much is too much? How do we balance patient lives versus patient data? How are decisions made within covered entities—many of which have large governance challenges? The answers to these questions are not easy and are the subject of our next chapter.

CHAPTER 17

A Matter of Life, Death, and Data

Security incidents have gone up 5–10 times during the pandemic, so there is an increased need for security operations risk management, identity and access management, data privacy and compliance.

—Ashok Soota

Throughout this book, we have talked about privacy, compliance, UL 2900, some basic considerations for protecting data from a cybersecurity perspective, and the overall role that IoMT plays within organizations. Clearly, the protection of human life is paramount, and protecting data related to IoMT is equally important. Many of the advanced cybersecurity certifications built into their values is the value of human life.

As you'll recall, the CIA triad encompasses the concepts of confidentiality, integrity, and availability. Confidentiality is the cornerstone of HIPAA; failure to protect sensitive medical data from exposure can result in fines. Integrity is important because in worst-case scenarios, poor data integrity can have catastrophic effects. For example, if there is no record that a patient is deathly allergic to a certain medication, that can result in loss of life. Availability is critical as well; if someone falls ill or has an emergency while traveling and their medical history is unavailable, that, too, can lead to loss of life.

Today we know that breaches are on the rise and ransomware is becoming rampant. Some of this has to do with how decisions are made within organizations. Who decides what IoMT products to purchase?

Does security have any say when it comes to those purchases? Once purchased, is adequate time allotted for security to assess and IT to implement recommended requirements? The answers to these seemingly simply questions can have a drastic impact on the security posture of organizations. In this chapter we will explore the decision-making processes, governance models, and some of the mindsets that create additional challenges within organizations.

Organizational Structure

Before moving into some of the challenges that organizations face, it is important to have a rough characterization of some of the forces that may be at play within organizations. The politics can create many different outcomes and can influence things in subtle ways that are not always immediately predictable from an external perspective. Keep in mind that every organization is a little different—there is no exact blueprint for success that fits all of them. Covered entities, like all organizations, are ever growing and ever changing in the ways they respond to the external world.

This section outlines the roles within organizations to give you a better perspective of how and why decisions are made. The titles and responsibilities of certain roles may differ somewhat, but this will give you a general sense of how organizations operate.

Board of Directors

The intent of the board of directors is to provide the strategic direction for an organization, but how involved they are in the day-to-day politics can differ among various companies. In some cases, C-level executives report directly to the board, while in others they report to various lines within organizations. Many people believe it is just the CEO who reports to the board, but larger organizations can have any of the positions reporting directly to them.

The people and the experiences that make up each board can be quite unique and can potentially have a large impact on the shape of the organization. For example, one of the gaping holes in many boards is the lack of a cybersecurity expert. Without that keen insight, non-cybersecurity experts cannot make a determination about what is or is not an appropriate level of cybersecurity. It could be that IT is calling all of the shots for security (which happens in some organizations), and although it may seem that IT and cybersecurity are similar disciplines, they are actually extremely different. Having a cybersecurity expert on a board of directors is absolutely critical to protecting the organization.

Chief Executive Officer

The Chief Executive Officer (CEO) is the person who helps with the visionary leadership of the covered entity. Their job is to weigh the balance of the various departments within organizations and determine the overall direction for the organization. In theory, the CEO is well balanced in understanding all aspects of the organization, but it all depends on their background. Some CEOs are really involved in IT, while others may be focused more on patient outcomes. The reality is everyone has their individual strengths and weaknesses that can permeate throughout the organization—the good and the bad alike—to different extents.

Chief Information Officer

The Chief Information Officer (CIO) is the technical lead of the organization—especially from an infrastructure perspective. Typically, the CIO oversees many different teams such as a networking team, Windows team, Linux team, database team, and so on. They are absolutely critical to the lifeblood of any larger covered entity. Without a technology department, most covered entities would not exist. The CIO is indispensable to an organization. They organize the various teams to interconnect and work together. They are also the liaison between the business and other parts of the organization. They are there to enable the execution of the business strategy. In many covered entities, they are also the public face of the organization.

From a cybersecurity perspective, they are there, in part, to enable an aspect of the vision of the cybersecurity department and close findings as a result of many of the various programs. For example, hardening systems is not typically performed by a cybersecurity program; that is performed by IT with sometimes a validation of the build by cybersecurity. A good example might be a vulnerability management program. Cybersecurity often owns the scanning of the systems and the architecture of the vulnerability scanning, but IT performs the builds of the systems, installs the agents (if applicable), sets up the access, and so on. There is a partnership that must be in place to determine when to scan systems, how to handle things in the rare event that a system might go down, and so on.

IT has its own mandates that are separate from security. They exist to work with the business—to enable their strategy and vision from a technological perspective. They determine the how, but sometimes they work with the business to determine the cost—which, in turn, can modify the goals of the business. Rome cannot be built in a day.

General Counsel

The General Counsel (GC) is the primary legal internal representative for the organization. Their role is typically much larger than just HIPAA as they can advise (or have specialists on their team or sometimes outside firms) on any legal consideration for the organization. Just as there are different specializations in IT, there are different specializations for legal. In today's ever-changing privacy world, it is important to understand not only HIPAA, but also the requirements for local state laws to ensure that data is appropriately protected.

Chief Technology Officer

The Chief Technology Officer (CTO) typically oversees the development of software within an organization. They can have one or more teams that focus on different aspects of development. They help to translate the business needs to developers to ensure they create the products the business needs. That may sound easy, but the reality is that software development is a profession of its own, and what may seem obvious from one person's perspective is not always as clear as one might think. There is an art to writing requirements and to ensuring that software code is written securely. The CTO quite often is the champion who takes charge of that to ensure that the full software development lifecycle is overseen with the appropriate level of consideration.

Chief Medical Technology Officer

The Chief Medical Technology Officer (CMTO) is the liaison between the medical staff and the IoMT staff. They work with the various doctors and medical experts to determine their needs and help them to select the best medical devices for the organization. In a healthy organization they have to take into account IT needs, security needs, and the needs of covered entities. Given the accelerated pace of technological innovation, that includes many of the modern IoMT and all of the directions of innovation. What was highly intelligent a year before may be folly the next year. Weaving that fine line is where the CMTO lives and breathes.

Chief Information Security Officer

The Chief Information Security Officer (CISO) is responsible for leading the organization's cybersecurity. For different organizations, this can mean different things, but generally it means at least some involvement in everything detailed in Chapter 9. In many cases it means ownership of many of those programs. In others, it means defining requirements or reiteration of those requirements from a legal perspective. They also need to understand the technology and all of the various processes that are being developed by IT in order to steer covered entities in the right direction. Many of them are also intimately familiar with different cybersecurity frameworks such as HITRUST—which can also be part of the overall maturity of organizations.

Chief Compliance Officer

The Chief Compliance Officer (CCO) is responsible for the compliance of the organization. In covered entities, that usually means HIPAA and HITECH, but sometimes this can mean meeting other compliance frameworks such as HITRUST. It just depends on the capabilities and mandates of organizations. In many cases, especially with covered entities, the CCO also acts as the Chief Privacy Officer (CPO), but typically the privacy activities remain focused on HIPAA/PII privacy and they may or may not focus on larger state privacy concerns (CCPA, for example). It all depends on many different factors within the organization.

There are many different types of CCOs. Some are focused specifically on non-technical legal requirements. Others are very technical and work alongside IT and security to help define requirements. In other cases, they are very contract focused and do not get involved in IT and/or security matters. These differences can have a profound impact on how the organization functions. A legal-oriented CCO may not understand what took place with an incident and thus may miss the legal implications of an incident. Really thinking through what kind of CCO is required within an organization is critical.

Chief Privacy Officer

The Chief Privacy Officer (CPO) generally looks at privacy across the board. With covered entities, they are sometimes merged with CCOs and even CISOs in some cases. They have the tough job of keeping up with all of the various privacy regulations and translating them into a clear direction for covered entities and their business associates. In many cases, drastic changes may be made to keep up with the state privacy landscape and then the associated BAA and contracts.

Reporting Structures

It should be obvious that each of these roles brings something extremely valuable to the table. With very few exceptions, the reporting structures within organizations can be about anything one can imagine. As this is a story about cybersecurity and protecting IoMT and thus covered entities, we will emphasize the cybersecurity part of the story. The reporting structures are a minor consideration in a healthy organization, but unfortunately (and unsurprisingly), organizations are not always at optimal health, so reporting structures become more important. Depending on the people and the personalities involved, this can greatly affect the organizational politics and the security of a covered entity if security is not prioritized appropriately.

As mentioned in the first chapter, the prominence of cybersecurity in covered entities is rising. Scarcely a day goes by without some story related to cybersecurity hits the news. As these stories hit closer and closer to home, covered entities (and other businesses) are moving cybersecurity up the chain of command and into the spotlight more and more.

That understood, cybersecurity is sometimes buried deep within the IT hierarchy, even a level or two below the CTO. That creates some interesting challenges for the CISO (if the covered entity even has a CISO or equivalent). As discussed in Chapter 9, part of cybersecurity's mandate is to monitor the practices of IT. However, IT might not always be willing to accept the advice of cybersecurity for a number of reasons. For example, IT might be hesitant to expose some of its own flaws because that exposure might be used against them and therefore IT may sweep them under the rug. Reporting lines matter in such cases because the business needs to understand those flaws so they can effect change.

The same thing can be true for many other roles. If HIPAA compliance is buried within another part of the organization such as communications, some of its effectiveness can be lost as other priorities take precedence. In the end, whether through the CEO, the board of directors, or other executives, it is critical to think about those reporting lines and ensure that the voices are heard throughout the organization.

Committees

To get around the challenges of rigid reporting structures, it is important to set an open forum for communication. There are lots of different terms, but having committees for open discussion is probably one of the most important things that business leaders can do. They need to hear unfiltered messages from rank and file employees. How they react to this information is of vital importance—business leaders need to create an atmosphere of trust so that people at every level can express their concern without fear of losing their jobs.

The types of committees that organizations have is equally important. Having a meeting just on IT prioritization where security is included is a good thing, but without understanding the context of the risks to an organization, a business leader will never prioritize cybersecurity over IT. If there is a committee to understand the cybersecurity risks in addition to an IT prioritization meeting, it helps to bring context to discussions that may be too abstract or possibly misunderstood when the point is to focus on IT goals and priorities.

Cybersecurity should be part of the business discussion, but not dominate it. There may be certain points to emphasize during an IT operations committee, but the focus should be on the direction of IT—including resolving cybersecurity issues. The same is absolutely true for privacy and HIPAA compliance issues. If the compliance officer and the privacy officers are not present in these discussions, key points of focus may be missed. The overall goal should be everyone working as a team. No one should always get their way. The business needs to help balance and prioritize the actions of other teams. The same types of meetings can take place that also discuss compliance, privacy, and other kinds of business risks.

The same can be true even of sales meetings. Say that someone wants to buy de-identified data from a company that has PHI data on California residents. Because of CCPA, that data falls under HIPAA once it's re-identified. The GC or the CCO may have something to say about that sales process, and considerations for California residents should be built into the contract—as well as possible limitations on the use of the data. These kinds of decisions are incredibly important for covered entities to consider. Having the right people, in the right place, at the right time, can make all the difference in the world for protecting organizations not only from cybersecurity considerations, but also legal data protection considerations.

All of the gaps here, and many more, are part and parcel of creating a healthy organization. Inattention to management styles and effects can result in reverberations throughout organizations that can have real-world, material impacts on not only the security of IoMT, but also covered entities and the associated data within those organizations. If any voice is not heard and understood by the business unit, it can mean larger pain down the road.

Risk Management

In the last section we started to talk a bit about risk management and where to apply it, but the reality is that risk management is absolutely critical within covered entities—and not just because HIPAA and OCR require it as part of their framework. If risk management is being used specifically to meet compliance and no more, cybersecurity practitioners are not doing what they need to do to protect the organization. Risk management, if used right, is the rudder for steering organizations in the right direction. The recommendations in the previous section are really related to how to apply the key risks. It is worthwhile exploring a bit more about the topic to help understand what some options are in relation to risk management.

Risk Frameworks

There are many different risk frameworks and approaches when it comes to risk management. At the heart of what is important from a risk management perspective is meeting the compliance requirements and communicating with the business. You should have enough differentiation to prioritize risks in a reasonable fashion so you don't leave the business wondering how to do it. For example, if your risk matrix had "big" risks and "small" risks as the only options, it is probably too binary to communicate effectively with the business and will probably create some frustration.

There are two centralized types of risk frameworks—qualitative and quantitative. *Qualitative* usually provides a more generalized, less specific, and a bit more of a ranged approach to risk management. For many risk practitioners this way makes more sense. *Quantitative*, on the other hand, is more focused on specific dollar amounts. One of the standard equations of quantitative risk assessments is Single Loss Expectancy (SLE) × Annual Rate of Occurrence (ARO) = Annualized Loss Expectancy (ALE). The SLE can be a specific dollar value. The ARO is how many times the event will probably occur over a period of a year. Multiply those numbers together to get a specific dollar value. Many Chief Financial Officers (CFOs) and CEOs love this framework because it provides a very specific dollar value and a very clear definition about prioritization. That isn't to say that qualitative assessments cannot have a dollar value, but that dollar value is usually a range that is built into risk management.

There are dozens of variations of these two themes, and many CISOs create their own frameworks to meet specific requirements. Some organizations take inherent risk and multiply that by a percentage—often based on key performance (some prefer key risk) indicators of various programs—to represent the overall risk to the organizations. All of these methods have pros and cons and are worthwhile. As mentioned back in Chapter 9, the important thing is to label the variables with confidentiality, integrity, and availability in order to help meet HIPAA compliance. A simple tag tied to each risk or each vulnerability related to the risk is an easy way of accomplishing this goal.

Determining Risk

Neither quantitative nor qualitative risk assessments are 100% accurate. In risk assessments, not letting the "perfect" be the enemy of the "good" is especially important to remember. It is also important to remember that risks change all the time. The SolarWinds breach greatly upset the risk assessments of a large number of CISOs. Companies that utilized SolarWinds all of a sudden had far more risk than they were aware of.

There are numerous places to go to source risk. Many vendors provide copious notes for assessing the risks to organizations. Risk assessors should not be focused on any one source because each vendor looks at things from slightly different angles and tells a slightly different story. The more sources of information, the better and broader the picture that can be painted surrounding risk.

Internal experiences and information should also be a driver for organizations. What is true for one organization may not be true for another. Even the size of an organization matters—a greater number of people potentially clicking on phishing emails makes the risks higher for larger organizations than for smaller organizations. Paying attention to the internal maturity and the internal controls is a critical part of assessing risk for long-term strategies. With the sheer volume of IoMT in many covered entities, that changes the risks for covered entities, too.

Other sources of information may be vulnerability management information. If there are thousands of unpatched vulnerabilities in a covered entity, the risks go up. The more PHI that a covered entity has, the greater the risks to that organization. All of these things need to be considered when performing a risk assessment.

Third-Party Risk

Third-party risk management programs have been around for quite a while, but the SolarWinds incident also demonstrates how important it is for covered entities to know their third-party security posture. In fact, that breach caused a flurry of activity amongst many companies so that they could better understand the security surrounding their third-party vendors. Common methods for doing this include using standardized tools such as Standard Information Gathering (SIG) questionnaire. While there are many variations available, they consist of a standard set of questions that can be used to assess an organization's security posture. They are often in Excel format, and the owner of the SIG can modify the questions to suit his or her needs. Organizations can utilize any number of these tools available on the market or choose to create their own tools to assess where a business associate or another covered entity may be from a security standpoint.

SIG questionnaires and similar assessment tools give cybersecurity an opportunity to work with compliance and/or privacy—especially given how quickly the privacy landscape is changing in the United States and globally. The compliance or privacy teams may have a list of their own questions they may be interested in for these kinds of questionnaires. Quite often cybersecurity acts in a silo without collaborating with other parts of the organization. Reached across the aisle to work with the privacy team can help to make a stronger organization. Partnerships such as these can help organizations protect itself from not only IoMT risks, but also associated privacy risks or risks of data loss. Often in organizations there are silos that prevent teams from cooperating the way they need to in order to maximize the protective mechanisms.

There are also a range of other tools for assessing an organization's security posture that are not related to an Excel spreadsheet or other questionnaire format. For example, sometimes vulnerability management tools are used to get a rough sense of where the posture is of organizations. Some use open-source intelligence tools such as Shodan, which is search engine that can provide a great deal of technical information—including clues for hackers to attack organizations. Yes, hackers also use information from Shodan to find vulnerabilities. There are commercial tools that are a step up from Shodan that are also available that perform some of the same tasks such as passively detecting information from a commercial entity. The challenge with all of these tools is that they are often old or sometimes wrong. While sometimes they are correct and remediation can take place, seeing a response to something old or wrong can be extremely revealing to the assessor. That understood, IT, security, and account teams can and do get frustrated from having to respond to some of the output from these tools.

Risk Register

One of the key mechanisms for organizations to look at their top risks is through the creation of a risk register, which is essentially a list of risks that organizations face. How they are organized depends on the type of risk assessment, the risk to vulnerability format, what is considered a risk, what the business tolerance for risk is, and so on. They can include information from almost any of the sources we have spoken about so far including third-party risks. In totality, organizations can take the high-priority risk items and use that as the focal point to reducing risks. That is not always the yardstick that covered entities work from. Sometimes it is very easy for organizations to focus on risk remediation based on ability to remediate rather than on the highest risk. There are many factors that can make this a more reasonable approach to risk remediation. Most companies work on risk remediation projects simultaneously and often continuously. Sometimes building of one cybersecurity program can reduce several risks for an organization. Whatever the strategy, the risk register is a great way for organizations to evaluate where they need to focus their collective efforts.

Enterprise Risk Management

In healthy organizations, enterprise risk management (ERM) is a natural outcome of risk assessments. While cybersecurity is certainly important, so is compliance, privacy, and legal. Everyone has some blinders when it comes to other professions, which is why it is so critical for everyone to work together to make a strong organization.

But ERM is bigger than this. IT, finance, other legal considerations, sales, the ability to save lives, new technologies, getting the best doctors, and so on are all extremely critical to covered entities—each to their own degree. ERM is a place where organizations can discuss their top risks and help organizations determine the best path forward. It is a way of democratizing top priorities to focus on the right path to get the work done. It is not always perfect, though. Like all democracies, it can be an ugly, messy, imperfect business, but it is better than not doing it at all and letting passing whims dominate the strategies of covered entities.

Final Thoughts on Risk Management

Risk management is another tool not only within cybersecurity, but also within many other professions. There are numerous ways of applying many different forms of risk management within IT and cybersecurity. Not all personalities handle those risks the same way. Some CEOs, as hard as this might be to believe, are willing to accept just about any risk. Some are interested in buying and selling covered entities, so ERM processes are just another cost to consider. In these cases, no ERM system in the world can change someone's mind. It is exceptionally challenging to work with these situations. In the end, we are all people. Understanding the risk management processes, the differing views of various teams, and how to prioritize risks are all critical to protecting organizations. At least with an appropriately delegated, thoughtful approach, doing the right thing is a bit more achievable.

Mindset Challenges

Mindsets are very interesting to deal with. Everyone within an organization has particular way of thinking about what's important, and base their decisions on what's relevant to their cause—whether that's cost, compliance, privacy, or whatever. This can sometimes be detrimental to doing security properly. However, security cannot be the only consideration in a business decision—the goal is to find the right balance among a sea of factors. Many leaders get caught up listening to only certain vantage points, which can pull their perspective away from cybersecurity. It may only move the needle a few degrees in one direction, but that can be enough to push the outcome away from protecting IoMT and covered entities, which can sometimes affect lives.

The Compliance-Only Mindset

For security professionals, with some exceptions, the compliance-only mindset is one of the most dangerous mindsets a company can have.

That is not to downplay the importance of compliance because it is critical, but the challenge that security professionals have with compliance is that it is insufficient to keep up with modern-day risks. Almost from the moment a compliance framework is released, it begins to become dated. The adversaries are constantly innovating and so is the technology designed to defend us from them. For example, the HIPAA Security Rule was released in 2003, and covered entities should have been compliant by 2005. It has been fifteen years since the rule was put into place—meaning it hasn't changed. While many of the requirements are still relevant and have value, new technologies have emerged that have more value than those used currently. Security practitioners will implement requirements because it is the smart thing to do from a legal perspective, but also strive for the stronger controls before they become compliance requirements.

Further, there are always particularities within organizations that warrant a more fine-grained approach than what compliance requires. The flat network discussed in Chapter 10 is one such gap. If compliance is the only goal of organizations, some compliance models have no requirement around protecting IoMT or having an unflat network. This is one area where a more risk-based approach is better than compliance—something that covered entities should be embracing. The extent of the approach depends on a number of variables. At the very least, having positive and ongoing discussions about, for example, what VLANs to put in place will result in some progress being made, even if its imperfect from some viewpoints.

Cost Centers

Sometimes accompanying the compliance-only mindset is the mindset that IT and cybersecurity are cost centers. Twenty years ago, this was the challenge that IT had and, in some ways, still influences organizations today. As security became more of a discipline, it was seen in much the same way as IT. Both compliance and cybersecurity require us to follow rules, such as changing our complex passwords, that provide little or no business value from the perspectives of some business leaders.

As a result of this attitude, IT teams are often extremely lean—they don't have the resources to do their jobs effectively, and budgets are tight. By the time cybersecurity is considered (if at all), it piles on more work for the IT teams, and things, unsurprisingly, get deprioritized.

The challenges of IoMT just amplify the overall problems in organizations. The lack of centralized management for the systems multiplies the number of things that simply cannot get done. It is very painstaking, detail-oriented work in many of these cases. Luckily, as CMTOs know the value of getting systems ready, they will often require centralized management—unless it is someone else's responsibility. This is why committee and team meetings are so critical. What is a small detail in one case can be tremendously important in another case.

In the end, seeing IT and cybersecurity as a cost center only makes the likelihood of a breach all the more possible. While defending against an advanced adversary such as a nation-state is almost impossible, adding enough security may make the incidents less likely to happen, thus saving covered entities in the long run.

Us Versus Them

Sometimes, the cost center mindset can result in hostilities between IT, compliance, privacy, or cybersecurity teams. IT has important work to do for organizations. If they are completely overwhelmed, the additional work added from the other teams can be seen as an annoyance, especially if senior management judges IT based on IT demands, but not security. Or worse, management has their own blinders on, not worrying about what gets dropped or assuming that everything gets done in a reasonable manner (when it is not). What sometimes happens in these cases is that cybersecurity, privacy, and compliance become the enemy because they get in the way of getting things done from an IT perspective.

While sometimes this only results in de-prioritization, it does illustrate the importance of free and open communication for all parties involved—especially with the business unit. In many cases, senior IT, security, or compliance leadership will shift their focus to whatever senior management wants. It is a delicate balance that needs to be well thought out. If the us-versus-them mentality does not rear its head, sometimes the shiny object syndrome is the challenge.

The Shiny Object Syndrome

The shiny object syndrome is another classic management flaw that many organizations succumb to. What typically happens is that every project becomes a priority, so nothing becomes a priority. All leaders, IT, security, CEOs, and so on sometimes fall into this trap. Some new issue comes up or something hits the news and they focus entirely on that issue while many other things get dropped in the meantime. Sometimes those issues are really urgent, while other times waiting a few days for more information is the best way to approach the problem. If there are too many of these shiny objects, the workload becomes too overwhelming and organizations lose focus of what is or is not important. In short, projects that would normally get done, get pushed off as a result.

Like many of the other challenges that organizations face, the shiny object syndrome can be very disruptive to goal setting. Good organizations take the time to talk about the impacts of new projects on the overall process, and good business leaders take note and will course correct. Again, having the discussion as a round table with all the leaders involved is critical to appropriate balancing. Bad leaders just assume everything will get done and continue to pile on more shiny objects—not realizing that resources get stretched thinner and thinner.

These kinds of activities can be accomplished, but at the cost of dropping other activities or needing extra resources. Sometimes new people are hired, but not always at the pace required to get work done in a reasonable time. In companies without the appropriate business communications, this can result in a number of problems. Again, communication is key.

Never Disrupt the Business

A common mantra within organizations "never disrupt the business." With healthcare, it takes on special meaning as lives are often on the line—especially for anything related to the emergency room. This mentality has a great deal of weight behind it in this scenario. It adds to the overall risk of organizations, but for good reasons. For those who ascribe to the same ideals across the whole organization as a result, it creates additional challenges to better protect standard systems and IoMT devices. Now organizations are having to weigh the business risks related to ransomware against human lives. Covered entities are having to make some hard choices—do they finally start to do something about security, or do they continually pay ransoms? The balance between the two is not always simple.

It's Just an IT Problem

CEOs, business leaders, and boards of directors often don't appreciate the full breadth of cybersecurity, compliance, and privacy. Nor should they. That is what the respective leaders are for. They are the experts in their field. There are many different disciplines that comprise cybersecurity, compliance, and privacy, and most business leaders do not understand these complexities. It is important to look at each of these different disciplines in turn to see how they relate organizationally.

Cybersecurity grew out of IT. The vision of IT's role traditionally has been that cybersecurity takes care of firewalls, antivirus, and a host of security products. The reality is that cybersecurity and IT are linked at the hip, but cybersecurity is a business challenge. Many of the cybersecurity activities that we have talked about through this book are designed to check on IT activities or as additional protection against threat actors. Most of the items in IT hygiene are designed the same way. Improving the configurations improves what IT is doing. Adding EDR and MDR improves the defenses of organizations against the threat actors. Identity governance helps to shore up unused accounts in organizations. Vulnerability management and penetration testing is all about finding the problems before the threat actors do in order to remediate the risks. Many of the data protection items are to limit or prevent the loss of data.

Most of this seems very reasonable on the surface, but the perspectives change drastically in fiscally tight environments. Those extra five thousand vulnerabilities that need to be focused on get in the way of doing the "real" IT work that the business cares about. To many of you this may seem subtle, but in the minds of many leaders, the shift can be seismic. Organizations that do not listen to IT leaders about the amount of work being done and fail to help them can result in animosity. In addition, the fact that many problems related to IoMT are simply unresolvable can make cybersecurity seem something of an annoyance.

Privacy and compliance are seen in a slightly different light in many organizations. The experts tend to be lawyers. In fact, many of the HIPAA and HITECH considerations are best suited to those with a legal background. A cybersecurity professional can read HIPAA and HITECH, but their background does not include understanding the significance and subtleties of the law. That said, the HIPAA Security Rule does have some cybersecurity requirements. Some lawyers have taken it upon themselves to learn what that means operationally and have become respected experts in their field, but many lawyers do not focus on or understand the complexities of IT. Depending on the organization and the people involved, organizations may need either or both type of professional.

What is interesting, though, is that both compliance and privacy were born well outside of IT and offer another much-needed perspective within organizations. Going back to the earlier discussion of IT and cybersecurity, if there is a committee that includes all of these different perspectives, the weight of that discussion changes—especially outside of IT.

What many leaders do is hyper-focus on IT and hear only one side of the discussion—not really understanding the complexities of other perspectives. It lends itself to insufficient emphasis placed on other disciplines. Extremes of this perspective move toward a form of myopia where the leaders are aware, but not sufficiently focused on, other disciplines.

Tools over People

Some leaders put an emphasis on tools without realizing that supporting the tools can take an enormous amount of time and effort. From a cybersecurity perspective, it is not just about the tool, but how that tool is governed. Is the configuration secure? Is it properly protected from a network perspective? Are logs being centrally managed, monitored, alerted on, and responded to? Are those requirements reviewed on a periodic basis? Where are things slipping?

If one of five thousand devices isn't reporting, is the reason for that followed up on? While that seems like a rather minor consideration from those monitoring the logs, turning off alerting is often one of the first things that hackers will do. With IoMT, that may be the difference between being aware of an attack or not. Not investing in the appropriate resources to support the tools or the processes often leads to people overlooking "minor" considerations. Tools are critical, but so is the appropriate level of support—both related to the tool and from a personnel standpoint. Seemingly disparate teams can be affected by insufficient resources in one area.

We Are Not a Target

Many business leaders feel that their organizations are too small to be a target. When it comes to breaches, small businesses are just as much targets as anyone else. In fact, even the smallest covered entity can be targeted. Some threat actors prefer to go after smaller businesses because they usually are not equipped to protect themselves nor do they respond appropriately to cyberattacks. While Verizon's 2020 Data Breach Investigation Report reported that 28% of breaches involved small business, the reality is that smaller business probably get hit more than reported. From an attacker's perspective, sometimes the lack of maturity of smaller companies makes them easier targets.

The end result is that small businesses are often the target of ransomware and other attacks—often because the vulnerabilities are there and they are easy to compromise. The ransoms may not be of the eye-catching multimillion dollar variety, but they can shut down a practice. The reality is, every covered entity is vulnerable—not just the larger hospitals and conglomerated practices.

The Bottom Line

The bottom-line mindset is about a large emphasis on dollars and cents that can cause issues with implementing cybersecurity properly. Leaders that report into CFOs often run into this philosophy—everything runs the risk of being reduced to cost. Why pay for a $100,000 tool when a $15,000 tool is exactly the same type of tool? The $100,000 tool might be 80% more effective, but that may not matter if the bottom line is the only consideration. Some covered entities have purchasing groups that have the same function even if they report into different arms of the business. It can take a tremendous amount of time and effort to work with the groups to fully understand the impact of decisions that may harm other organizations. Let's take IoMT devices. As mentioned in Chapter 2, some have multiple device management capabilities, while others do not. If the CTO or purchasing groups do not understand the complexities and importance of device management, that can make the difference between having secure or unsecure devices, which can affect the security of the organization as a whole.

But amplify this across a hundred details for organizations that are extremely focused on the bottom line and it can be a real challenge to make changes. While device management is important, there may be numerous other considerations. When you are talking about the difference between saving lives and not, sometimes the IT or cybersecurity considerations are pushed to the side—and it is hard to argue with that perspective.

Final Mindset Challenges

Very rarely are any one of the mindset challenges discussed the only consideration within covered entities. Most covered entities have a blend of different personalities, issues, or emphasis. Usually flavors of the issues show up in varying degrees in different covered entities. Each one has a unique impact on organizations that can influence the thinking of leaders in different ways. These can slow or create challenges within organizations when it comes to protecting IoMT, data, and occasionally human life.

Decision-Making

How decisions are made varies greatly depending on the covered entity. Some covered entities are very informal. A quick discussion around the water cooler may be as much thought as is put into a decision. Other covered entities are more formal in their decision-making process, but most have a blended approach. Small decisions may be made around the water cooler, but larger decisions require more discussion or often escalation parameters. There are always course corrections that need to take place.

What is important to remember is that decisions are rarely made in a vacuum. They require communicating appropriately from many perspectives within an organization. The communication of risk is especially critical. Say the business does not want to pay for a firewall (a basic cybersecurity tool) due to cost. It is really important to have accountability in place. Maybe the CIO is asking for a firewall, but the business is saying no. What are the risks in that case? Who signs off for the fact that the firewall was not purchased? Who signs off on the risk? Are the denial and the sign-off on not purchasing a tool aligned with one another? How can alignment be achieved in the decision-making processes?

A Measured View

From many perspectives, the important things to focus on are facts and data. Blow things out of proportion and people remember that. Take a measured view with data to back up a viewpoint, and that starts to earn credibility. Credibility is absolutely key. Fortunately for IoMT, cybersecurity has a built-in tool to help with reasonable measuring of risk.

Today there are many different ways of measuring risk, but as mentioned earlier, the two primary types of risk measurements are qualitative and quantitative. Both have their pros and cons, and each appeals to different types of leaders. From a HIPAA standpoint, tying the risk into confidentiality, integrity, and availability is a critical aspect. If an IoMT device is facing the open internet with no firewall ACLs, no password requirement to gain full access to all hospital data through an EHR, and no patching or security software installed, most cybersecurity professionals would call that a critical risk. The likelihood of the system being hacked is high, and the impact would also be high. More than likely, if OCR found out about that situation after a breach, stiff penalties would be applied, and it would be an indicator of governance problems within an organization.

While that particular scenario is obviously extremely risky if not downright negligent, many other scenarios have shades of gray. Both quantitative and qualitative risk assessments can help with this. In some cases, the risks outlined on the risk resister may be tied to multiple vulnerabilities. In some cases, the risks may be tied to multiple vulnerabilities.

Whatever the format, most organizations pick top risks/vulnerabilities to focus on first and work their way to lower risks from year to year.

The reason that risk assessments and risk registers are so important is that they are a structured, written, repeatable process within the organization. Even external assessments that take a different format can be translated and integrated into the overall format to more accurately capture the risks that organizations face. They can also serve as a foundation for discussions in other committees throughout a covered entity. This may seem trivial to those outside of organizational politics, but it is absolutely essential. Let's take an IT steering committee as an example. If no one in the meeting understands the risks that IoMT devices often pose, merely stating that it is an issue is not going to go anywhere. On the other hand, if the weak security of poor IoMT devices is the cause of a top-five risk in an organization, the weight of that discussion takes on a very different tone.

Communication Is Key

As mentioned, communication is key. How that communication is made is extremely important. The more communication between the various entities, the more cohesion the senior leadership team is going to have. The more involved with the cross decision-making of various teams, the better the communications between different groups.

Trying to right size the various communication structures is extremely important. What is right for one covered entity may not be right for another. That said, there should be ample communication between all of the organizational teams discussed in this chapter and many more. Committees with the right people are very critical. If IT has operational meetings only within IT and does not include the business in the decision-making process, they head off in a direction not in line with the business. If the CFO has major sign-off in organizations, it is really important for the IT and cybersecurity leaders to justify what they are doing with the CFO. In fact, being in lockstep with them can be critical to the success or failure of a whole department.

While that is a tiny portion of what can go on, it may be important to include the CFO in many of the committees within a covered entity so they can buy into some of the initiatives. This may not always be appropriate depending on the governance framework of organizations, but getting that visibility across key players (which are different in each covered entity) is helpful. If decisions are made without the key players present, there is no way for the business to understand the dynamic for what is going on within their organization. This is where trust becomes incredibly important. Too much or too little trust from a business unit can make or break an organization a layer down from the key communication sources.

In the end, this can greatly impact the security of IoMT. In turn, this can influence how the data related to IoMT is disseminated, sanitized, tracked, or used. If key players are not present in the communication process, important observations can be missed by senior leadership that can greatly impact things. Let's say the business talks to IT about the technical feasibility of selling anonymized data, but not the privacy officer. They may not be aware that if the data is re-identified for California residents, it becomes PHI. That affects the contracting team—who may be fantastic at creating contracts but may not know about the finer points of California law.

While this is but one small example, these are the kinds of oversights that many organizations face to a greater or lesser extent. It takes active thoughtfulness on the part of business leadership to overcome these blind spots and not be over-reliant on any one part of the business. Without open communication, at several different levels within the organization, covered entities will continue to be compromised.

Enterprise Risk Management

In healthy organizations, enterprise risk management will emerge out of the various groups. It can grow from all of the different committees and points of discussion throughout the organization. Usually there is a formalized risk framework that the business utilizes, but quite often ERM boards (or committees) are much looser, where the top issues of covered entities are discussed holistically. Human resources, IT, the CMTO, and the CCO may bring their top concerns. While some business leaders are opposed to this kind of board, it is actually very critical to have these discussions because the types of challenges can really bring to light the health of different parts of the covered entity.

The more formalized the ERM process, the better things can be tracked. Maybe it is the case that cybersecurity has far too much staff or the challenges are trivial and compliance is completely overrun with extreme concerns. While those are hypothetical examples, they do serve to illustrate that each company has its own interesting challenges to overcome, and ERM is a great place to see how all of this works out and how everything translates to risk. If that risk reduces over time, that gives business leaders (and sometimes boards of directors) a sense that the business is improving.

ERM is a critical business function that larger covered entities should be engaging in to determine the overall health of their organizations. They help to see if key problems are being resolved over time, or at least that the challenges are identified and progress is being made in the long run. It may seem silly, but very large organizations have personality conflicts—some of which can be dealt with by utilizing better governance. ERM is one such place to depersonalize some of the issues and help move the needle in the right direction.

Writing and Sign-Off

The weight of the word is sometimes considered more important to leaders from a due diligence perspective, but from a legal standpoint, written words are better. In written form, a company could be held liable for not acting to address an issue because they cannot deny their knowledge that the problem exists. As a result, CEOs tend to take formal written communication more seriously. From a cybersecurity perspective, that written form is the risk register. If the CEO signs off on that strategy, all the better.

But signing off on a hundred vulnerabilities and risks is not always feasible in an organization. If even the high-risk items in the organization are signed off on by the CEO (or even the board of directors), it can be a huge win. Getting them involved with the push to reduce that risk within an organization can be a huge win from a cybersecurity perspective. Every single thing that can be done to move the needle in the right direction is a positive step.

Not all business leaders are willing to do this or even see the importance of doing so. There are business leaders that sign off on critical risk and still decide to do absolutely nothing. Doing all the right things is not a guarantee of a perfect outcome. The important thing is to strive to do the right thing.

Data Protection Considerations

Data protection is a major part of our overall story. It is also why protecting IoMT is so critical to covered entities and their business associates. However, having the right governance in place is important. Some organizations rely too heavily on the legal team to protect them if data happens to be stolen from a business associate.

The challenge with this overreliance is that they often do not take into account the cybersecurity of the organization they are sharing information with. It may come as a surprise to some of you, but some organizations are willing to sign BAA despite the fact they have very little security in place—not really realizing the severe gaps in their own cybersecurity that can, in turn, put not only themselves in legal jeopardy, but also the covered entities that the PHI originated from. The best way to handle this is for the legal team and the cybersecurity team to work together to create a better BAA or have a separate assessment process for those organizations. Let the legal team do what they are good at, and let the cybersecurity team do the same. Together, they can make a very powerful team for protecting organizations. They just need the time and the space to get the work done.

The same idea is true for many of the privacy laws. Whether it is around the selling of anonymized data or taking into account how California's laws affect data and the way contracts are written is of vital importance for organizations. Keeping one group out of a discussion puts organizations at a big disadvantage. The know-it-all mentality is not conducive to protecting data—especially from boards or CEOs.

In Summary

Organizational politics play a huge role in the ability of covered entities to defend themselves from IoMT, data-related risks, compliance risks, and occasionally human life. Every organization has its challenges, but governing an organization in the right way is absolutely critical to its overall success.

The goal is to bring to light some of the challenges of modern-day covered entities. It takes long hours and an interdisciplinary approach to protect organizations. Cybersecurity professionals often lack the nuance for understanding the effort it takes to do the work that IT engages in. It really does take a village to protect IoMT, data, and the associated covered entities.

If it was not clear before, we'll state it one last time: the key to a successful organization is communication, communication, communication. Senior leadership needs to communicate, up, down, and sideways. They need to give time to their senior leaders to communicate and perform not only the due diligence, but also the due care—to be thoughtful and research the best means to protect their organizations. Today's world is so complex and has changed so significantly from 20 years ago that many more technologies and solutions are needed to accomplish the goals. Once upon a time, simple legal agreements and simple cybersecurity practices were enough to protect covered entities. The solutions of yesterday cannot be held onto as the beacon of light for organizations—in fact, those solutions can lead to problems.

Being nimble and adapting, both from a management perspective and from a structural perspective, can completely change the foundation of how organizations are formed. Business leaders need to listen to the key players who report to them and realize that everyone has an important perspective to bring to the table. Listening to all voices is critical to overcoming today's challenges. With the appropriate leadership, we can better protect IoMT, our data, covered entities, and perhaps more than a few lives along the way.

Part

III

Looking Forward

So far, we have defined the challenges related to IoMT and many of the solutions. For some, things may seem extremely bleak and there is simply no hope for protecting covered entities and IoMT devices. While there are reasons to be concerned, the darkest hours often are the catalysts for the most important and fundamental changes within organizations.

With cybercrime growing so rampantly across the globe, the question is when and how will cybersecurity be adopted as part of the process—at least enough to reduce the fundamental risks? The purpose of this part of the book is to examine what changes are underway, how we can move toward doing no harm, and what further changes we need to better protect IoMT, covered entities, and human life.

These fundamental questions are often more about the people, processes, and technologies—not just on an organizational level, but on a global level. What is in motion to change the laws that allow global threat actors to act with impunity? How can we stop our data from being sold around the globe? How can we make changes to IoMT devices that allow for innovation yet still be secure? How should covered entities respond to these mix of challenges, and how are things changing?

Whether we like it or not, things are changing. In some cases it is for the better, and some cases not. Sometimes there are simultaneous steps forward and backward, depending on your point of view. This part explores the changes happening all around. It provides a lens for decision-makers to decide on better paths forward. Each change starts with a change of perspective, because having a bit more understanding of the context helps to elucidate a better way to move forward.

Seeds of Change

*The secret of change is to focus all of your energy, not on fighting
the old, but on building the new.*

—Socrates

Despite all the challenges that IoMT devices bring to the table, there
are many reasons to be hopeful—many of which we have discussed
throughout this book. Yes, most IoMT have poor security—the effects
of which are a significant drag on the security of covered entities. That
said, we have talked about two important strategies for covered entities
related to IoMT cybersecurity—UL 2900 and the cybersecurity approach.
Both of them have drawbacks that companies will have to navigate their
way through, but there is an answer for organizations. More awareness
needs to be drawn to the issue at the right level within organizations
to effect change.

As IoMT innovators make changes, so too are changes being made on
the technological front that are shifting how we approach. More solutions are being developed and/or integrated into existing technology
to deal with the challenges of IoMT.

From a legal perspective, there have been changes that will help to
increase the security of IoMT, but will also affect how we handle and
work with the data. As individual states start to make changes, there
is some movement on the federal level to make significant changes in
how we do or do not protect data.

One of the key pain points that needs far more attention is international cooperation to fight cybercrime. We discussed the challenges caused by poor international cooperation in Chapter 7, but it is not all doom and gloom. We have a very long way to go, but some of the seeds of change are already in place. We'll discuss some of these in this chapter.

Of course, all of these challenges affect how organizations think about cybersecurity, IoMT, and data security. The challenge is in creating the right kind of awareness at the right level within organizations to effect the right kind of change. Let's explore how all these ideas are affecting the interplay between protecting IoMT, covered entities, our data, and sometimes human life.

The Shifting Legal Landscape

In some respects, the United States has some catching up to do with other countries in terms of where our legal focus is. Europe's GDPR regulation demonstrates that they are leaps and bounds ahead of the United States in terms of privacy regulation. There have been several instances of the larger technology companies facing potential fines for gaps in their privacy practices. Quite often, but not always, companies take the approach of acting first and then asking for forgiveness later if they get caught. The level of fines that Europe is leveraging is beginning to make changes to how organizations operate—some companies going so far as to block Europe from accessing their systems.[1]

Attention on Data Brokers

Data brokers serve many legitimate purposes and are crucial for identity validation in many different contexts, though there are some challenges related to data brokers as discussed in Chapter 3. As pointed out in that chapter, Vermont's H.764 was the first law in the United States to focus on the challenges that data brokers bring to the table. California passed the second law in 2019 (A. B. 1202 Privacy: data brokers).[2] The number of laws that are proposed is obviously much higher—including proposals

---

[1] "GDPR: Tech firms struggle with EU's new privacy rules," May 2018, https://www.bbc.com/news/technology-44239126.
[2] Consumer Data Industry Association, "The California Data Broker Law," January 26, 2020 https://www.cdiaonline.org/the-california-data-broker-law/.

from Washington State, Illinois, and so on. New York has also passed (but not yet signed as of this writing) Senate Bill S6848 for data brokers to register their business with the state of New York.[3]

For those seeking protection from the risks that data brokers pose to sensitive data such as HIPAA data, the registration of data brokers may seem like a small step, but it takes some time to identify who is operating in a particular state and to understand, at least at a high level, what the business practices are related to the data. New York's Senate Bill S6848 defines personal information as "any information concerning a natural person which, because of name, number, personal mark, or other identifier, can be used to identify such natural person."[4] This is important because it is much broader than a strict definition of personal information used in other contexts. We, as a nation, are starting to realize that many of the data points identified previously are woefully inadequate to today's data mining techniques.

Senate Bill S6848 also informs the state if the data broker offers consumer and opt-in or opt-out option regarding the collection of personal information. The same holds true for the sale of personal information. If 99% of the data brokers had an opt-out model for the sale of information, that would help inform lawmakers of the types of challenges they face. If the data brokers had neither an opt-in nor an opt-out model, that demonstrates a whole different set of challenges. Armed with that kind of information, lawmakers can make better laws regarding how data brokers ought to use our personal information.

While more and more states are starting to create data broker legislation, these are patchwork solutions to a national issue; for example, someone in California could opt out, but someone in Oregon might not have that option. In the end, these are very positives steps, but it could take decades to get legislation across all 50 states to determine the extent of the data privacy challenges and appropriately strategize a response. There have been calls for a national registry. For example, the *New York Times* published an opinion article that said just that. Essentially, it stressed the need to have a national registry in order to help us determine how to distinguish between good and bad practices in regards to actions that data brokers may take.[5] For example, if a global data broker sold data

---

[3] November 13, 2019, https://legislation.nysenate.gov/pdf/bills/2019/S6848.

[4] Ibid.

[5] Jordan Abbott, "Time to Build a National Data Broker Registry," https://www.nytimes.com/2019/09/13/opinion/data-broker-registry-privacy.html.

on American citizens to China, we have to determine if that is in our best national interest or not. The answer to that question may depend on a large number of factors and may not be easily intuitable. Certainly collecting more information about the practices that data brokers have is a worthwhile endeavor. While things are far from perfect in the data broker space, at least laws like this are building awareness and helping us define the extent and the scope of the data privacy challenges.

While each state focuses on the data broker issues in a slightly different way, having the solid information and facts about data brokers will help us to build a reasonable response to many of those challenges. Data has been referred to as the new gold. Not regulating how that data is used has caused numerous harms that need a higher level of attention. If we want to do no harm, more and better universal regulation is required.

Data Protection Agency

The United States is one of the few democracies that does not have a data protection agency of some kind. We have elements of privacy and data protection on the national level through HIPAA, but nothing that is holistic in its approach. However, in 2020, Senator Kirsten Gillibrand proposed a Data Protection Agency for the United States that would have the power and authority to tackle the immense privacy challenges regarding the sharing of our data by data brokers.[6] While the focus is obviously much larger than the concerns of HIPAA (as it should be), such an agency could have a profound impact on the utilization of HIPAA data. Right now, foreign governments can purchase data on American citizens—including re-identified (HIPAA) data (except for California residents). The United States is clearly not equipped to handle these kinds of challenges. Whether or not Senator Kirsten Gillibrand's proposal becomes law, it does clearly illustrate that we need to make some federal-level changes in how we handle data. We cannot have all-encompassing and draconian laws related to data because there are always exceptions that need to be considered—especially as technology and data science grow and change over time.

---

[6] "Confronting A Data Privacy Crisis, Gillibrand Announces Landmark Legislation To Create A Data Protection Agency," February 13, 2020, https://www.gillibrand.senate.gov/news/press/release/confronting-a-data-privacy-crisis-gillibrand-announces-landmark-legislation-to-create-a-data-protection-agency.

IoT Legislation

In late December 2020, the United States passed the IoT Cybersecurity Improvement Act.[7] Part of the impetus for this act is to improve the abysmal security of IoT in general so that IoT devices destined for the federal government have to minimally meet NIST IoT cybersecurity standards. From an IoMT perspective, what is positive about this bill is that companies that wish to sell medical devices to the federal government have a bar that is set for them that is not as stringent as UL 2900, but still far in excess of the almost no standards now. From a non-governmental perspective this is important because some of those security precautions will affect the security of IoMT as well. The reportability criteria will hopefully mean that there is a public record of vulnerabilities that will provide greater clarity around their exact nature. In short, if covered entities choose IoMT devices that are compliant with NIST, they can better respond to the vulnerabilities that exist within organizations.

But the IoT Cybersecurity Improvement Act also requires secure development of the software that is part of IoT. This means that there should be fewer vulnerabilities in those devices. Manufacturers will have to focus on vulnerability reduction rather than simply features and time to market. NIST also requires stronger identity management within IoT devices, which means that stronger controls will be put into place. Patching and configuration management are also part of the requirements. Devices that meet the NIST standards must have security patching related to those devices.[8]

These along with many other provisions are destined to make things better. Of course, not all manufacturers sell to the federal government nor do they need to comply with the IoT Cybersecurity Improvement Act, but the act will provide greater options than permitted under UL 2900. It is an excellent middle-of-the-road option for covered entities that choose not to go with the full protection of UL 2900.

---

[7] Maria Henriques, "IoT Cybersecurity Act Improvement Act signed into law," December 9, 2020, https://www.securitymagazine.com/articles/94123-iot-cybersecurity-improvement-act-signed-into-law.

[8] 116th Congress (2019-2020) H.R. 1668—IoT Cybersecurity Improvement Act of 2020, https://www.congress.gov/bill/116th-congress/house-bill/1668/text.

Privacy Legislation

The 2020 state legislature meeting stated that 24 states are considering consent requirements prior to collecting information from or disclosing information to third parties. Other rights under considerations by various states include:

- The right to delete personal information
- The right to correct personal information
- The right to opt out of collecting information
- The right to opt out of sharing information
- The right not to be discriminated against for exercising rights

That said, there are numerous state bills under consideration for changing the privacy rights. There could be whole books set to explore the impact of how privacy will be changing the landscape in the near future. As discussed in Chapter 6, California has been leading the charge to better protect PHI from the various data brokers, but also to protect privacy in general. These kinds of legal remedies are not perfect, but they do change the risk landscape from a business perspective to nudge data brokers and others to be more careful about how they approach data. As each state adopts its own standard, covered entities will have to be extremely careful about the impacts within their organizations.

Obviously, companies that are in nations around the globe have to comply with the slew of international privacy regulations. This radically shifts the international landscape and incentivizes companies to think more carefully about their data governance practices. In the end, privacy will have a very large impact on protecting our data—whether it be PHI, PII, or other such data.

A Ray of Legal Light

In the end, we have a patchwork of improvements across the legal landscape that are changing IoMT, cybersecurity, and privacy for everyone in the United States, but we clearly have a long way to go in terms of meeting the requirements comprehensively. Still, every step we take means we get closer to a better situation overall. Take CCPA. Some companies, like Microsoft, have decided to assume that CCPA is a national requirement and apply it throughout the United States.[9] While many covered entities will not take this stance, even a few adopting the practice is a positive step forward.

International Agreements

As discussed in Chapter 7, the fact that many countries provide a relative safe zone for cybercriminals by not cooperating with law enforcement is not just a pain, but actively encourages cybercriminals to carry out their attacks. The reasons for this are multifold, and this should not be construed as blame; it is more of an unfortunate consequence of resource constraints and the capabilities of the host country. There are hundreds of other influences that can have an impact on countries being able to respond effectively.

Despite the challenges, the need is quite high for international cooperation. Cybercriminals sometimes hop from system to system in order to hide their tracks. These hops can be in multiple countries that provide the cybercriminals with a degree of anonymity. If the chain is broken in even one country, that creates attribution challenges for law enforcement. Sometimes these can be overcome, but other times, this broken link can make attribution impossible. Universal global cooperation is the best way to maximize attribution.

Public-Private Partnerships

Cybercrime is an interesting challenge for organizations to deal with because it is typically targeted at a private company, so they need to work hand in hand with law enforcement to collect the evidence. When considering covered entities, they can have a range of forensic capabilities or even awareness. Quite often attacks are recognized from external law enforcement. The Mandiant M-Trends report for 2020 still demonstrated that in the Americas companies found out they were compromised external to their own capabilities 48% of the time. Conversely, internal

---

[9] Julie Brill, "Microsoft will honor California's new privacy rights throughout the United States," November 2019, https://blogs.microsoft.com/on-the-issues/2019/11/11/microsoft-california-privacy-rights/.

detection of a compromise was 52%.[10] This means that many companies (which does include covered entities) are not detecting the attacks in their environment.

Law enforcement is dependent on private cooperation and vice versa. If law enforcement detects an attack, they need to work with private companies to handle the challenges. Conversely, private organizations typically do not have the power to handle law enforcement actions. Cross collaboration between public and private organizations is the best way to achieve the maximum chance of convicting cybercriminals.

But sometimes, there are activities that private corporations can do. For example, in the famous SolarWinds case, Microsoft, through the courts, gained control of the domain name that the malware was using to control other systems. They turned it into a "sinkhole" to prevent the owners of the malware from using it in a malicious fashion.[11] Part of the reason Microsoft did this is to discover all the firms that were affected by the attack. It is not the first time that Microsoft engaged in such a formal response, and this was also done against botnets.[12]

In the end, these extraordinary measures can help the larger private organizations in the fight against global cybercrime in these severe cases. Sometimes these monolithic corporations can reach beyond the short arm of the law to work with courts around the globe more quickly than local law enforcement, while at the same time being dependent on that law enforcement for more individual responses.

Better National Coordination

The United States has been working toward better cybersecurity intelligence since 1998 when the federal government asked each sector to share information about threats and vulnerabilities. By 1999, the first Information Sharing Analysis Centers (ISACs) were formed. Two ISACs related to healthcare specifically are the Health ISAC, which covers threat intelligence and best practices, and Healthcare Ready, which focuses

---

[10] FireEye Mandiant, "M-Trends 2020 Report," https://content.fireeye.com/m-trends/rpt-m-trends-2020.

[11] "Microsoft unleashes 'Death Star' on SolarWinds hackers in extraordinary response to breach," December 2020, https://www.geekwire.com/2020/microsoft-unleashes-death-star-solarwinds-hackers-extraordinary-response-breach/.

[12] Catalin Cimpanu, "Microsoft and industry partners seize key domain used in SolarWinds hack," December 15, 2020, https://www.zdnet.com/article/microsoft-and-industry-partners-seize-key-domain-used-in-solarwinds-hack/.

more on the healthcare supply chain. They provide invaluable insights about attacks that are occurring in the sector.

A standard format was needed for sharing this information without exposing the companies that were attacked. The language for modeling and representing cyber threat intelligence is known as Structured Threat Information Expression (STIX). It can include things like the attack pattern, the threat actor, geographic information, metadata, and so on. Accompanying STIX is TAXXI (Trusted Automated eXChange of Indicator Information). The purpose of TAXXI is to share the information of STIX from a cross-organizational perspective. Through these formats (and others), ISACS can share data without giving away information about the organizations that determined the intelligence. It makes it more likely to suss out the attacker's location outside the organization, which makes us better able to defend ourselves from would-be attackers.

Of course, threat intelligence is far from perfect, and the value depends on the type of information and the techniques and tactics the threat actor employs. If the hash of a file is used in STIXX, generally it is of less value today than it was 15 years ago, which is why the antivirus of yesteryear is simply not as effective as today's next-generation antivirus with EDR and MDR—they are not even in the same league. If you are talking about the point of origin for an attack, that can be much more valuable if the threat actor is reusing that domain or IP address on the network to launch their attack from. With each threat actor, the value will be different.

While these kinds of activities are fantastic and have definitely had an impact on the security of organizations, they often are not enough—SolarWinds definitively proved that. In fact, as a result of this single attack against this single organization, the FBI, the Cyber Unified Coordination Group (UCG), CISO, and ODNI—with support from the NSA—all started working together to look at the ongoing effects of the attack throughout many of the compromised organizations.[13] This coordination of US Government interagency work is uncommon, but it does help to illustrate how serious this kind of attack is. It also points to how federal agencies can work together and how those agencies can work with private companies to help thwart the damage of known cyberattacks. While the event that led these agencies to work together was reprehensible, it does show the positive that can be inspired as a result. Hopefully this will inspire more cooperation between government and private enterprises.

---

[13] Cybersecurity & Infrastructure Security Agency, January 2021, https://www.cisa.gov/news/2021/01/05/joint-statement-federal-bureau-investigation-fbi-cybersecurity-and-infrastructure.

International Cooperation

Despite all of the problems the world has, many nations have started to realize the impact of global cybercrime and have started to take steps to reduce it. Already, 55% of the members of Budapest convention have domestic legislation in place to criminalize cybercrime.[14] This may seem low, but even stepping back to 2013, only 71% of the Americas had cybercrime laws underway or undertaken on the books compared to 91% in February 2020.[15] These are positive steps forward in the fight against cybercrime. They are also a step forward for international cooperation because nations need to have laws in place prior to legally going after cybercriminals in their own countries.

That said, there are still a large number of hurdles before we achieve parity between physical crimes and cybercrimes. If there are even a handful of countries that are non-cooperative, they become relative safe havens for cybercriminals. But what do countries do when traditional espionage actors turn to cybercrime? That is exactly what happened with Chinese espionage group APT27. They changed their methodology to ransomware.[16] Espionage by itself is tolerated between nations, but when those traditional actors turn to financially motivated crimes, it shifts the balance of power. Imagine the cybersecurity damage that can be done when slow, methodical threat actors turn away from espionage and begin draining companies through ransomware. Russia's involvement in the SolarWinds attack was not detected for months. This may be the beginning of a whole new set of crimes.

In the end, we have large setbacks and a long way to go in the international arena. Some solutions will require diplomacy, some will require furthering cooperation between nations, and still others will require better technology. It is that relationship between technology and law enforcement that is absolutely critical for protecting IoMT and covered entities.

---

[14] "Global state of cybercrime legislation: Update!" March 20, 2020, https://www.coe.int/en/web/cybercrime/-/global-state-of-cybercrime-legislation-update-.

[15] "The global state of cybercrime legislation 2013 - 2020: A Cursory overview," March 20, 2020, https://rm.coe.int/3148-1-3-4-cyberleg-global-state-feb2020-v1-public/16809cf9a9.

[16] Global Threat Center, "APT27 Turns to Ransomware," December 2020, https://shared-public-reports.s3-eu-west-1.amazonaws.com/APT27+turns+to+ransomware.pdf.

Technology Innovation

While some of the technology changes recommended in this book are decades old, there has been a growing interest in cybersecurity as companies invest more and more in a range of products. In 2004, the global market was a mere $3.5 billion. In 2017 it was worth more than $120 billion. In 2021 it may exceed $1 trillion.[17] While traditional products such as antivirus and firewalls are still mainstays of cybersecurity, the numbers and types of products that exist today far outstrip what existed in 2004. The fact that threat intelligence had only been on the scene for a few years meant that the market had room to expand and change radically. This would not only apply to forensic investigations, but also the creation of file integrity tools, virus signatures, and sandboxes (for safely detonating threats).

Threat Intelligence

Threat intelligence has also focused on what is happening on the dark web. People and companies monitor the deep and dark webs for unusual domains, attack signatures, compromised passwords, and so on. Many companies offer services where they have people join criminal organizations posing as threat actors. This gives a more complete picture of attacks that may be imminent against covered entities and a forewarning of possible zero-day attacks that may be unknown on any given day.

Machine Learning Revisited

In the last few years, we have seen the advent of machine learning and the beginning of artificial intelligence built into an array of products, which greatly improves the success rate of detecting and/or stopping attacks in our environments. Without these technologies, covered entities would be almost completely defenseless against adversaries. Machine learning can also include behavior analytics (user and machine) to detect new or unusual behavior in an array of contexts—intrusion detection, email, network, and so on. Many companies are realizing the limiting nature of looking at logs alone and are starting to examine packets to

---

[17] Steve Morgan, "Global Cybersecurity Spending Predicted To Exceed $1 Trillion From 2017-2021," June 2019, https://cybersecurityventures.com/cybersecurity-market-report/.

detect behavioral anomalies. Many products today can also block newly formed domains, discussed in Chapter 3, which are a huge source of problems for organizations.

Zero Trust

Also, in the last few years the concept of zero trust has been gaining a lot of traction. Zero trust, as its name implies, means not trusting anyone or anything. In part, it is an extension of the principle of least privilege—people and machines have only the access they need and no more. This extends to many different parts of IT, but the first place that most people tend to think of is the network. The network ACLs discussed in Chapter 10 are a really good start and are effective in a static network, but the reality is there are many other tools and technologies on the market today. One technology can "hide" all operating systems and environments unless you have the agent installed on the system and the specific user is authorized to see that system. Others create dynamic ACLs that incorporate access based on who the individual person is on the network. This can have huge advantages for international organizations because network ACLs are created on the fly to reflect the access requirements of that person-ultimately saving network administrators time. PAM, too, can be a great way to establish zero trust. Today, there are many options based on the network alone.

Astute observers or experienced cybersecurity practitioners have probably realized that inherent in the last few options presented is a powerful shift toward the user. This is far from accidental and part of the design of zero trust. In the old-school network ACLs, if someone logged in to a computer that was from a different location, they would have the access of the computer they were at and not necessarily have the access for that specific user. It is an older way of setting up networks, but not necessarily ideal from a zero-trust perspective. It is not a business-flexible design.

Look at it from another standpoint. The data is not protected. If that user from another location had access to a shared drive on the computer, in the old-school model, that user could read all the files and information. Many of the enterprise encryption tools discussed in Chapter 15 lend themselves to that zero-trust model. In that same chapter, we also discussed tokenization. Since tokenization can allow data to be seen based on the specific user, that too can be part of a zero-trust model.

From an identity perspective, the example of allowing a user to access a computer they do not normally have access to could also be a violation of zero trust. Giving people the minimal access they need to do their jobs is another great way of moving toward that zero-trust model. Separating normal user accounts from administrative accounts when tied to network access completely enhances the zero-trust capabilities.

Zero trust may seem extreme to some of you, but from an IoMT perspective, many of these capabilities (and there are many other options) is the perfect way to help defend those systems. In a zero-trust environment, depending on the solution, hackers may be slowed down significantly. It is completely the opposite of the open network so common in covered entities from 20 years ago. Everything that we have been talking about these last several chapters lays the foundation for protecting IoMT, covered entities, our data, and sometimes our very lives. In the spirit of doing no harm, these approaches are some of the better ones for protecting today's systems.

Final Technology Thoughts

We have barely begun to scratch the surface of the kinds of innovation available on the market today for protecting IoMT systems. Each tool can be set up and utilized in a unique way to help organizations. What may seem useless from one person's perspective can be a fantastic tool from another's perspective. Today there are so many different types of products on the market that can be used in so many different ways that we need to be thoughtful about our approach to protecting IoMT and its associated ecosystem. If IT or cybersecurity were easy, we would not be facing the challenges we have today. Systems would not be breached, ransomware would not exist, and we would be living in a fairytale. To truly protect ourselves, we need to focus on these next-generation technologies and solutions to protect us.

Leadership Shakeups

As companies experience more and more breaches and as the amount that ransoms demand grow year after year, the way business is done is changing. Cybersecurity used to be an IT activity where antivirus was installed and firewalls were configured. Comparatively, that seems like the golden age of technology from a risk perspective. Today, cybersecurity is a board-level issue (or should be). There is a problem if the board of directors is not hearing part of the cybersecurity story and the business is not actively engaged with it.

Cybersecurity is complicated. It's far too complicated for either the CEO or board of directors to understand how every single risk ties into every little detail. Information needs to be conveyed to senior management in bite-sized messages in order for them to understand. Today's business is often dependent on having a strong cybersecurity program. Many organizations will refuse to work with or share data with companies that have weak cybersecurity programs. It is built into many of today's contracts. This applies to covered entities as well. If cybersecurity is not in lockstep with the business or vice versa, contracts can be signed that should never be signed.

That said, humble leadership is absolutely essential. Giving a fair shake to everyone on the team from the privacy officers to the compliance officers to the CIO and CISO is absolutely essential. It takes fair and balanced teamwork with everyone working together to ensure that organizations are protected properly. The compliance checkbox approach of yesteryear is no longer sufficient to defend against today's threats. Agile leadership that listens to the strengths and weaknesses of the various disciplines that work for them is essential in today's world. The successful companies are the companies that listen to everyone on their team.

Blended Approaches

In business, covered entities need to make choices and trade-offs between protecting the patient and protecting data. A draconian approach on one side of the needle or the other can lead to failure. As we saw in Germany, with the ransomware that prevented a hospital from operating, a patient was diverted to another hospital and subsequently died. The hospital was arguably too lax on cybersecurity. It focused more on human life. No one would ever argue that there should be less focus on protecting human life. Rather covered entities should focus more on cybersecurity. That is often easy to say and hard to do. With resource limitations, often decisions need to be made about where to focus resources. Hiring one extra resource for cybersecurity may mean not hiring an additional resource for the emergency room. Taking a balanced, blended approach is probably the right thing to do—recognizing that each choice has a consequence. The answers to protecting organizations are not black and white, but a blend of gray.

Unfortunately, the current threat landscape is in favor of the attackers. This is why many of the basic controls are so critical to put into place, along with new technologies. It is also important to remember that weak security in IoMT can mean downtime because of ransomware or other attacks. These are not easy decisions that covered entities need to make—especially with human life potentially hanging in the balance on both sides of the equation. The cybersecurity team working with the medical device team to evaluate the pros and cons of various solutions from both perspectives is absolutely critical to protecting today's IoMT and covered entities. Including everyone in the decision-making process means better decisions can be made overall.

Other options are on the table, too. For example, for life-sustaining IoMT, sometimes the best approach may be UL 2900, while for other less important systems, UL 2900 may not need to be the standard. There are so many paradigms that the leadership within covered entities can take to best create a balance between human life and cybersecurity. Providing the appropriate time to get all of this done is absolutely critical.

In Summary

What often accompanies adversity is an array of possible solutions. The challenges that both the threat landscape and the vulnerabilities of IoMT pose are no different. Countries around the world are starting to see the value of international cooperation when it comes to cybercrime—it simply makes every company, every government, and every person a little bit safer. There is no one solution to fit every crisis, but creating a balance and blend of different practices, management styles, technologies, and strategies will help us to create a better tomorrow. The seeds of change have very much been planted and will continue to grow with each new challenge.

Much of what we have focused on throughout this book are solutions that have been around for years, if not decades, in some cases. Of course, there are new twists on old technologies and innovation for blending and balancing the needs of people with advanced IoMT technologies with the safety and security of new technologies and strategies. There is no one-size-fits-all approach as IoMT is not a one-size-fits-all technology.

By utilizing legal, compliance, risk, IT, governance, and process strategies, a dent can be made in the processes we utilize to protect IoMT, data, and overall privacy. We have to be flexible and push forward on multiple fronts in order to defend the modern covered entity in the face of poor IoMT security.

CHAPTER

19

Doing Less Harm

Don't let perfect be the enemy of the good.

—Voltaire

It is important to remember that not all IoMT devices and all covered entities are the same. When striving to deal with the challenges that IoMT devices present, not every challenge is worth equal attention. It depends on the context. Doing no harm in one area means allowing harm to be done in another. To make that clearer, in some cases the risks are very low from poor security and the innovation can save lives, so it may be worthwhile to introduce minor risks. For example, an ingestible IoMT device presently poses very little risk from cybercriminals harming an individual or covered entities and can provide powerful diagnostic capabilities for medical practitioners. As a result, spending valuable resources to secure that disposable device is not a prudent use of time—nor is it the best way to do less harm.

The goal of doing no harm is admirable, but with limited resources and a race against time to save lives, we have to be realistic about which challenges we are going to deal with. Risk can never be completely mitigated, but being thoughtful about the approach is absolutely critical to maximizing the reduction of risk.

But each group can offer their own approach to doing what they can to do less harm. This chapter explores what manufacturers, covered entities, manufacturers of cybersecurity products, and even you can

329

do to do less harm overall. We all have our part to play in solving the challenges that IoMT devices bring to the table.

What IoMT Manufacturers Can Do

It would be easy to say that all manufacturers should follow UL 2900 and get their devices certified, but the reality is that sometimes strict requirements get in the way of much needed innovation. When Silicon Valley works alongside the men and women who work in hospitals to see the challenges that existing products have in real-world scenarios, that truly makes a difference. The information gleaned from those meetings allows companies to innovate faster and better design new tools and systems to help doctors and patients alike. It really is a cornucopia of innovation. The challenges of each innovation spawn the next level of innovation in a never-ending improvement cycle.

That said, it does not mean that a cybersecurity on/off switch must be utilized. We do not have to choose between having UL 2900 or no security in place. There is room for a whole spectrum of gray—even for innovative startups. Even taking the time to have the system connect to Active Directory (it is bigger than this, but think of it as a central repository for logon accounts in this case) means that at least there is the possibility of centralized account administration—one of the cornerstones of cybersecurity.

If software development is being performed, take advantage of free resources available on the web. OWASP has more than just the IoT top-10 security risks. Have the software developers read up on the resources available on OWASP's website to at least reduce some of the risks they may be developing into the IoMT products. There is also a whole range of open-source tools on the market for doing basic security checks. Yes, mature security practitioners would be quick to point out that these tools are insufficient to completely protect organizations or that sometimes these tools have deficiencies or malware built into them. Remember, though, we are looking at creating a path rather than simply doing nothing. Many startups cannot afford to develop mature cybersecurity programs or pay for external companies to help them with it. Even a little bit can help reduce the cybersecurity challenges that IoMT brings to covered entities.

As startups go through their funding stages (if applicable) and grow, they can begin to increase both their internal cybersecurity and their software development cybersecurity. They can begin to either move away from freeware tools and use their own, or depending on what they can afford, they can begin to outsource at least a few checks against their software. (DAST) is one such tool that can be utilized for analyzing vulnerabilities in software in a live environment. While not as thorough as a code review or penetration testing, at least it is a step in the right direction.

As pointed out in Chapter 4, the larger manufacturers are often moving in a more Silicon Valley direction in terms of their IoMT development. They are taking the time to develop their products hand-in-hand with covered entities to make the products better on the fly as doctors, nurses, and others are working on the floor. In turn, they change the design of the product to make it easier to use. Each tiny innovation is an important step. It helps those larger manufacturers interconnect with other products and often help save lives.

What is great about these larger organizations is they often have the ability to invest in the tools to ensure a more secure development process—even if those changes are happening relatively quickly. In some cases, UL 2900 is not an out-of-reach dream, but a must have for their markets.

This is not the only advantage these larger companies have. They often have more influence on chip manufacturers related to the security of chips. They can focus on cybersecurity as a point of leverage when choosing the manufacturer to use.

Some manufacturers use older operating systems in their IoMT devices because they are less expensive. For some markets, in some contexts, this makes perfect sense. For organizations that are striving to save money, a few dollars off per device can save hundreds of thousands of dollars or more. The question is, is it really worth it when considering the risks to organizations and to data?

Two other key problems that IoMT manufacturers can focus on is supporting patching and the installation of cybersecurity protective software. Some small manufacturers cannot support updates natively, but even if they partnered with a company to do the testing and support for covered entities, it would go a long way toward alleviating the pains associated with unprotected IoMT devices. Extra costs and support plans may need to be factored in, but given the overall prevalence of threat actors, this is a small price to pay. Conditions can be built into the process that if functionality is broken by companies patching IoMT devices prior to authorization, it is not the responsibility of the manufacturer.

Opponents of this perspective are quick to point out that this creates operational overhead for the already overworked IT teams, as patching schedules will be different based on different kinds of systems—which can be especially challenging in the case of IoMT. Testing each type of IoMT that may be within an organization prior to rollout of the patches can be costly. However, patching can be a less expensive alternative to installing new software. Some organizations will have to choose which is the most palatable option.

Cybersecurity as Differentiator

As the importance of cybersecurity continues to grow, it can, and should, be a differentiator for organizations. As CISOs become more involved in the IoMT decision-making process, manufacturers are starting to move the needle more in the direction of cybersecurity. The sales departments are starting to add security into their overall sales strategy—and becoming more specific about what that means. It also means that CISOs (or someone on his or her team) are becoming part of the sales discussions for many manufacturers.

As covered entities, and in particular hospitals, are the targets of an increasing number of attacks, they are becoming more careful about the solutions they purchase. Not all covered entities require UL 2900 from their IoMT devices, but taking strong steps to ensure a secure SDLC process would go a long way in securing IoMT. In fact, remediating everything in the OWASP IoT Top 10 list would also be a big help for many companies. It is obvious that not all startups in the IoMT space can afford to do security the right way, but even small steps are a big help.

What Covered Entities Can Do

Covered entities are caught between a rock and a hard place. We have already covered the medical staff verses cybersecurity debate, but another challenge they may have is the innovative fast-paced designs that can be cheaper than the UL 2900- or NIST- compliant devices. Both options have costs associated with them. These conundrums are slowly dragging cybersecurity out of the technical discipline and into spotlight for both business executives and the board of directors. The challenge they now face is how to communicate with people who quite often have no cybersecurity training nor a means of understanding the plethora of technologies and strategies that cybersecurity professionals have to offer.

Luckily, there are strategies that can help, such as the NIST Cybersecurity Framework (CSF). It's a risk framework that breaks things down into five functional areas: Identify, Protect, Detect, Respond, and Recover. Even those not overly versed in cybersecurity will instantly have a rough idea what those words mean. Organizations can choose to rate a company's effectiveness in each of those areas on a scale of 1 to 5 (5 being the highest), so if any of them receives a 1, it's clearly a cause for concern.

While there are many other ways to communicate the various types of problems, this is probably about the right level to give a general sense of the challenges within organizations. The ratings, although unrefined, can act as a general compass for organizations to move in the right direction when it comes to cybersecurity—as long as cybersecurity is given a voice.

Cybersecurity Decision-Making

CEOs and boards of directors have a fiduciary responsibility within covered entities. Toward that end, it is absolutely critical that they become involved in the decision-making process for security—not in the day-to-day minutia, but in the overall trends. Oftentimes, the needs of doctors and IT take the limelight—with no one really understanding how security is doing. Giving cybersecurity an unfiltered voice within organizations is critical from the top down. If IT or other voices are allowed to mute that conversation, there is far less hope of achieving the right balance within the organization from a cybersecurity perspective.

That said, cybersecurity is beginning to have more influence across organizations. If covered entities are serious about doing no harm, then cybersecurity has to have a larger influence. In fact, many businesses outside covered entities are heavily investing in cybersecurity. In many instances the cybersecurity spend will be more than 40% of the IT budget,[1]

---

[1] Steve Zurier, "Security spending will top 40% in most 2021 IT budgets," February 2021, https://www.scmagazine.com/home/security-news/security-spending-will-top-40-in-most-2021-it-budgets/#:~:text=Some%2056%25%20of%20IT%20leaders,budgets%20to%20cybersecurity%20in%202021.

whereas the healthcare currently spends anywhere from 4% to 7% of their budget on cybersecurity.[2] With numbers like these combined with IoMT devices, it is no wonder that healthcare is in such dire straits from a cybersecurity perspective. They need to do more to protect themselves in many cases. In fact, cybersecurity needs to be a continually improving process. The only way to get there is to give cybersecurity the latitude to do the right thing—with everyone cooperating.

Compliance Anyone?

HIPAA compliance, although dated, has a large number of cybersecurity requirements that are worthwhile for today's covered entities. The challenge is that there is no HIPAA certification for organizations. There are HIPAA risk assessments that can bring risk into the equation, but that is far from saying a company is HIPAA certified. An attestation letter of compliance is about the best companies can do aside from HITRUST. IoMT brings a number of challenges when it comes to HITRUST, though. IoMT balloons the number of records that covered entities have and thus the risk increases from a HITRUST perspective. With increased risk comes an increase in the number of requirements.

But this isn't the only impact that IoMT has on HITRUST. As many of the IoMT devices are devoid of basic controls, the operational overhead required to maintain the IoMT controls can be quite significant. HITRUST at least has some flexibility built into it so that if a control fails in one area, covered entities can compensate by increasing the controls in another area. For some hospitals, though, the challenges that IoMT brings to the table are so severe that meeting the requirements can be impossible or near impossible for many organizations.

Where this is the case, many covered entities are turning to another compliance model—SOC 2 Type 2. The requirements of SOC 2 Type 2 are very similar to both HIPAA and HITRUST, but the depth of the requirements are nowhere near the same, nor are they as onerous to meet because the reporting styles are quite different. For example, SOC2 is about reporting the controls and noting identified gaps. HISTRUST has a scoring rubric that a percent for not only each cybersecurity domain, but also a specifically identified score for overall compliance. Further, IoMT can be that black

---

[2] Steve Morgan, "Healthcare Industry To Spend $125 Billion On Cybersecurity From 2020 To 2025," September 2020, https://cybersecurityventures.com/healthcare-industry-to-spend-125-billion-on-cybersecurity-from-2020-to-2025/.

box that gets covered entities past pesky IoMT deficiencies. The challenge with the SOC 2 Type 2 certification is that the requirements may change a bit depending on the company that is giving the assessment, but for many covered entities, it is the best path forward to maintain security. While it has some glaring holes, it does give some level of assurance that cybersecurity is reasonably in place.

In the end, compliance can offer a measure of assurance of cybersecurity maturity. It isn't perfect, though, which is why risk assessments are such an important part of the governance process—why CEOs need to be at least tangentially involved in the decision-making process. We need to think about those compliance requirements and what the impact is of IoMT on compliance mandates. There are risks that need to be considered. The more out of place compliance is, even for IoMT, the greater the fines from OCR may be.

The Tangled Web of Privacy

Privacy, from a HIPAA standpoint, is complex enough, but as state and global laws continue to expand, the legal web of interdependencies related to data will only grow. Striving to bridge the gap between the legal requirements and IT will continue to be a bigger and bigger challenge. IT and cybersecurity will need to work with legal to ensure that the appropriate stewardship is taking place. As we saw in Chapter 3, the ability of data brokers to pierce the veil of anonymized data takes us clearly outside the realm of pure law and into the realm of data analytics when it comes to protecting data.

It is only exposing each branch of an organization to new ideas and continuing to learn that we can hope to keep up, not only with the privacy/legal landscape, but also with our moral responsibilities as defenders of the data. The legal/privacy angle is a critical part of the governance of today's organizations and needs to be included as part of the overall governance process.

Aggregation of Influence

All of the influences within organizations are critically important to protecting the modern covered entity. They all need an equal voice and need to be on a level playing field when talking with the CEO and the board of directors. Everyone's voice is important and needs to be heard and understood, because without that, it can be potentially disastrous for the organization. It is important for both the CEO and the board of directors to reach out beyond the reporting lines and work with all the key players on the team, so they should be asking to talk to all of the leaders within their organization.

Many times, knowing what the right level of communication is for a CEO or board of directors is challenging. They grew up with less cyber-security guidance than what is available in today's classrooms. Many of them are aware of cybersecurity incidents, but not what the impact is of, say, a poor risk management program. While it is great to have a CFO on the board, there also needs to be a privacy expert, a compliance expert, an IT expert, a cybersecurity expert, and so on. Lacking a holistic group of experts on the board and not understanding the environment well enough can be very problematic because it can mean that the right kinds of questions will not be asked.

The other side of the equation is that businesses in general, not just covered entities, are often afraid of the board, so they may not reveal that things are not perfect. Getting the board involved means that actions must be taken, and the leaders then become accountable for what must be done. The obvious challenge for organizations in these situations is *how* things get done. If there is no knowledge about these issues, there is no accountability. Corporate risks, including risks for covered entities, will remain higher than they should be. It does not matter if that issue is a CCPA/HIPAA violation, or highly risky IoMT devices. Risks exist that may or may not be mitigated.

What the board of directors should ask for is risk assessments—enterprise risk assessments for the whole organization. What are the top risks that covered entities face? Those risks may be cybersecurity risks related to IoMT, but they also could be market risks, demographic risks, or reputational damage. These all need to be taken into account. Everyone's voice needs to be heard. Enterprise risk management (ERM) is the place to do that. ERM provides much needed background for everyone to understand the challenges and contexts. Getting everyone on the same page coalesces them around the covered entity's mission so that everyone understands the goals as a team. It creates more cohesion to build that buy-in that may take much longer to build without a cohesive, centralized methodology. Sometimes a single meeting with all of the players on equal footing, with an equal voice, can accomplish more in one hour than could be accomplished in ten hours of separate meetings.

What happens as a result of these meetings is the trickle-down effect, meaning that the direction that people take are a bit more on target and people know that they have the backing of everyone around them. In the end, if everyone is given an equal voice and appropriate transparency in the decision-making process, there is a greater chance that a more optimal goal may be achieved.

Of course, the challenge is that not all boards are created equal, and like all human endeavors, there may unintended imbalances within a group of people. Some board members are quirky and full of perspectives that may or may not be aligned with the risks, which is why influencing these groups is so important. As humans, as speakers, as presenters, we need to make the best arguments we can from a certain perspective. From a cybersecurity perspective, risk is one of the best communicators. Every covered entity and every organization has risks that need to be balanced against other risks.

The other challenge is how to handle scarcity of resources. In the absence of knowledge, it is easy to say why one decision is bad or another decision is more important. Sometimes the bigger picture needs to be assessed. Part of team building incudes getting everyone on the same page and making a decision collectively as part of the overall process. Although this is sometimes painful, it adds the ownership of everyone involved in the decision-making. While not everyone might agree on the outcome, being part of that process is part of collective team building and aggregates influence across the organization.

Maybe the right decision is to keep a five-million-dollar piece of equipment three more years, even if it increases the cybersecurity risk. Knowing it is a risk means that the cybersecurity team can plan around the risks related to those devices. Maybe the money saved can allow for building the unflat network—the valleys, mountains, rivers, and oceans that can slow down the attackers. Regardless of the reasons why a particular decision is made, being thorough and diligent about the options for dealing with IoMT is at the heart of cybersecurity for covered entities, but always keep in mind that every organization is different.

Cybersecurity Innovators

The number and types of tools available has grown over the last 30 years. We used to be fine with simple firewalls and antivirus, but since then there has been an explosion of interconnected devices. Cell phones and other mobile devices connect to computers in a variety of different ways. The cloud has completely changed the innovation strategy. Now, new vectors of weaknesses need to be considered in the approach to cybersecurity as the attack surface has become a large sprawling mess.

To handle these kinds of challenges, cybersecurity vendors have risen to the occasion with a plethora of new tools and techniques. Cell phones can now have next-generation antivirus on them and be managed from the cloud. It is now possible to integrate login capabilities and add multi-factor authentication to those cloud resources—all while aligning to principles of identity management and governance.

A system firewall can be managed from remote tools without having anything installed on it. This is part of the work innovators can do. The same can be true for many of the automation tools. They can access and reset systems on a periodic basis to ensure that systems maintain their configurations.

Industrial Control Systems Overlap

Many industrial control systems (ICSs) that are used to manage massive devices have a degree of overlap with IoMT challenges, in that they will sometimes allow small kinds of security software on IoMT devices, but not antivirus. One way for cybersecurity to overcome this is to use a tool that freezes the operating system so that anything outside of basic parameters is automatically blocked. If IoMT manufacturers were to allow these kinds of software on their systems, the risks to some of the IoMT devices would be reduced drastically—even attacks from nation-state adversaries.

Whether ICS or other systems, the number of tools on the market designed to compensate for the IoMT cybersecurity inadequacies is growing and will continue to grow. Where there is a will, there is an innovator trying find a way. It may not be as perfect or as fast as is needed, but changes are happening, and innovation is taking place to solve for these kinds of problems. The challenge is learning about the kinds of tools and capabilities that are available. Many of them are not mainstay products as they are specifically designed for that niche market. They typically do not get the kind of attention that, say, a firewall manufacturer would have. There is just more profit in that space. It is also full of competitors.

The companies that are working to protect IoMT and healthcare should continue to innovate. Sometimes the niche markets have fewer competitors and thus provide better opportunity because they are not fighting to stand out in an overcrowded market. As IoMT requirements continue to change, keeping on top of new innovations is paramount.

What You Can Do

If you are not connected to the IT or cybersecurity fields, nor connected to the medical field in any way, many of the issues brought up in this book are perhaps too abstract for you, as an individual, to address. You cannot independently assess a hospital for its cybersecurity to know if it is safe, any more than you can know if using a credit card related to a specific institution is safe. For the average person, much of this is beyond what they can do anything about. It just is not a reasonable ask. When it comes to health concerns, unless you live in a large metropolitan area you cannot, for example, realistically choose what hospital to go to—if you even have a reasonable option for the circumstances. A doctor cannot be expected to understand the intricacies of cybersecurity when prescribing IoMT devices. In many cases, the doctor is the only person who can reassure you about the relative safety of a device. To be honest, it is daunting for cybersecurity professionals to keep up with those challenges, too. It just isn't reasonable for anyone to know thousands of products and what the specifics are. Even experts have to look at reports and trends to see the big picture rather than focusing on the minutia of individual IoMT devices. And those that do look at the minutia often have a hard time seeing the big picture. This is true not only in medicine, but also in engineering, architecture, and, of course, cybersecurity.

It is important to keep in mind that, despite everything, there have been very few deaths caused by cybersecurity and IoMT devices themselves. On an individual level, the risks to IoMT are presently unlikely to manifest, but the potential exists. The rewards of using IoMT devices far outweigh the risks to any individual, and their value is undeniable. It is the hospitals and other large covered entities that presently have the bulk of the risk. That said, there are some basic things that each of us can do to reduce the risks related to IoMT security if you care about IoMT security. We will explore those in the following sections.

Personal Cybersecurity

Real cybersecurity is complex, but there are a number of things you can do to protect yourself and your home. It is important to ensure that your home network is secure. Always use encrypted communications when using wireless. Ensure that the password is complex. You do not want someone to easily guess your passwords and gain access to your devices. If you are using a wired network, strive to keep your IoT devices off of the same network as your IoMT device(s). IoT devices having as many vulnerabilities as they do can greatly increase risks. Also, continuing to patch the IoMT in your house is critical to keeping the devices secure.

I highly recommend using OpenDNS. OpenDNS is a free DNS service that helps to block malware and other bad traffic for free. It blocks bad traffic well before it reaches your computer. IoT and IoMT devices can also utilize OpenDNS.

If you have teenagers, it may be wise to keep them separated from your devices. They often download software that can easily infect other systems and ultimately cause problems for other computers in the household—just as IoMT devices can. If you allow your kids to use your computer, give them their own profiles to use and not use your profile. It may be wise for you to do much of your important work in a virtualized computer rather than directly on the computer—at least it offers a bit of a buffer against some malware.

Some of the next-generation antivirus programs that use machine learning are becoming available to consumers instead of just the commercial markets. Moving in this direction can help against some of the other strains of malware that have not yet been created.

Always keep your home systems up to date and patched. The better patched you are, the better protection you would have against possible attackers. Patching is not just for operating systems but also phones and applications. These need to be updated on a regular basis.

Beware phishing scams whether they be via email or text message to your phone. If you don't know the user, do not click on link. Do not connect to sites by clicking on links. It is better to go to the site you know directly and log in that way. Another good practice is keeping your apps on your devices to a minimum and try to go with ones that have greater trust. This is easier said than done, but as a general rule, stay away from unknown apps in your mobile devices and only use those from a trusted source. Using a minimal number of applications wherever possible and keeping up to date with patches is critical. Not allowing apps access to your microphone is also wise. Anything you can do to help protect yourself is going to be a value add in the long run.

Back up your computer and files to the cloud or to physical hard drives. This way if your computer is compromised, you will have all of the major files you will need. This way you will never have to pay the ransoms if you click on a link and accidentally infect a computer. If you do become infected, wiping your computer and starting from scratch is the safest course of action.

Politics

It may seem strange to talk about politics in a book on IoMT, but it is wise to think about many of the items brought in this book as part of your voting strategy. Do you care that your personal information can be sold to third- and fourth-party firms by almost any government around the world? If so, find a political candidate that supports your viewpoint. Maybe building an agency to help us cope with this age of data is worth considering.

Other considerations include securing of IoMT devices that are critical to personal health. If you are concerned with a heart monitor being hacked, it may be worthwhile to support candidates that push for UL 2900 or the creation of other standards that will accomplish similar objectives, but not be as onerous on the manufacturers.

No matter what side of the political fence you are on, being active in politics and letting candidates on all sides know what your preferences are can be useful. If a candidate is in office, even if you disagree with their central politics (however you define that), letting them know that you want legislation to protect IoMT can make a difference in aggregation. They are dependent on you and your voice to understand the central issues.

While IoMT cybersecurity is not typically the hot issue of an election, it is starting to affect us more and more. Hospitals have to increase their premiums to deal with IoMT challenges and improve their cybersecurity. It is too costly not to focus on cybersecurity—especially with multi-prong ransoms that not only steal data, but then ransom both the system they stole data from and the data itself. Hospitals and other covered entities cannot afford to continue with the status quo. Insurance is starting to react to ransom attempts as well—significantly increasing their premiums and becoming smarter about cybersecurity in general. Ultimately, we all have to pay more through higher premiums and higher prices—even if the attack did not affect us directly.

Another key component is voting for candidates that support greater international cooperation from a law enforcement standpoint. No country can embrace the digital age and really afford to deal with the growing challenges related to cybercrime on its own. Law enforcement agencies working together across the globe is becoming a greater and greater necessity—no matter your other politics.

Ultimately, though, putting aside political differences and focusing on some of the core issues of international cybercrime is going to be one of the best ways to move the needle in the right direction. No one solution will solve the problems that IoMT has, but a range of solutions and people investing in the right options can help align the political discussion with your viewpoints. We will never completely solve the problems, but at least reducing them can go a long way toward protecting all of us.

In Summary

Doing less harm is not a one-size-fits-all endeavor. There is no one approach that will magically solve all our problems related to IoMT devices. There are obviously different types of risks related to different IoMT devices, and each type of device—and even each device, in some cases—must be treated differently. Some IoMT devices have corresponding apps for cell phones. Making those apps secure can really help protect not only individual patients, but the IoMT manufacturer and the covered entity that is using the device as well. An interconnected world requires an interconnected set of solutions. For the manufacturers that utilize the cloud, making sure that the cloud is secure is obviously paramount.

Doing less harm also means not giving up. Covered entities are scanned, probed, and attacked every hour of every day. It may seem hopeless, but many of the recommendations in this book can be used to defend IoMT and covered entities from attacks from organized crime to nation-state attackers. What is important is to adequately assess the risks to IoMT and ultimately to organizations and act accordingly. Doing less harm means listening to the expertise of others and striving to do the right thing. No organization can make the right choices all the time, but creating an equal playing field for everyone can help them work toward making better choices. The more the individual players' voices are heard, the better chance at success each organization will have.

CHAPTER

20

Changes We Need

Security is always too much until the day it is not enough.
—William Webster, Former Director of the FBI

In this book we have talked about a whole range of interconnected subjects related to IoMT and the context for which IoMT weaknesses add to the existing privacy and cybersecurity challenges. Unfortunately, many covered entities only see the importance of cybersecurity after they have suffered an attack. Sufficient money and resources come through only after a breach has occurred. There is an almost daily deluge of news about companies being breached, but still many companies do not give cybersecurity the resources to sufficiently accomplish their goals. We have almost become inured to the fact that these kinds of events happen.

While the situation is grim and is becoming even more grim day by day, accepting the status quo does not help to resolve the challenges that IoMT and covered entities face. It allows the problem to fester. The organizations that are not taking cybersecurity seriously need to start down the cybersecurity path, taking into account the risks they really face. If they don't, it is only a matter of time before they are compromised and have to deal with the fallout of a large variety of incidents.

International Cooperation

If there is one universal truth that should be agreed upon when striving to protect IoMT and covered entities it is that we need greater international cooperation in dealing with cybercrime. We have already pointed out the nations that are starting to enact their own cybercrime laws to make it illegal to hack organizations. These are fantastic first steps, but we definitely need to go further.

We also need to figure out how we are going to handle countries that tacitly attack other countries. China moving to ransomware attacks as a means of achieving their country's strategic vision means that covered entities will soon see even more nation-state attacks. Russia is a growing concern when you consider how devastating the SolarWinds attack was on our nation's strategic infrastructure. It may not be surprising to see similar attacks against IoMT manufacturers that could end up affecting hospitals in a similar way as SolarWinds. Threat actors that act with relative impunity because of where they live are strategic challenges for the United States. The result is that covered entities are up against sophisticated threat actors on their own.

Each attack has a cascading set of costs associated with it. The cost of cyberinsurance is rising along with the rising ransom demands. Each attack against our covered entities means an increased cost in doing business—whether that's increased premiums for insurance or a greater investment in cybersecurity, it adds to the overall costs of healthcare. We, as members of a common planet, of a common communication platform (the internet), have to find ways of working together to protect us all.

Covered Entities

Not all of the problems can be solved by looking to a national strategy. Covered entities need to develop their own strategy for dealing with cybercrime. Not to beat a dead horse, but the covered entities that have not fully prioritized cybersecurity as part of their organizational strategy will be hit with a breach sooner or later. Having a vision about what cybersecurity prioritization means is exceptionally important. Business leaders often do not know what a vision should look like. Often CISOs, when they first start out, don't have a complete vision of what this means because every organization is a bit different. That understood, there are some resources that organizations can use as benchmarks. For example, the Enterprise Strategy Group created a Security Maturity Model, which touches on some high-level considerations when thinking about cybersecurity.[1] It is far from the definitive model, but CEOs and other business leaders using this as a template might begin to think about cybersecurity differently by using resources such as this as a starting point for discussions within organizations. The Security Maturity Model may not fit entirely within your organization, but it is worthy of a serious conversation.

If organizations prefer a different approach, performing external assessments of the security program might be worthwhile. There are many different ways to accomplish this such as risk assessments, mapping to any of the frameworks, or using a CISO as a service for the person to sit in the organization for a while and come up with their own assessment model are all excellent options. Getting an outside assessment, free of the internal biases, is always a worthwhile endeavor. Whatever covered entities choose, thinking very hard and long about the options is absolutely critical to protecting organizations effectively.

Another key consideration that all covered entities should do is ensure that a cybersecurity expert is on the board is absolutely critical. A CIO is not sufficient because they are looking at risk through the lens of IT management—a wholly different discipline than cybersecurity. This blends well into the next section to enable those who are part of a board of directors to ask the pertinent questions.

Questions a Board Should Ask

It may be helpful for people who are on the board of directors of covered entities to address a few basic questions to the CEO, CIOs, and CISO as the board of directors has a fiduciary responsibility for the governance of the covered entities they work with. Here are a few questions that are worth considering:

- What is the risk tolerance or risk appetite of the organization?
- Are we aligned with our risk tolerance or appetite?
- Where do we deviate, and why is there a deviation?

---

[1] Brian Krebs, "What's your security maturity level?" April 27, 2015, https://krebsonsecurity.com/2015/04/whats-your-security-maturity-level/.

- How many vulnerabilities are related to IoMT devices?
- What percentage of the vulnerabilities are related to IoMT devices?
- Do we have adequate compensating controls for the IoMT vulnerabilities?
- How far do we deviate from HIPAA or other compliance models?
- Do we have the appropriate contractual requirements to protect ourselves from risks related to HIPPA, CCPA, CPRA, and other privacy frameworks?
- Since we sell anonymized data, how are we taking into account CPRA or other privacy considerations?
- Do our contracts cover all the CPRA considerations for anonymized data?

These questions are very basic, and CEOs and other C-level executives should know the answers off of the top of their heads. They need to be aware of the challenges within their organizations and not just leave it to others to manage. Where there is misalignment, business leaders need to make decisions about how to best reduce the risk within their organizations. Chances are, with competent people in place, people underneath them can answer many of these questions, but sometimes the answers to questions the board of directors may ask companies are not prepared for, and there may be more surprises under the hood that companies need to think about more carefully.

The purpose of the board is to help protect and guide organizations on their journey. They cannot do so without understanding what the inherent challenges are. They have a responsibility to ask relevant questions to make the changes to the organization based on input provided to them.

More IoMT Security Assurances

Security is hard. Assessing the level of security related to IoMT is even harder. We almost have an on/off switch when it comes to IoMT security—UL 2900 or bust. Sure, we have government requirements for patching IoMT, which is a good start, but beyond that, what are the real assurances? We have many cybersecurity standards and regulations to assess the overall security of an organization, but compliance models don't address the security of a specific device. The cloud portion is relatively addressed (though imperfect) with most compliance frameworks, but the overall IoMT portion is not. Let us take a look at some of the changes we need for many of our IoMT devices.

Active Directory Integration

Like many things in IT, it is far easier to say an IoMT device has Active Directory (AD) integration than to talk about the specifics related to AD integration. Some manufacturers use an older version of AD that might be inherently insecure by today's standards. As a result a company that purchases IoMT might have to degrade the cybersecurity of their whole AD infrastructure to add new IoMT devices. This can set AD/Windows back in terms of the cybersecurity posture. Most reputable companies will not do this, but in the world of startups, the startup may not fully understand the intricacies of AD or what the impact is of using an older AD system. Challenges like this are not uncommon when working with startups. While this issue may not be present, there are often other issues that pop up as improvements are made. There are ways of working around these issues, but they become costly and time-consuming to support.

Software Development

For local IoMT devices, the manufacturer software development process is one of the key ingredients for protecting IoMT systems. How do you judge how successful a software development program is in terms of creating secure code? Some programs are demonstrably better than others. There are many software development tools on the market that are great for developers, but just okay when it comes to real software security. The developers may be following all the requirements of their tools, but miss a large number of software development bugs that a more mature product could catch. This creates a number of challenges in assessing security. You not only have to look at the security products being used, but also at the process and the remediation activities of the company creating the IoMT systems—not an easy task.

A company can invest in the best tools but have a very poor process in place that makes having the tool almost useless. This is usually assessed in a questionnaire, but how do you capture that in a questionnaire in a manner that another company will answer honestly? You can ask about the tool and whether it is integrated into the program, but the answer could be yes, even if it is only 5% integrated. You can ask how often the tool is used and what the remediation processes are, but even those kinds of questions can be dodged or stretched, so a questionnaire is not always a sufficient tool.

Yet another area that needs to be considered is how vulnerabilities are managed. A company may have a very mature strategy and process around vulnerabilities, but they may remediate only critical vulnerabilities, and nothing else. Another company could have the exact same strategy, but they remediate everything from critical to low vulnerabilities. Knowing the extent that the process is carried out is also important. It should be painfully obvious which company's process would be better from that very specific perspective. Both companies are being diligent; it is just a matter of *how* diligent those companies are being.

The only way to truly get around some of these challenges is for organizations to do a proof of concept and perform a penetration test of the devices themselves. This can be an expensive and time-consuming process for organizations that need to be agile when making IoMT device selections, so for many covered entities, this is an undue burden.

Independent Measures

There will always be a demand for independent innovation that will help save lives. This is a critical part of the innovation process. That said, each company striving to come up with an independent assessment of their security provides an undue financial or resource strain on organizations. There is room for independent measures of software security—something objective and easily recognizable. Even having an external penetration test against a specific device is helpful, but on a certain level, the pen tester may have a limited time to perform the penetration test in order to cut the cost of the penetration test. Companies can ask for penetration test results (or even the executive summary), but sometimes companies will not show if they remediated the findings or not. While there are ways to work through these challenges, these do underscore some of the challenges related to using independent measures.

In Summary

Some of the themes that have been straddling different parts of this book are those of thoughtfulness, due diligence, communication, and risk—all of which are important for creating a general strategy around protecting both IoMT and covered entities. Without transparency and thoughtfulness at the senior leadership level, there is no hope of doing the right thing. Each group within covered entities needs the freedom to talk about improvements that need to be made, and the gaps that need to be resolved.

To that end, who is to say that cybersecurity is more important than saving lives? No cybersecurity practitioner would make that claim if they care about human life. That said, as cybersecurity risks begin to pile up around IoMT and related systems, human lives will become more and more at stake—especially as profits grow for the cybercriminals and nation-states willing to come after covered entities despite the risks to human life. There is a balance between the two that is shifting day by day—and not for the better, as cybercriminal organizations emulate big business tactics with almost no regard or concern for the short arm of the various laws they operate within or often beyond.

Privacy is the cousin of cybersecurity. While there are marked differences between the two disciplines, they are intertwined. Failure to protect data from a cybersecurity perspective represents legal risks, as OCR has the power to leverage fines against companies for failures of compliance. Today many of the fines are often due to simple oversights in IT activities such as allowing simple passwords on external connections.

The various parts of the organization need to work together to achieve balance among the needs of today's covered entities. Cybersecurity cannot simply be subservient to IT. The conflict of interest is too high, as are the concerns that cybersecurity may simply represent too much risk to the organization to keep the concerns buried underneath an insecure CIO.

What makes protecting IoMT and covered entities so challenging is not so much all of the technical weaknesses, but the processes that provide a skewed version of what is happening in organizations. It's important for businesses to listen all voices within their organization, including the legal and cybersecurity professionals, to come up with processes that work for everyone.

In the end, protecting IoMT and covered entities is about understanding the business, understanding IoMT, having strong communication across the various divisions, and focusing efforts across the organization in the right way. Every organization always has too much to do. What matters is focusing the priorities so that perspective is gained. Adding things like IT Steering Committees to organizations helps leaders to understand that prioritization process and focus on the critical items. Determining priorities based on the risk they pose is absolutely essential. It is 100% okay to have moderate-level vulnerability in an IoMT device if the appropriate controls are in place to protect it, but higher-level vulnerabilities should be priority one.

These kinds of issues get to the heart of what modern governance can and should be about. A laissez-faire attitude about what needs to be focused on will not get to the goals needed to cross the bridge. It may mean that some issues are not addressed, or are pushed off for months (or even years), but without this kind of prioritization and discipline, we'll never hope to protect our IoMT devices or our covered entities. Focusing on the governance process is the best way to protect IoMT. Cybersecurity is as much about education as is it is all the tools and gizmos available to protect those devices. The cybersecurity professionals need to communicate to senior management how important it is to implement these tools as well.

Ultimately, it takes the right communication, at the right level, with the right people and the right strategy at the senior management level to get everything done in the right way. There is no better way to accomplish protecting IoMT and covered entities in general.

Clearly, though, everyone needs to be involved in their own way to help protect our covered entities and IoMT from harm. Politicians have to create better laws and focus internationally to create strong liaisons across our tiny planet to stop cybercriminals in any country and find a way to work with countries that are not as cooperative with law enforcement. There is a reasonable balance to protecting both covered entities and IoMT. We just need to find that balance between saving lives, compliance, privacy, cybersecurity, enforcement, and within our institutions and our laws.

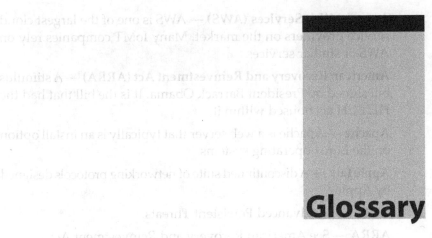

Glossary

AB-713 — California Consumer Privacy Act of 2018.

Access Control List (ACL) — There are many types of ACLs, but in this book the context is primarily around a firewall ACLs, which can block traffic.

Accountable Care Organizations (ACO) — ACOs are healthcare organizations that tie prover reimbursements to quality metrics and reduction in cost.

ACA — See Affordable Care Act.

ACO — See Accountable Care Organizations.

Advanced Encryption Standard (AES) — AES is an encryption cipher used to encrypt data.

Advanced Persistent Threat (APT) — An APT is a threat actor that is well funded and trained, such as a nation-state or organized crime.

Advanced Research Project Agency Network (ARPANET) — ARPANET is the first wide area network whose fundamentals created the foundation for the internet.

AES — See Advanced Encryption Standard.

Affordable Care Act (ACA) — Also referred to as Obamacare, the ACA is a comprehensive healthcare reform bill signed into law in 2010.

Amazon Web Services (AWS) — AWS is one of the largest cloud service providers on the market. Many IoMT companies rely on AWS or similar services.

American Recovery and Reinvestment Act (ARRA) — A stimulus bill signed by President Barrack Obama. It is the bill that had the HITECH act housed within it.

Apache — Apache is a web server that typically is an install option on the Linux operating systems.

AppleTalk — A discontinued suite of networking protocols designed by Apple.

APT — See Advanced Persistent Threats.

ARRA — See American Recovery and Reinvestment Act.

Artificial Intelligence — Artificial intelligence is intelligence demonstrated by machines and not people or animals.

Availability — In the context of this book, availability is part of the CIA triad that represents the need to keep data and systems available for use.

Big Data — Big data is the term used to describe data sets that are too large to be handled by traditional software. In this book it refers to the fact that anonymized data can be re-anonymized as a result of combining anonymized data with large data sets.

Black Hat Hacking — Black hat hacking is unauthorized hacking. Often it is with malicious intent.

Bluetooth — A short-distance radio communication band. The created network is referred to as a personal area network.

Breach — A breach is an unauthorized release of information. The exact definition and implication will change based on the laws, data types, etc., that will govern the process. This is true even for HIPAA data.

Breach and Attack Simulation (BAS) — BAS is a new class of vulnerability management tools that utilize the ATT&CK framework to find vulnerabilities in operating systems so they can be reported on.

Bring Your Own Device (BYOD) — BYOD is a movement where companies have their employees and/or contractors use their own phones rather than receive corporate paid phones.

Business Associates Agreement (BAA) — BAAs protect covered entities and business associates by requiring business associates to protect data in a somewhat similar fashion as the covered entities. Under HIPAA, a business associate is directly liable under the HIPAA rules.

California Consumer Privacy Act (CCPA) — CCPA is a California law designed to protect privacy rights of California citizens.

Center for Internet Security (CIS) Benchmarks — The CIS Benchmarks are instructions for configuring systems so they will be harder for attackers to compromise.

Center for Medicaid and Medicare Services (CMS) — The CMS is a federal agency within the US Department of Health and Human Services that focuses on partnering with state and local government related to health programs.

Chief Compliance Officer (CCO) — The CCO is responsible for handling the compliance within organizations — typically HIPAA and HITECH.

Chief Executive Officer (CEO) — A CEO is the highest-level officer in a company ultimately responsible for making managerial decisions.

Chief Financial Officer (CFO) — A CFO is responsible for the company's budgeting and the financial health of an organization.

Chief Information Officer (CIO) — A CIO is responsible for overseeing the IT strategy for an organization.

Chief Information Security Officer (CISO) — A CISO is a role within an organization that leads cybersecurity initiatives.

Chief Medical Technology Officer (CMTO) — A CMTO is responsible for evaluating the medical technology within an organization, including IoMT.

Chief Privacy Officer (CPO) — A CPO is the person responsible for privacy within an organization.

Chief Technology Officer (CTO) — The CTO is the person responsible for the software development process within an organization.

CIA Triad — The CIA triad is one of the tools that cybersecurity uses to assess the types of risks in a plain fashion. HIPAA requires that risk assessments include an assessment of CIA.

Clinical Monitor — A clinical monitor is a device used for monitoring and oversight of a patient.

Cloud — Cloud refers to IT resources that are available over the internet.

Cloud Access Security Broker (CASB) — Now referred to as a SASE, a CASB is a cybersecurity tool for helping to manage and monitor cloud-based threats and capabilities.

Common Vulnerabilities and Exposures (CVE) — CVE is the common reference for identifying public vulnerabilities.

Common Vulnerability Scoring System (CVSS) — The CVSS is the public means of scoring the severity of a known vulnerability.

Common Weakness Enumeration (CWE) — CWE is the standard for determining weaknesses and vulnerabilities in software.

Communications Assistance to Law Enforcement Act (CALEA) — CALEA is a US law that allows law enforcement to intercept telecommunications that are slightly outside the scope of their investigations.

Compensating Controls — A compensating control is a backup control that is not in place. A control requirement might be for a network intrusion detection system. The compensating control might be the utilization of a threat intelligence gateway instead.

Compound Annual Growth Rate (CAGR) — CAGR is the rate of return that would be required for an investment to grow.

Computer Fraud and Abuse Act (CFAA) — CFAA is the US law that addresses hacking and other unauthorized access to computer systems.

Confidentiality — Confidentiality is about allowing information only to authorized users.

Confidentiality, Integrity, Availability (CIA) Triad — The CIA triad is one of the many tools that cybersecurity professionals use to define types of threats, risks, etc.

Configuration Drift — Configuration drift refers to the changes in the configurations of machines over time.

Contact Tracing — Contact tracing attempts to identify people who have recently been in contact with someone diagnosed with an infectious disease.

Cooperative Research and Development Agreement (CRADA) — A CRADA is a cooperative research agreement between a government agency and a private company or university.

Crowd-Sourced Penetration Testing — Crowd-sourced penetration testing leverages a large group of people to find vulnerabilities in systems.

CVE — See Common Vulnerabilities and Exposure.

CWE — See Common Weakness Enumeration.

Cybersecurity & Infrastructure Security Agency (CISA) — CISA is a US agency with the mission to manage physical and cybersecurity risk to our critical infrastructure.

Cybersecurity Assurance Program (CAP) — CAP is a UL program designed to help organizations manage their cybersecurity risks.

Data Analytics — Data analytics is the process of inspecting and modeling data with the goal of discovering useful information.

Data Brokers — Data brokers are companies that specialize in collecting information from a wide variety of sources.

Data Governance — Data governance means the act of oversight related to data. What that entails changes depending on the rights and regulations surrounding the data. It covers legal obligations and practices surrounding that data.

Data Loss Prevention (DLP) — Also called Data Leak Prevention, these are tools and processes designed to prevent the loss of data.

Data Mining — Data mining is the process of discovering patterns within data sets.

Data Privacy Impact Assessments (DPIA) — A DPIA is a process whereby a system is assessed from a cybersecurity and privacy standpoint to assess what the privacy impact will be.

Data Science — Data science is the interdisciplinary field that uses scientific methods and processes to gain insights into various forms of data.

Data Tokenization — Data tokenization is the process of replacing data with a token with the goal of keeping it restricted to authorized users only. It is more effective than encrypting a database.

DDOS — See Distributed Denial of Service.

Deep Learning — Deep learning is a subset of machine learning that requires a large quantity of data.

Deep Packet Inspection (DPI) — DPI tools look at the network from a packet-level perspective to determine if there are any attacks on the network.

Demilitarized Zone (DMZ) — A DMZ is a network location between the internet and internal systems.

Distributed Denial of Service (DDOS) — A DDOS attack is designed to make a system or network resource unavailable by utilizing a number of systems to overwhelm the target so it cannot operate.

DLP — See Data Loss Prevention.

DMZ — See Demilitarized Zone.

DNS Security (DNSSEC) — DNSSEC is a set of internet Engineering Task Force specifications for securing DNS.

Domain Name Service (DNS) — DNS is a technical tool to translate an IP address into a domain name.

DPI — See Deep Packet Inspection.

Dynamic Application Security Testing (DAST) — DAST is a tool set and process for testing applications or software while it is in an operating state.

Electronic Communications Privacy Act (ECPA) — ECPA is a US law that protects oral, wire, and electronic information while in transit or stored in computers.

Electronic Health Record (EHR) — An EHR is a system to capture and store health information (PHI) in bulk.

Encryption — Ideally, encryption is the process of encoding information so it cannot be read by unauthorized parties.

Encryption Gateway — An encryption gateway is a gateway through which information is encrypted. Information gathered outside the gateway is encrypted.

Endpoint Detection and Response (EDR) — EDR is software that detects and responds to attacks. Not all responses are complete, however.

Enforcement Rule — The enforcement rule is the part of HIPAA that regulates liability and fines under HIPAA.

Enterprise Risk Management (ERM) — ERM is a tool of governance where each department contributes to overall risk discussions within an organization.

European Union (EU) — An international organization of countries and governance that works toward common economic, social, and other policies.

FDA — See Food and Drug Administration.

Federal Information Processing Standard (FIPS) 140-2 — FIPS 140-2 is a NIST validation of an encryption module to provide assurance around the build of the cryptographic module.

File Integrity Management (FIM) — FIM is a type of tool that monitors files for unauthorized changes.

File Transfer Protocol (FTP) — FTP is a network protocol for the transfer of computer files. Since it is unencrypted, it is considered insecure by cybersecurity professionals.

Final Omnibus Rule — Passed in 2012, the HIPAA Omnibus rule has edits and updates to all previously passed HIPAA rules. It is intended to implement the HITECH Act.

Firewall — A firewall is a network device designed to protect networks from an array of network-based attacks.

Flat Network — A flat network is a network that does not have "obstacles" in it such as VLANS, VLAN ACLs, etc.

Food and Drug Administration (FDA) — The FDA is the US agency responsible for protecting public health, including IoMT.

FTP — See File Transfer Protocol.

General Counsel (GC) — A GC is head of a legal office within an organization.

General Data Protection Regulation (GDPR) — GDPR is a European law designed to protect the data of European citizens.

GLBA — See Gramm-Leach Bliley Act.

Government Accountability Office (GAO) — The GAO provides the legislative branch of the government with auditing, evaluating, and investigative services for the US Congress.

Gramm-Leach Bliley Act (GLBA) — GLBA is the act that helped to modernize the financial service industry, and includes cybersecurity and privacy requirements.

Hard Tokens — Hard tokens are authentication tokens that are not installed, messaged, or scanned. They contain a series of numbers and are considered the most secure form of authentication because they are much more difficult to hack.

Health and Human Services (HHS) — HHS is the US Agency responsible for the oversight of human health.

Health Information Exchanges (HIE) — HIEs are designed to allow healthcare systems to share information.

Health Information Technology (HIT) — HIT is information technology related to healthcare. Its scope is larger than IoMT.

Health Information Technology for Economic and Clinical Health Act (HITECH Act) — The HITECH Act was designed to modernize the healthcare ecosystem, which helped to foster the IoMT revolution.

Health Insurance Portability & Accountability Act (HIPAA) — HIPAA is the foundational law that governs how healthcare data should be reviewed.

HIPAA — See Health Insurance Portability & Accountability Act.

HITECH — See Health Information Technology for Economic and Clinical Health Act.

HITRUST — HITRUST is a company that created a "common" security framework for meeting multiple regulations — the foundation of which is HIPAA.

HTTP/S — See Hypertext Transfer Protocol.

Hypertext Transfer Protocol (HTTP/S) — HTTP is the protocol for transferring information over the internet. The /S is an indicator that HTTP is secure.

Identity and Access Management (I&AM) — Identity and Access Management is the people, processes, and technology of managing identities, usually accounts, within an organization, including the connected and interconnected systems. The goal is to provide people with the access they need to do their jobs.

Identity Governance — As I&AM processes are far from perfect, it is important to validate the process to ensure that it is functioning properly. For example, to ensure people who have been terminated from a company no longer have access. Reviewing I&AM helps organizations find issues and correct flaws in I&AM processes. It helps to reduce the vectors of attack.

Information Sharing Analysis Center (ISAC) — ISACs are non-profit organizations that help to gather information on cyberthreats and provide two-way sharing between the public and private sector.

Information Technology (IT) — IT is the discipline of using technology to store, transmit, and process information. There are many disciplines that comprise all of these functions.

Infrastructure as a Service (IaaS): — IaaS is a cloud service to provide network infrastructure to organizations.

Integrity — Integrity is part of the CIA triad that focuses on ensuring the data has not been altered in an unauthorized fashion.

Internet of Medical Things (IoMT) — IoMT are any of the medical devices that are connected to the internet.

Internet of Things (IoT) — IoT are things that are connected to the internet such as refrigerator, a toaster, a television set, etc.

Internet Protocol (IP) — Internet Protocol is the foundation for the internet. It provides the common basis for networks to communicate with one another.

Internet Services Provider (ISP) — An ISP is any service provider that provides internet access to homes.

IoMT — See Internet of Medical Things.

IoT — See Internet of Things.

ISAC — See Information Sharing and Analysis Center.

IT Hygiene — IT hygiene is hygiene for computers. It can take on different definitions, but generally it includes things like patching a system, removing vulnerabilities, and securely configuring the systems.

Keyloggers — Keyloggers are a type of malware that captures every keystroke on a computer. Usernames and passwords can be captured this way.

LAN — See Local Area Network.

LDAP — See Lightweight Directory Access Protocol.

Leet — One of any number of systems to modify the spelling of a word. It is primarily used on the internet.

Leetspeak — Also known as leet, leetspeak is one of many different systems, often informal, for modifying spellings. Usually it has some resemblance to the actual spelling. For example, a 1 can be used instead of the letter *l*.

Lightweight Directory Access Protocol (LDAP) — LDAP is the free cousin of Microsoft's Active Directory.

Linux — An open-source operating system that is based on Unix. Many variants of Linux are popular today.

Local Area Network (LAN) — A LAN is a network that has a limited area.

Machine Learning — Machine learning is a process where an application learns through experience. It is considered a stepping-stone toward artificial intelligence.

Malvertising — Advertising with malware hidden in it.

Malware — Software designed to disrupt, damage, or gain unauthorized access to a computer and related systems.

Managed Detection and Response (MDR) — MDR is an outsourced security service designed to remove threats in an environment.

Managed Security Services Provider (MSSP) — MSSPs are services for aggregating, correlating, enhancing, and alerting on cybersecurity issues within an environment. MSSPs are primarily based on network devices and operating systems, but have been expanding out from there.

Medical Device User Fee and Modernization Act of 2002 (MDUFMA) — MDUFMA is the act that provided the FDA with the resources to better review medical devices.

Medicine 2.0 — Medicine 2.0 is the idea that we have IoMT devices providing constant feedback about the health and status of people in order to collect information to further refine the current understanding and treatment of patients.

Meltdown — Meltdown is an attack that circumvented the fundamental isolation between applications on systems. It was discovered at roughly the same time as SPECTRE.

MITRE ATT&CK Framework — The MITRE ATT&CK framework is a globally accessible source for adversarial tactics and techniques related to cyber threats.

Mobile Device Management (MDM) — MDM is a type of solution that allows IT to manage mobile devices.

Multi-factor Authentication (MFA) — There are generally three factors for authentication: something you have, something you know, and something you are. Using two or more of these factors creates greater security.

National Institute of Standards and Technology (NIST) — NIST is a non-regulatory agency of the US Department of Commerce designed to promote innovation and competitiveness.

National Institutes of Health (NIH) — A US agency that is a medical research center.

Near Field Communications (NFC) — NFC is a short-range (about 1.5 inches) wireless connectivity.

NetBEUI — NetBEUI is a LAN-based communication protocol not typically in use anymore.

Network Address Translation (NAT) — This is a method of mapping a public IP space to a private IP space.

Network Intrusion Detection Protection (NIDPS) — NIDPS is a system that can either detect or protect a network on the network level.

Network Intrusion Detection System (NIDS) — NIDS is similar to NIDPS except that it only has the ability to detect.

Nevada Senate Bill 220 — Nevada's Senate Bill 220 is a privacy bill that provides a way for residents to request their information not be sold.

New York SHIELD Act — The SHIELD Act requires businesses to maintain reasonable safeguards to protect private information.

Office of Civil Rights (OCR) — Related to the OCR for HHS, OCR is responsible for the enforcement of HIPAA.

Open Source Web Application Security Project (OWASP) — OWASP is an open-source foundation for application security.

Open Systems Interconnection (OSI) Model — The OSI model is a conceptual model to characterize how web traffic traverses the internet.

OWASP — See Open Source Web Application Security Project.

Patient-Centers Outcomes Research Institute (PCORI) — PCORI is a nonprofit company devoted to bridging the gap between government and the private sector for helping with evidence-based patient outcomes.

Patient Protection and Accountable Care Act (PPACA) — The PPACA is the former name for the Affordable Care Act.

Payment Card Industry Data Security Standard (PCI-DSS) — PCI-DSS, sometimes called PCI, is a set of standards that companies who collect, store, or transmit PCI data must follow.

PCI — See Payment Card Industry Data Security Standard.

Penetration Testing — A penetration test is an authorized attack against an organization for the purpose of finding vulnerabilities before hackers find them.

Personal Health Information (PHI) — This is the type of sensitive information as defined by HIPAA. It includes PII and health information.

Personally Identifiable Information (PII) — PII is information relating to an individual person. It is a type of sensitive information. It includes such specifics as name, address, phone number, etc.

Petabyte (PB) — A PB is equal to 1024 Terabytes of data or 1 million gigabytes.

Pharming — Pharming is the process of setting up a fake website to look like a legitimate one. It usually involves getting people to visit fraudulent websites through any number of scams, advertising, or even typosquatting.

Phishing — Phishing is a social engineering technique that involves sending emails out to people in order to get them to respond, click on links, or download documents for any number of malicious purposes.

Platform as a Service (PaaS) — PaaS is a type of cloud service where the provider provides management up to the operating system within the cloud.

Privacy Impact Assessments (PIAs) — PIAs are an assessment of the overall privacy related to new projects.

Privacy Rule — The privacy rule is the part of HIPAA that protects PHI.

Privileged Access Management (PAM) — PAM is a type of product that helps with people and processes for managing privileged access on a system — access that is above and beyond ordinary access.

QR Codes — A label that links to known information that can be scanned with cell phones, etc.

Quality Assurance (QA) — A QA process is a process to ensure product and/or service performance.

Rainbow Books — The Rainbow series of books are cybersecurity books that are not usually referenced today.

Ransomware — Ransomware is a malware used to lock up a computer or system to hold it hostage, in theory, until an individual or organization pays the ransom. It can have a profound impact on organizations.

RE&CT — Based on MITRE's ATT&CK framework, RE&CT defines responses to the ATT&CK attacks.

Regional Health Information Organization (RHIO) — RHIOs are organizations designed to facilitate the exchange of health information.

Remote Desktop Protocol (RDP) — RDP is a Microsoft tool built into its operating systems for connecting to other Microsoft systems.

Risk Register — A risk register is essentially a list of risks that an organization may face. In health organizations it is used as a governance tool to prioritize actions.

S3 Bucket — An S3 Bucket is the name AWS uses for its cloud native database.

Scytale — An ancient Greek baton used to encrypt information.

SDLC — See Software Development Life Cycle.

Secure Access Secure Edge (SASE) — SASE is the term coined by Gartner to refer to tools that interconnect with cloud-related services.

Secure Email Gateway (SEG) — A SEG is a set of tools and services designed to protect email from a range of attacks.

Secure Shell (SSH) — SSH is a network protocol for operating network services over an unsecure network.

Secure Web Gateway (SWG) — An SWG is a set of tools and services designed to protect web traffic (HTTP/S) from a range of attacks.

Security Information Event Management (SIEM) — SIEMs are monitoring tools used to aggregate, correlate, and alert on significant events in a log system.

Security Operations Center (SOC) — An SOC is a centralized unit that deals with security issues on a technical level.

Security Orchestration Automation and Response (SOAR) — SOAR is a set of tools designed to automate incident response tasks within an organization.

Security Rule — Within HIPAA, the Security Rule requires administrative, technical, and physical safeguards to protect information.

Separation of Duties (SoD) — SoD is a fundamental principle of cybersecurity where more than one person is required to complete a task. It is especially important for developers.

Service Set Identifier (SSID) — SSID is a natural language identifier for users to know what network they are connecting to in a wireless context.

Short Message Service (SMS) — An SMS is a text message on a phone.

SIGTRAN — SIGTRAN is a technical term for transport signaling.

Single Sign-On (SSO) — SSO is a tool that allows users to log in to a single environment, yet gain access to disparate resources without needing to log in again.

Smishing — Smishing is a form of phishing that takes place over an SMS message.

SOC — See Security Operations Center.

Soft Tokens — Soft tokens are authenticators that are installed on an operating system — either a phone, a pad, or other computer.

Software as a Service (SaaS) — SaaS is a cloud service model where a provider owns all of the infrastructure, hardware, software, etc. The SaaS is a service that is used by other organizations.

Software Development Lifecycle (SDLC) — SDLC is a process for software development, for programming an environment while ensuring the fundamentals are in place.

Spear Phishing — Spear phishing is phishing targeted at a specific person.

Spectre — Spectre is a vulnerability on a system that allow attackers to trick programs into leaking information. It was discovered near the same time as Meltdown.

SS7 — SS7 is a telephony signaling used to set up and tear down phone calls.

SSID — See Service Set Identifier.

Static Analysis Security Testing (SAST) — SAST is part of a secure SDLC process where software is used to scan the code to look for defects that could result in security vulnerabilities.

STIX — STIX is a format for storing threat information.

Stop Hacks and Improve Electronic Data Security (SHIELD) — A New York law requiring any person or business to maintain reasonable safeguards to protect private information.

SweynTooth — This vulnerability affects the Bluetooth capabilities in the device. In some cases it can be used to crash devices or otherwise bypass the security in the device.

TAXII — TAXII is the exchange process for sharing threat information.

Telehealth — Telehealth is a means of attaining healthcare from a distance.

Telemedicine — Telemedicine is similar to telehealth, but is a bit broader to include intervention, monitoring, and remote admissions.

Threat Intelligence — Threat intelligence, related to this book, is information about threat actors whether it be specific IP addresses, hashing information, tools, techniques, or practices.

Threat Intelligence Gateway (TIG) — A TIG is a device that uses threat intelligence to monitor and often block potentially malicious traffic.

TOR — TOR, also called the Onion Router, is software that allows one to have their traffic concealed from the internet. It is a hotbed for criminal activity.

Typosquatting — Typosquatting is the practice of buying domains that are slightly off from another domain that people may accidentally type. Cybercriminals do this for nefarious purposes.

UL 2900 — UL 2900 is a cybersecurity standard for IoMT that is much more secure than other options.

Unified Threat Management (UTM) — UTM is a philosophy where a single device is used to perform multiple security functions on a system.

Uniform Resource Locater (URL) — A URL, also called a web address, is a reference to a location on a network.

Veterans Affairs (VA) — The VA is a US agency designed to provide life-long healthcare to eligible military veterans.

Virtual LAN — A virtual LAN is a logical network set up on a network device known as a switch.

Virtual Private Network (VPN) — A VPN is a way of setting up a secure connection over an insecure network such as the internet.

Vishing — Vishing is similar to phishing except that it involves directly talking to someone.

VLAN — See Virtual LAN.

Web Application Firewall (WAF) — A WAF is a firewall specifically designed to protect web applications.

Whaling — Whaling is similar to spear phishing, but it goes after extremely important targets like the C-suite of an organization.

Wi-Fi — Wi-Fi is a networking technology that allows computers and other devices to connect to the internet wirelessly.

Windows Internet Name Service (WINS) — A legacy protocol for resolving NetBIOS names to IP addresses. It has been replaced by DNS.

WINS — See Windows Internet Name Service.

Wired Equivalent Privacy (WEP) — WEP is a wireless encryption protocol designed to protect transmissions over wireless networks. It has been replaced with WPA as the encryption is far less than perfect.

World Health Organization (WHO) — WHO is an organization within the United Nations designed to deal with health issues around the world.

WPA, WPA2, WPA3 — WPA is a set of encryption algorithms typically used to encrypt wireless communications.

XDR — XDR is a solution that works with a range of sources and log types across security and IT solutions.

Zero-Day Vulnerabilities — Zero-day vulnerabilities are vulnerabilities that are not recognized by any system.

Zero Trust — Zero trust is a ubiquitous set of cybersecurity requirements that revolve around not trusting anyone or any system in any environment. It involves limiting the access of each person to the minimal required to do their job and no more.

Index

A

AB-713, 110
Accenture, 60
account hijacking, as a risk of internet-connected medical devices, 8
Accountable Care Organizations (ACOs), 56–57
AccuDoc, 46
ACLs, 220
actions on objectives, 90
Active Directory (AD), 234, 347
advanced persistent threats (APTs), 138
Advanced Research Project Agency Network (ARPANET), 90
adware, 145–146
Affordable Care Act, 16, 55, 56–57, 86–87
aggregation, 278
aggregation of influence, 335–337
aging population, 15
aging systems, 240
alerts, 278–279
Alvi, Baset and Amjad Farooq, 143
amateur hackers, 136
Amazon Alexa, 205
Amazon Web Services (AWS), 44–45
America Recovery and Reinvestment Act (ARRA, 2009), 58
Americans with Disabilities Act, 103
anonymized health data, 66–67
antivirus
about, 210–211, 215
alternate solutions, 213–214

evolution of, 211
future of, 215
IoMT and, 214
as a key discipline in cybersecurity, 161
solution interconnectivity, 211–212
uses for, 212–213
Apache Struts, 192
Apple, 103, 121, 122, 145
application architecture, as a key discipline in cybersecurity, 162
Application layer (layer 7), in OSI model, 174
APT27, 322
artificial intelligence (AI), 69–70
Ashton, Kevin, 28
asset exposure, as a strategy for vulnerability management, 251–252
asset management, 31
Atrium Health, 46
authentication
about, 233, 239
aging systems, 240
multi-factor, 236–238, 240
passwords, 233–236, 239–240
authenticator applications, 238
automation, 283–284
AV-Test Institute, 147–148

B

behavior, bad, 121–122
big data, 63–68
biosensors, 16

Bit9, 16
black box, 76
Black Hat, 168
black-box testing, 255
black-hat hackers/hacking, 93–94, 127
Blockbuster Entertainment Inc., 20
Blue Cross Blue Shield, 66
Blue Health Intelligence, 66
BlueSnarfing, 41
Bluetooth, 29, 41
board of directors, 288–289, 345–346
bottom-line mindset, 304
Brazilian Data Protection Law, 113
Breach and Attack Simulation (BAS), 259–260
breaches
  about, 85, 281
  anatomy of, 89–95
  black-hat hacking, 93–94
  internet of medical things (IoMT) hacking, 94–95
  locations for, 95
  pharming, 90–92
  phishing, 90–92
  smishing, 90–92
  statistics on, 13–14, 86–88
  vishing, 90–92
  web browsing, 92–93
Bring Your Own Device (BYOD), 209–210, 221
brute-force attacks, as a risk of internet-connected medical devices, 8
Budapest Convention, 131, 322
Business Associate Agreements (BAAs), 105, 260

C

Cable Communications Policy Act (1984), 102
California Consumer Privacy Act (CCPA), 108–111, 116–117, 119, 318–319
category 5 (CAT 5) cable, 173
The Cathedral and the Bazaar (Raymond), 191
cellular systems, 40
Center for Internet Security (CIS), 166–167
Center for Medicaid and Medicare (CMS), 12, 58
changes, needed, 343–348
Chief Compliance Officer (CCO), 291
Chief Executive Officer (CEO), 289
Chief Information Officer (CIO), 289–290
Chief Information Security Officer (CISO), 291

Chief Medical Technology Officer (CMTO), 290
Chief Privacy Officer (CPO), 291–292
Chief Technology Officer (CTO), 290
Children's Online Privacy Protection Act (COPPA), 103
Chile Privacy Bill Initiative, 113
China, 130, 131
Churchill, Winston, 100
CIA Triad, 104, 155, 287
cipher device, 98
CISO Compass (Fitzgerald), 23–24
clinical monitors, 47–48
Cloud Access Security Broker (CASB), 194
cloud connections
  challenges related to services, 193–194
  cloud accounts, 231
  for medical devices, 43–46
  penetration testing and, 258–259
Coalfire, 125
command and control, 90, 145
committees, 293–294
Common Vulnerability Scoring System (CVSS), 250–251, 253
Communications Assistance to Law Enforcement Act (CALEA), 103
compensating controls, as a strategy for vulnerability management, 252
compliance, 158–160, 334–335
compliance-only mindset, 298–299
Comprehensive Crime Control Act (CCCA), 127
Computer Fraud and Abuse Act (CFAA), 126–127
configuration management
  about, 215–216
  applications, 219–220
  change process, 216–217
  databases, 221–222
  drift, 222
  enterprise considerations, 224
  exception management, 223–224
  firewalls, 220
  IoMT, 218
  as a key discipline in cybersecurity, 166–168
  Linux systems, 219
  mobile devices, 220–221
  strategy for, 217–218
  tools for, 222–223
  Windows system, 218–219
consultant accounts, 232
contact tracing, 106–107
Content Disarm and Reconstruction (CDR), 214

contextual challenges/solutions, 151–152
contractor accounts, 232
Cooperative Research and Development
    Agreement (CRADA), 81
Corbin, Bethany, 25
corporate temperature screenings, 107
cost center mindset, 299–300
Council of Europe's Convention of
    Cybercrime, 131
covered entities, 332–337, 344–345
COVID-19
    big data and, 64
    cloud connections and, 43–46
    contact tracing, 106–107
    corporate temperature screenings, 107
    evolving enterprises and, 198–199
    HIPAA Privacy Rule and, 104–107
    importance of data and, 56
    Medicine 2.0 and, 54
    QR codes and, 238
    ransomware and, 4–5
    telemedicine and, 29–30
    trending influences after, 12–13
    web browsing attacks and, 92–93
    wireless technologies after, 39
crowd source penetration testing, 260
Cyber Unified Coordination Group (UCG),
    321
cybercrime, enforcement of, 128–131
cybersecurity
    about, 153–154
    antivirus, 161
    application architecture, 162
    basics of, 154–156
    compliance, 158–160
    configuration management, 166–168
    digital forensics, 166
    evolution of, 156–158
    identity and access management (I&AM),
        163–164
    incident response, 165
    insurance industry, 132
    key disciplines in, 158–169
    monitoring, 164–165
    network architecture, 161–162
    patching, 160–161
    personal, 339–340
    risk management, 168–169
    threat and vulnerability, 162–163
    training, 168
Cybersecurity and Infrastructure Security
    Agency (CISA), 155
Cybersecurity Assurance Program (CAP),
    82
Cybersecurity Framework (CSF), 333

D
dark web, 141–143
data
    accuracy of, 62
    big, 63–68
    importance of, 55–57
data access, 267–268
data aggregation, 57–59
data analytics, 30–31
data at rest, 118
data brokers, 60–63, 314–316
data governance, 264–268
data in motion, 118
Data Loss Prevention (DLP), 268–270
data mining, 64–65, 68–70
Data Privacy Impact Assessments (DPIA),
    115
data protection
    about, 263–264
    data governance, 264–268
    Data Loss Prevention (DLP), 268–270
    data tokenization, 272–273
    decision-making and, 308–309
    enterprise encryption, 270–272
Data Protection Agency, 316
data risks, as a risk of internet-connected
    medical devices, 7–10
data tokenization, 272–273
data transfer and storage, internet of
    medical things (IoMT) and, 33–34
databases, 221–222
data-centricity
    about, 53
    big data, 63–68
    data aggregation, 57–59
    data brokers, 60–63
    data mining automation, 68–70
    importance of data, 55–57
    non-HIPAA health data, 59–60
    volume of health data, 53–55
Datalink layer (layer 2), in OSI model,
    173–174
decision-making
    about, 304–305
    cybersecurity, 333–334
    data protection and, 308–309
    enterprise risk management (ERM),
        307–308
    importance of communication, 306–307
    "in writing," 308
    measuring risk, 305–306
Deep Packet Inspection (DPI), 179
deep web, 141–143
default settings, internet of medical things
    (IoMT) and, 34

de-identified PHI, 109–110
demand, escalating, 10–13
De-Militarized Zone (DMZ), 161–162, 189
deprecated services, challenges related to, 197
device management, internet of medical things (IoMT) and, 34
Diameter, 41
digital forensics, as a key discipline in cybersecurity, 166
disclosure, 104
dissolvable agent, 249
distributed denial of service (DDoS) attack, 35, 137
"do no harm," 3
Domain Name Service (DNS), 195–197
domain/directory accounts, 229–230
Drucker, Peter, 19
Dynamic Application Security Testing (DAST), 249, 331

E
eavesdropping, as a risk of internet-connected medical devices, 8
ecosystem interfaces, internet of medical things (IoMT) and, 32–33
electronic boards, 36–37
Electronic Communications Privacy Act (ECPA, 1986), 102–103, 128
Electronic Health Records (EHRs), 47, 55, 58, 70
embedded internet, 28
encryption
  about, 45
  of data, 265–267
  enterprise, 270–272
  history of, 98
  with Wi-Fi, 182
encryption gateways, 271–272
Endpoint Detection and Response (EDR), 211, 284
enforcement, of cybercrime, 128–131
Enigma Code, 100
enterprise encryption, 270–272
enterprise risk management (ERM), 297–298
escalating demand, 10–13
evidence handling, 282–283
exception management, 223–224
Experian, 60
Extended Detection and Response (XDR), 279

F
Facebook, 67
Fair Credit Reporting Act (1970), 101
false positives, 162, 165
Federal Trade Commission (FTC), 62
Federal Wiretap Act (1968), 128
file encryption, 271
File Integrity Monitoring (FIM), 223
File Transfer Protocol (FTP), 189–190
FIPS 140-2-compliant cryptographic modules, 82
firewalls, 181, 220
Fitzgerald, Todd
  CISO Compass, 23–24
5G cellular service, 40–41
flat network, 48, 175–178
flavors, of Linux, 191
Food, Drug, and Cosmetic Act, 78
Food and Drug Administration (FDA), 77–81
forensic tools, 283
4G cellular service, 40–41
Foursquare, 106
Fourth Amendment, 101
frameworks, risk, 294–295
freeware, 190–191

G
GE Healthcare, 49–50
General Counsel (GC), 290
General Data Protection Regulation (GDPR), 108
Gillibrand, Kirsten, 316
Google, 62, 67, 121, 122, 145
Government Accountability Office (GAO), 128
Gramm-Leach-Bliley Act (GLBA), 103–104, 111
gray-box testing, 255
gray-hat hackers, 125–127
grep, 282

H
hackers/hacking, 94–95, 124–127
hacktivists, 137
hard tokens, 236–237
hardcoded, 18
Healey, Jason, 128–129
Health and Human Services (HHS), 61, 105
Health Information Exchanges (HIEs), 58

Health Information Technology for Economic and Clinical Health (HITECH) Act (2009), 55, 73–75, 86–87, 302

Health Insurance Portability and Accountability Act (HIPAA, 1996), 66–67, 73–77, 103–104, 155, 159, 171, 264, 266, 268–270, 302, 316, 334–335. *See also* non-HIPAA health data

health regulation
  about, 73–77
  Food and Drug Administration (FDA), 77–81
  internet of medical things (IoMT) and, 73–83
  UL 2900 standard, 81–83
  Veterans Affairs (VA), 81–83

Healthcare Ready, 320–321

heart devices, patient deaths related to, 21–22

high availability, 186

HIPAA Privacy Rule, 75, 104–107

HIPAA Security Rule, 299

Hippocrates, 3

HITRUST, 74, 160, 334–335

home healthcare, 15

I

IBM, 63, 68

Identity and Access Management (I&AM)
  about, 227–228
  authentication, 233–240
  cloud accounts, 231
  consultant accounts, 232
  contractor accounts, 232
  domain/directory accounts, 229–230
  identity governance, 232–233
  IoMT accounts, 230
  as a key discipline in cybersecurity, 163–164
  local accounts, 229
  minimal identity practices, 228–233
  physical access accounts, 231
  Privileged Access Management (PAM), 240–242
  service accounts, 230
  technologies for, 243–245
  vendor accounts, 232

identity centralization, 243

identity governance, 232–233, 244

identity management, 244

implanted medical devices, 30

importance, knowing, as a strategy for vulnerability management, 252

incident response and forensics
  about, 275–276, 281–282
  alerts, 278–279
  automation, 283–284
  breaches, 281
  defining context, 276–281
  EDR, 284
  evidence handling, 282–283
  forensic tools, 283
  incidents, 280
  IoMT challenges, 284–285
  as a key discipline in cybersecurity, 165
  lessons learned, 285
  logs, 277–278
  MDR, 284
  SIEM alternatives, 279–280

incident response plan, 165

incidents, 280

India Personal Data Protection Bill, 113

Individually Identifiable Health Information (IIHI), 104

industrial control systems (ICSs), 338

Information Sharing Analysis Centers (ISACs), 320–321

innovation, importance of, 19–25

innovators, cybersecurity, 337–338

insiders, 136–137

internal servers, as Internet servers, 197–198

international agreements, 319–322

international cooperation, as a needed change, 344

International Mobile Subscriber Identity (IMSI) catchers, 40

international privacy regulations, 113

internet of medical things (IoMT)
  about, 9, 27–29, 48, 202
  accounts, 230
  antivirus and, 214
  assurances for, 346–348
  challenges related to, 189
  clinical monitors, 47–48
  cloud, 43–46
  combined with IoT, 204–206
  configurations, 218
  current challenges with, 48–50
  data analytics, 30–31
  electronic boards, 36–37
  hacking, 94–95
  health regulation and, 73–83

historical challenges with, 31–36
incident response challenges, 284–285
increase in workflow efficiency from, 54
interconnection of technologies in, 49
life span of technology, 203
manufacturers and, 330–332
mobile devices/apps, 46–47
network infrastructure and, 171–182
operating systems, 37–38
patching, 208
selecting, 203–204
software development, 38–39
technology and, 36–48
telemedicine, 29–30
vulnerability challenges, 249–250
websites, 48
wired connections, 43
wireless connections, 39–42
as workstations, 204
Internet of Things (IoT)
    combined with IoMT, 204–206
    legislation for, 317
Internet Protocol (IP) address, 174, 178
internet service providers (ISPs), 186
Internet services
    about, 185–186
    challenges with, 194–198
    cloud services, 193–194
    deprecated services, 197
    Domain Name Service (DNS), 195–197
    evolving enterprise, 198–199
    internal servers as Internet servers,
        197–198
    internet of medical things (IoMT)
        services, 189
    network services, 186–187
    open-source tools, 190–193
    operating system services, 189–190
    websites, 187–189
internet-connected medical devices
    compound annual growth rate (CAGR)
        of, 13
    risks of, 4–10
    types of, 11–12
    updating, 16–19
IoT Cybersecurity Improvement Act (2020),
    317
IT hygiene
    about, 201–202
    antivirus, 210–215
    configurations, 215–224
    internet of medical things (IoMT) and,
        202–206
    patching, 206–210
It's just an IT problem mindset, 301–303

J
Jha, Paras, 35

K
Kamkar, Samy, 126
keyloggers, 145
kill chain, 89–90
Kreb, Brian
    Spam Nation, 139

L
leadership, 325–327
legal issues
    about, 123–124
    black-hat hackers, 127
    cybercrime enforcement, 128–131
    future of, 314–319
    gray-hat hackers, 125–127
    with hacking, 124–128
    shortcomings, 131–132
    white-hat hackers, 125
less-documented vulnerabilities, as a
        strategy for vulnerability management,
        253
lifecycle, of data, 265
Linux
    about, 191–193
    configuration management, 219
    patching in, 209
local accounts, 229
Local Area Network (LAN), 173–174, 175
locations, for breaches, 95
Lockheed Martin, 89
logs, 277–278

M
machine learning, 323–324
Maine, 112
malvertising, 93
malware
    construction kits, 148
    evolution of, 143–144, 146–147
    types of, 144–146
Managed Detection and Response (MDR),
    211, 284
Managed Security Services Provider
        (MSSP), 279–280
man-in-the-middle attacks, as a risk of
        internet-connected medical devices, 8
manufacturing, 119–120, 330–332
McKinsey, 60, 69–70
Medical Device User Fee and
        Modernization Act (MDUFMA, 2002),
        78

Medicine 2.0, 54, 172
MedTronic heart valve, 21–22
Meltdown, 18
Merlin@home Transmitter, 36
Microsoft, 24–25, 318–319, 320
MimiKatz, 142
mindset challenges, 298–304
MITRE ATT&CK framework, 259
MITRE corporation, 41–42
mobile device management (MDM),
    209–210
mobile devices/apps
  configuration management, 220–221
  patching, 209–210
  use of in medicine, 46–47
Mobilewalla, 62–63
monitoring, as a key discipline in
    cybersecurity, 164–165
Morris worm, 145
Mougalas, Roger, 63–64
multi-factor authentication (MFA), 163,
    236–238, 240, 242
MyLife, 100

N
Nachi worm, 126
nation-states, 139–141
Near-Field Communication (NFC), 29, 39,
    42, 54
Network Address Translation (NAT), 178
network infrastructure
  alternate defensive strategies, 178–181
  flat network, 175–178
  internet of medical things (IoMT) and,
    171–182
  as a key discipline in cybersecurity,
    161–162
  Open Systems Interconnection (OSI)
    model, 173–175
  wireless connections, 181–182
Network Intrusion Detection Protection
    Systems (NIDPSs), 179, 213
Network Intrusion Detection System
    (NIDS), 164
Network layer (layer 3), in OSI model, 174
network security, adding in PAM, 242
network services
  challenges related to, 186–187
  internet of medical things (IoMT) and, 32
Nevada, 111–112
never disrupt the business mindset, 301
New York, 111, 315
New Zealand Privacy Bill, 113
Nigerian Prince scam, 90–91, 168

NMAP tool, 256–257
non-HIPAA health data, 59–60
non-IT considerations, 115
Nuspire, 8–9

O
Obama, Barack, 131
Office of Civil Rights (OCR), 74, 105, 118
Onion Router, 141–142
Open Source Web Application Security
    Project (OWASP), 32, 187–188
Open Systems Interconnection (OSI)
    model, 173–175
open-source intelligence tools (OSINT),
    190–193, 256–257
operating systems
  challenges related to, 189–190
  firewalls for, 181
  internet-connected medical devices and,
    37–38
  vulnerability of, 17–18
operational privacy considerations, 114–115
Oracle, 60
organizational structure
  about, 288
  board of directors, 288–289, 345–346
  Chief Compliance Officer (CCO), 291
  Chief Executive Officer (CEO), 289
  Chief Information Officer (CIO), 289–290
  Chief Information Security Officer
    (CISO), 291
  Chief Medical Technology Officer
    (CMTO), 290
  Chief Privacy Officer (CPO), 291–292
  Chief Technology Officer (CTO), 290
  committees, 293–294
  General Counsel (GC), 290
  for reporting, 292
organized crime, 138–139
ownership, of data, 264–265

P
passwords
  about, 233–236, 239–240
  internet of medical things (IoMT) and, 32
  rotating in PAM, 242
  tools for, 244–245
patching
  about, 206–207, 210
  IoMT, 208
  as a key discipline in cybersecurity,
    160–161
  Linux, 209

mature process, 207
mobile device, 209–210
Windows, 208–209
Patient Protection and Accountable Care Act (PPACA), 10
Patient-Center Outcomes Research Institute (PCORI), 10
Payment Card Industry Data Security Standard (PCI DSS), 113, 159–160
penetration testing
about, 254–255
box color, 255
cloud considerations for, 258–259
phases of, 256–258
strategies for, 258
team color, 255
personal cybersecurity, 339–340
personally identifiable information (PII), 98, 137, 268–270
petabyte, 55
pharming, 90–92
phishing, 90–92
physical access accounts, 231
physical hardening, internet of medical things (IoMT) and, 34
Physical layer (layer 1), in OSI model, 173
pirating software, 143
playbooks, 165
politics, IoMT and, 341–342
polymorphicity, 144, 146
portals, for clouds, 45
Presentation layer (layer 6), in OSI model, 174
privacy
about, 97–98
bad behavior, 121–122
challenges with, 117–118
covered entities and, 335
importance of, 98–101
legislation for, 318
manufacturing and, 119–120
regulations, 108–113
security and, 115–119
technical and operational considerations for, 114–115
technology and, 115–119
US history of, 101–107
Privacy Act (1974), 101
privacy gaps, 106–107
Privacy Impact Assessments (PIA), 115
privacy protection, internet of medical things (IoMT) and, 33
Privileged Access Management (PAM)
about, 240–241
MFA access, 242

network security, 242
password rotation, 242
roles, 241
processors, vulnerability of, 18
Protected Health Information (PHI), 60, 98, 109–110, 136–137
public-private partnerships, 319–320

Q

QR codes, 238
qualitative risk frameworks, 294–295
Quality Assurance (QA) environment, 207
quality system regulations (QSRs), 79
quantitative risk frameworks, 294–295
QuintilesIMS, 66

R

rainbow tables, 235
ransoms, 132
ransomware, 4–7, 146
Raymond, Eric S.
The Cathedral and the Bazaar, 191
real time telemedicine, 30
reconnaissance phase, of penetration testing, 256–257
Regional Health Information Organizations (RHIOs), 58
Remote Desk Protocol (RDP), 189–190
remote patient monitoring, 16
replay attacks, as a risk of internet-connected medical devices, 8
reporting phase, of penetration testing, 258
reporting structures, 292
Right to Financial Privacy Act (1974), 101–102
risk assessment, HIPAA and, 76–77
risk management
about, 294, 298
determining risk, 295–296
enterprise risk management (ERM), 297–298
frameworks for, 294–295
as a key discipline in cybersecurity, 168–169
risk register, 297
third-party risk, 296–297
risk register, 297
risks, to data, 7–10
roles, in Privileged Access Management (PAM), 241
Roosevelt, Franklin, 63
rootkits, 90, 145
Russia, 131
Rutgers University, 35

S

S3 bucket, 44–45
scope phase, of penetration testing, 256
scytale, 98, 103
Secure Access Secure Edge (SASE), 194
Secure Email Gateways (SEGs), 91, 212
Secure Shell (SSH), 189–190
Secure Sockets Layer (SSL), 266
Secure Web Gateways (SWGs), 180
Security Information Event Management
    (SIEM) system, 165, 278–280
security operations center (SOC), 279,
    334–335
Security Orchestration Automation and
    Response (SOAR), 283–284
Senate Bill 220 (Nevada), 111–112
Senate Bill S6848 (New York), 315
Separation of Duties (SoD), 38–39
service accounts, 230
session hijacking, as a risk of internet-
    connected medical devices, 8
Session layer (layer 5), in OSI model, 174
shiny object syndrome, 300–301
Shodan, 296–297
Short Message Service (SMS), 238
SIGTRAN, 40–41
smart systems, 12
smishing, 90–92
Smith v. Maryland, 121
social engineering, 90
Social Security Act, 63
soft tokens, 237
software
    development of, 347–348
    internet-connected medical devices and
        development of, 38–39
    pirating, 143
software development lifecycle (SDLC), 38,
    187–189
Software-as-a-Service (SaaS), 39, 46
SolarWinds, 207, 280, 295, 320, 322
Spam Nation (Kreb), 139
spear phishing, 91
Spectre, 18
"The Spectrum of state responsibility,"
    128–129
Spokeo, 100
spyware, 145–146
SS7, 40–41
St. Jude, 36
stalkerware, 146
Standard Information Gathering (SIG), 296
state privacy laws, 111–113
static analysis security testing (SAST), 80

stationary medical devices, 31
statistics, on breaches, 86–88
Stingrays, 40
Stop Hacks and Improve Electronic Data
    Security Act (SHIELD Act), 111
store and forward telemedicine, 30
strains, of viruses, 147–148
streaming data, 64
Structured Threat Information Expression
    (STIX), 321
surface web, 141
SweynTooth, 41–42
switch, 173–174
Symantec, 147, 148

T

tampering, as a risk of internet-connected
    medical devices, 8
technical privacy considerations, 114–115
technology
    common, 118–119
    innovation in, 323–325
    internet of medical things (IoMT), 36–48
    lifespan of, 203
    privacy and, 115–119
    security and, 115–119
telehealth, 15
telemedicine, 29–30
third-party risk, 296–297
threat actors
    about, 135–136
    advanced persistent threats (APTs), 138
    amateur hackers, 136
    dark web, 141–143
    hacktivists, 137
    insiders, 136–137
    malware, 144–148
    nation-states, 139–140
    nation-states' legal posture, 140–141
    organized crime, 138–139
    tools for, 143–148
threat and vulnerability
    about, 247
    as a key discipline in cybersecurity,
        162–163
    new tools, 259–261
    penetration testing, 254–259
    strategies for vulnerability management,
        251–254
    vulnerability management, 248–251
threat calculation, 260–261
threat intelligence, 323
Threat Intelligence Gateways (TIGs),
    180–181

threshold, 278
tooling, 38
tools over people mindset, 303
Tor, 141–142
traditional application vulnerability scans, 249
traditional infrastructure vulnerability scans, 248–249
training, as a key discipline in cybersecurity, 168
Transmission Control Protocol (TCP), 174
Transport layer (layer 4), in OSI model, 174
Trojan horses, 145
Truffle Security, 45
Trusted Automated eXChange of Indicator Information (TAXXI), 321
typosquatting, 196

U

UL 2900 standard, 81–83, 125, 126, 189, 204, 206, 317, 331, 346
Umbrella, 195
Unified Threat Management (UTM), 213
Uniting and Strengthening America by Providing the Appropriate Tools Required to Intercept and Obstruct Terrorism Act (USA PATRIOT Act), 107
Universal Health Services (UHS), 5–6
universities, cybersecurity failings in, 23
update mechanisms, internet of medical things (IoMT) and, 33
up-to-date components, internet of medical things (IoMT) and, 33
us versus them mindset, 300
User Datagram Protocol (UDP), 174

V

value, business perception around, 24
variety, of data, 64
velocity, of data, 64
vendor accounts, 232
Verizon Data Breach Investigation Report, 14, 86, 130
Veterans Affairs (VA), 81–83
Video Privacy Protection Act (1988), 103

virtual LAN (VLAN), 175–176, 177–178
virtual private network (VPN), 176, 179
viruses, 143, 144
vishing, 90–92
volume, of data, 64
vulnerabilities, rating, 250–251
vulnerability assessment phase, of penetration testing, 257
vulnerability management. See threat and vulnerability

W

Watson, 68
Wavenet, 39–40
we are not a target mindset, 303
wearable devices, 30
Web Application Firewall (WAF), 188
web browsing, 92–93
web filters, 180
websites
    challenges related to, 187–189
    internet of medical things (IoMT) and, 48
Welchia, 126
whaling, 91
white-box testing, 255
white-hat hackers, 125
Wi-Fi Protected Access (WPA), 40
Windows systems
    configuration management, 218–219
    patching, 208–209
Wire Equivalent Privacy (WEP), 40
wired connections, for medical devices, 43
wireless connections
    for medical devices, 39–42
    network infrastructure and, 181–182
workstations, IoMT as, 204
worms, 145

X

Xi Jinping, 131

Z

zero trust, 324–325
zero-day vulnerabilities, as a strategy for vulnerability management, 252–253